THE CORE REQUISITES

BREAST IMAGING

The Core Requisites Series

Series Editor

James H. Thrall, MD
The Core Requisites Series Editor
Chairman Emeritus
Department of Radiology
Massachusetts General Hospital
Distinguished Taveras Professor of Radiology
Harvard Medical School
Boston, Massachusetts

Titles in the Series

Breast Imaging
Cardiac Imaging
Emergency Imaging
Gastrointestinal Imaging
Genitourinary Imaging
Musculoskeletal Imaging
Neuroradiology Imaging
Nuclear Medicine
Pediatric Imaging
Thoracic Imaging
Ultrasound
Vascular and Interventional Imaging

BREAST IMAGING

FOURTH EDITION

Bonnie N. Joe, MD, PhD

Professor
Department of Radiology and Biomedical Imaging
University of California
San Francisco, California

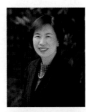

Amie Y. Lee, MD

Associate Professor
Department of Radiology and Biomedical Imaging
University of California
San Francisco, California

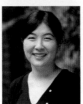

ELSEVIER

Elsevier
1600 John F. Kennedy Blvd.
Ste 1800
Philadelphia, PA 19103-2899

BREAST IMAGING, FOURTH EDITION

ISBN: 978-0-323-75849-9

Previous editions copyrighted 2017, 2011 and 2004.

Content Strategist: Melanie Tucker
Senior Content Development Manager: Somodottta Roy Choudhury
Senior Content Development Specialist: Malvika Shah
Publishing Services Manager: Shereen Jameel
Project Manager: Janish Paul / Haritha Dharmarajan
Design Direction: Patrick Ferguson

Printed in India

Last digit is the print number: 9 8 7 6 5 4 3 2 1

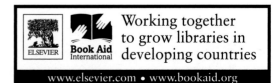

This book is dedicated to Dr. Edward A. Sickles, who has taught the science and art of breast imaging to so many of us at UCSF and around the world. He has mentored numerous breast imaging leaders and helped shape the specialty of breast imaging. In this book, we have tried to capture the fundamental lessons he has been teaching UCSF trainees for decades.

Contributors

Beatriz Adrada, MD
Radiologist
Breast Imaging
MD Anderson
Houston, Texas, United States

Shadi Aminololama-Shakeri, MD, FSBI
Professor
Department of Radiology
University of California Davis
Sacramento, California, United States

Dana Ataya, MD
Assistant Professor
Division of Breast Imaging
Department of Diagnostic Radiology
Moffitt Cancer Center
Tampa, Florida, United States
Assistant Professor
Department of Oncologic Sciences
University of South Florida College of Medicine
Tampa, Florida, United States

Debbie L. Bennett, MD
Chief of Breast Imaging
Mallinckrodt Institute of Radiology
Washington University School of Medicine
St. Louis, Missouri, United States

Sonya Bhole, MD
Assistant professor
Northwestern University, Feinberg School of Medicine
Lynn Sage Comprehensive Breast Center
Chicago, Illinois, United States

Maggie Chung, MD
Breast Imaging Fellow
Radiology & Biomedical Imaging
Breast Imaging Fellow of California, San Francisco
San Francisco, California, United States

Peter R. Eby, MD, FACR, FSBI
Section Head of Breast Imaging
Department of Radiology
Virginia Mason Franciscan Health
Seattle, WA, United States

Mohammad Eghtedari, MD, PhD
Associate Professor
Radiology
University of California San Diego
San Diego, California, United States

Amy M. Fowler, MD, PhD
Assistant Professor
Radiology
University of Wisconsin School of Medicine and Public
  Health
Madison, Wisconsin, United States

Sarah Friedewald, MD, FACR, FSBI
Vice Chair of Clinical Operations and Women's Imaging
Chief of Breast Imaging
Associate Professor, Department of Radiology
Northwestern University
Feinberg School of Medicine
Medical Director, Lynn Sage Comprehensive Breast Center
Chicago, Illinois, United States

Kimberly Funaro, MD
Assistant Member
Department of Diagnostic Imaging and Interventional
  Radiology
H. Lee Moffitt Cancer Center
Tampa, Florida, United States

Sujata V. Ghate, MD
Associate Professor
Radiology
Duke University Medical Center
Durham, North Carolina, United States

Julie Gibbons, MD
Residency Associate Program Director
Department of Radiology
Virginia Mason Franciscan Health
Seattle, WA, United States

Heather Ilana Greenwood, MD
Associate Professor
Radiology & Biomedical Imaging
University of California, San Francisco
San Francisco, California, United States

Mary S. Guirguis, MD
Assistant Professor
Department of Breast Imaging
University of Texas MD Anderson Cancer Center
Houston, Texas, United States

Anne C. Hoyt, MD
Professor of Radiological Sciences
Radiological Sciences
David Geffen School of Medicine at UCLA
Los Angeles, California, United States

Debra M. Ikeda, MD, FACR, FSBI
Professor of Radiology (Breast Imaging), Emerita
Stanford University School of Medicine
Stanford, California, United States

Bonnie N. Joe, MD, PhD
Professor
Chief of Breast Imaging
Radiology & Biomedical Imaging
University of California, San Francisco
San Francisco, California, United States

Andrew Nicholas Kozlov, MD
Staff Radiologist
Diagnostic Radiology
Radiology Associates of Florida
Tampa, Florida, United States
Assistant Professor of Radiology
Diagnostic Radiology
University of South Florida Morsani College of Medicine
Tampa, Florida, United States
Chief of Nuclear Medicine
Department of Radiology
Tampa General Hospital
Tampa, Florida, United States

Amie Y. Lee, MD
Associate Professor
Radiology & Biomedical Imaging
University of California, San Francisco
San Francisco, California, United States

Christine S. Lo, MBBS, FRCR, FHKCR, FHKAM (Radiology)
Radiologist
Department of Diagnostic and Interventional Radiology
    Hong Kong Sanatorium & Hospital
Hong Kong, China

Jing Luo, MD
Breast Imaging Fellow
Breast Imaging
Radiology
University of Washington
Seattle, Washington, United States

James Gordon Mainprize, PhD
Research Associate
Physical Sciences Sunnybrook Research Institute
Toronto, Ontario, Canada

Elizabeth S. McDonald, MD, PhD, FSBI
Assistant Professor
Radiology
University of Pennsylvania
Philadelphia, United States

Hannah S. Milch, MD
Assistant Clinical Professor
Radiological Sciences
David Geffen School of Medicine at UCLA
Los Angeles, California, United States

Kanae Kawai Miyake, MD, PhD
Program-specific Assistant Professor
Advanced Medical Imaging and Research
Kyoto University Graduate School of Medicine
Section Chief, Nuclear Medicine
Kyoto University Hospital
Kyoto, Kyoto, Japan

Linda Moy, MD
Associate Chair of Research Mentoring,
    Professor of Radiology
NYU Grossman School of Medicine
Center for Advanced Imaging Innovation and Research
    Faculty
Vilcek Institute of Graduate Biomedical Sciences
Laura and Isaac Perlmutter Cancer Center
160 East 34th Street, New York, NY 10016
New York, United States

Ramanjyot K. Muhar, MD
Associate
Radiology
Radiology Associates
San Luis Obispo, California, United States

Bethany Lynn Niell, MD, PhD
Section Chief of Breast Imaging
Department of Diagnostic Imaging and Interventional
    Radiology
H. Lee Moffitt Cancer Center and Research Institute
Tampa, Florida, United States
Professor
Department of Oncologic Sciences
University of South Florida
Tampa, Florida, United States

Haydee Ojeda-Fournier, MD
Professor
Division Chief of Breast Imaging
UC San Diego Health
University of California San Diego
La Jolla, California, United States

Dakota Orvedal, MD
Resident
Department of Radiology
Virginia Mason Franciscan Health
Seattle, WA, United States

Molly Peterson, MD
Radiology Resident
Department of Radiology
University of Wisconsin
Madison, Wisconsin, United States

Habib Rahbar, MD
Associate Professor
Vice Chair of Clinical Operations
Radiology
University of Washington
Seattle, Washington, United States

Jocelyn Rapelyea, MD
Professor and Vice Chair of Education
Department of Diagnostic Radiology
The George Washington University Hospital
Washington, District of Columbia, United States

Gaiane M. Rauch, MD, PhD
Professor
Departments of Abdominal and Breast Imaging
Division of Diagnostic Imaging
The University of Texas
MD Anderson Cancer Center
Houston Texas, United States

Kimberly M. Ray, MD
Associate Professor
Radiology & Biomedical Imaging
University of California, San Francisco
San Francisco, California, United States

Samantha P. Zuckerman, MD, MBE
Assistant Professor
Department of Radiology
Division of Breast Imaging
Hospital of the University of Pennsylvania
Philadelphia, Pennsylvania, United States

Congratulations to Drs. Bonnie N. Joe and Amie Y. Lee for producing *The Core Requisites: Breast Imaging, 4e*, now the third publication in the reimagined *Core Requisites series*. Drs. Joe and Lee have again successfully pivoted from a traditional narrative style to the new outline format. The new format brings out and immediately highlights the key points and concepts for each topic while minimizing the time required to sift through the text. An additional benefit of the new format is the ease of searching for information. Moreover, the books come in both print and online versions so that readers can access the information from wherever they are.

In the tradition of the *Requisites in Radiology* series, *Breast Imaging: The Core Requisites*, this book builds on the prior editions while bringing the information up to date and covering new topics that have come to the fore between editions. In that regard, *Breast Imaging: The Core Requisites, 4e* is a tour de force by Drs. Joe and Lee and their contributors because breast imaging has evolved rapidly, as much as or more than any subspecialty area of radiology. The evolution has progressed across multiple dimensions, all of which are reflected in this book. The diversity of imaging methods continues to grow. From a singular orientation to plain film x-ray mammography years ago, breast imaging requires knowledge of digital methods including digital tomosynthesis, multiple types of ultrasound applications, and diverse concepts in magnetic resonance imaging (MRI). Also, the need for standardized, guideline-based approaches and accreditation has been unequivocally recognized. The challenge of harmonizing radiology interpretations with clinical information needs has been more clearly recognized and defined. Better knowledge of breast pathology has brought with it new insights into the significance of image findings and how to report them:

the radiologic–pathologic correlation. The number and complexity of interventional methods continue to grow. These important trends and others find excellent coverage in *Breast Imaging: The Core Requisites, 4e*.

While the format of the *Core Requisites* series differs substantially from the traditional *Radiology Requisites* series, the philosophy remains the same—a series of richly illustrated books covering the core material required across the spectrum of what radiologists need to know, from their first encounters as residents with subject material in different subspecialty areas to studying for board examinations and later for reference during clinical practice. We hope that radiologists, whether in training or practice, will find the books useful, as well as trainees and practitioners in the related fields of medical and surgical oncology. The books in the *Core Requisites* series are not encyclopedic; they are intended to be practical and focused on material expected on board certification examinations.

Congratulations again to Drs. Joe and Lee and their contributors for adding an excellent new resource to the *Core Requisites* series. I hope that this and the following books in the series will be regarded with the same fondness as earlier books in the *Radiology Requisites* family that have been used by radiologists at all career stages for over 30 years.

James H. Thrall, MD
The Core Requisites Series Editor
Chairman Emeritus
Department of Radiology
Massachusetts General Hospital
Distinguished Taveras Professor of Radiology
Harvard Medical School
Boston, Massachusetts

Preface

In keeping with the philosophy of the new *The Core Requisites* series, the chapters in this book are relatively short, with focused, straightforward, and high-yield content. Our goal is to allow the reader to efficiently review core information and key concepts. We hope this book serves as a useful guide to breast imaging whether you are a new resident or a seasoned radiologist looking for a concise yet comprehensive overview of the fundamentals of breast imaging.

Thank you to all of the authors who wrote and edited chapters for this book amid a global pandemic. Thank you to Dr. Deb Ikeda, editor of *Breast Imaging: The Requisites*, third edition, for your sponsorship and support throughout this process.

And thank you Ed ("Dr. Sickles") for your continued mentorship and support.

Bonnie N. Joe, MD, PhD
Professor
Chief of Breast Imaging
Radiology and Biomedical Imaging
University of California, San Francisco
San Francisco, California, United States

Amie Y. Lee
Associate Professor
Radiology & Biomedical Imaging
University of California, San Francisco
San Francisco, California, United States

Contents

1 Introduction to Mammography: The Basics

MAGGIE CHUNG, BONNIE N. JOE AND AMIE Y. LEE

OVERVIEW | *This chapter is a basic introduction to the fundamentals of mammography, including standard and special views, technical adequacy, and normal anatomy.*

Breast imaging is integral to the diagnosis and evaluation of breast cancer and other breast pathologies. While ultrasound and magnetic resonance radiology (MRI) also play important roles, mammography is often considered the foundation or workhorse of breast radiology. Mammography is versatile with ubiquitous roles in breast imaging, including breast cancer screening, diagnostic evaluation, and procedural guidance. It is an efficient method for evaluation of the entire breast and offers excellent visualization and characterization of breast calcifications.

Screening mammography is key to early breast cancer detection. Breast cancer is the most common non–skin-related malignancy among women, affecting approximately one in eight women in the United States. It is also the second leading cause of cancer-related death in women and the leading cause of cancer-related death in women younger than 60 years old. Screening mammography has been consistently shown to be a cost-effective screening modality and is the only screening test that has been shown in randomized controlled trials to significantly reduce breast cancer mortality. As a result, mammography is a staple in modern medicine preventative care.

Refined by decades of technological advancements and now assisted by complementary ultrasound and MRI, mammography serves as an essential tool in the breast imager's toolbox. This chapter will cover the basics of standard two-dimensional (2D) digital mammography. Subsequent chapters will provide more in-depth review of specific applications of mammography, including a chapter devoted to tomosynthesis.

How Is a Mammogram Performed?

COMPRESSION

When a mammogram is performed, each breast is placed on a support plate and compressed by parallel compression plates. Breast compression spreads superimposed normal parenchymal tissue for better visualization of underlying lesions (Box 1.1). Breast thickness is decreased by compression, thereby decreasing the radiation dose to the breast. Compression helps achieve more uniform thickness throughout the breast to avoid overexposure of the thinner anterior breast and underexposure of the thicker

Box 1.1 Roles of Breast Compression in Mammography

- Reduces parenchymal superimposition for better visualization
- Decreases radiation dose
- Ensures adequate x-ray penetration throughout the breast
- Reduces image blurring by decreasing patient motion and exposure time
- Reduces geometric blur and improves spatial resolution by reducing the distance between the breast tissue and the image receptor
- Improves image contrast by reducing scatter production and allowing selection of lower kV x-rays

posterior breast. It reduces geometric blur by reducing the distance between the breast tissue and the image receptor. Compression improves image contrast by reducing scatter production and allowing for selection of lower energy (kV) x-rays. Compression also immobilizes the breast and decreases exposure time, minimizing image blurring due to motion.

Patients may experience breast pain during compression. Methods to mitigate patient discomfort include performing the mammogram during day 7 to 10 of the menstrual cycle, adding foam padding between the breast and compression plates, and taking analgesics prior to receiving the mammogram.

STANDARD VIEWS

The routine mammogram consists of two complementary standard views for each breast: the craniocaudal (CC) view and the mediolateral oblique (MLO) view (Table 1.1). Based on standard mammographic terminology, each projection describes the direction of the x-ray beam. The first letter in the projection refers to the location of the x-ray source and the second refers to the location of the image receptor. For example, in the CC view the x-ray beam travels superior to inferior, from the cranial to caudal direction.

When performing the CC view, the patient faces toward the mammography unit, and the image receptor is placed inferior to the breast. The inferior breast is relatively mobile and allows the inframammary fold to be elevated when the technologist lifts and pulls the breast forward onto the positioning platform. This maneuver allows greater visualization of the posterior and superior breast tissue. The breast is then compressed in the axial plane, perpendicular to the x-ray beam (Fig. 1.1). The CC view includes most of the breast tissue except for the far lateral and far posterior breast.

In the MLO projection, the x-ray beam travels from superomedial to inferolateral. The breast compression plane is along the angulation of underlying pectoralis major muscle, usually at 45 degrees (Fig. 1.2). However, angulation of the compression plane varies with patient anatomy and may range from 40 to 60 degrees; thinner body habitus may need a slightly steeper obliquity, and shorter or heavier body habitus may need a slightly flatter obliquity. The course of the pectoralis muscle can be approximated by drawing an imaginary line between the ipsilateral shoulder to the mid sternum. When properly positioned, the MLO view includes nearly the entire breast including the axillary tail.

These two standard views are complementary. The MLO view visualizes the most amount of breast tissue. It is the best for viewing the posterior, upper-outer quadrant, axillary tail, and lower-inner quadrant of the breast. However, there may be considerable breast tissue overlap, often with limited compression of the more anterior structures. Also, the far superior-medial breast tissue (upper-inner quadrant) may sometimes be excluded from the MLO view. The CC view allows for better visualization of the medial and posteromedial tissue, as well as better compression of the subareolar and central breast.

Standardized Labeling

Standardized image labeling is important for consistency, allowing mammograms to be accurately identified and interpreted even outside of the performing institution. According to the Mammography Quality Standards Act (MQSA), the patient identification label is required to include the patient's name, unique identification number and/or date of birth, facility name and location, examination date, technologist's initials, cassette (screen) number for screen-film and computed radiography images, and mammographic unit identification (if there is more than one unit in the facility) (Box 1.2). The view and laterality label should be placed near the axilla on all mammograms. The laterality should be listed first, followed by technique (e.g., magnification, implant displacement) and projection (e.g., CC).

What Is Acceptable Quality?

Before interpreting a mammogram, it is important to first assess whether the mammogram is technically adequate (Box 1.3). Suboptimal image quality compromises mammographic evaluation and may lead to missed cancers.

IMAGE QUALITY

Each view should demonstrate adequate compression with dispersion of breast tissue and adequate x-ray penetration

---

Box 1.2 Mammogram Standardized Labeling Requirements

- Patient name
- Unique identification number and/or date of birth
- Facility name and location
- Examination date
- Technologist's initials
- Cassette/screen identification (for screen film or computed radiography; not for digital mammography)
- Mammographic unit (if there is more than one unit)
- Laterality and view placed near axilla

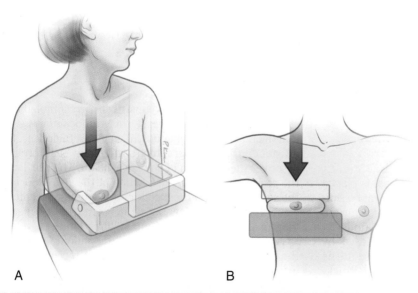
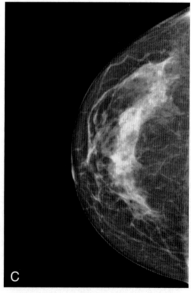

Fig. 1.1 The craniocaudal (CC) view. (A–B) The breast is compressed in the axial plane (at a 0-degree angle), perpendicular to the x-ray beam. (C) Example of a CC mammogram image.

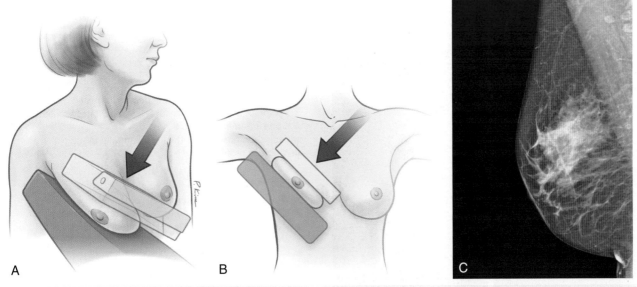

Fig. 1.2 The mediolateral oblique (MLO) view. (A–B) The breast is compressed along the angulation of the underlying pectoralis muscle (usually at 45 degrees). The x-ray beam travels from superomedial to inferolateral. (C) Example of an MLO mammogram image.

Box 1.3   Evaluation of Image Quality

- Compression: Look for adequate compression with dispersion of breast tissue
- Contrast: There should be sufficient contrast to differentiate breast tissues
- Exposure: Look for adequate exposure throughout the breast
- Sharpness: Check that the breast trabeculae and skin edge are sharp and free of motion
- Noise: Noise should be minimized as it can interfere with detection of small findings such as microcalcification
- Artifacts: Images should be free of artifacts, which may obscure or mimic pathology
    - Motion
    - Hair
    - Skin folds
    - Antiperspirant
    - Chin or other body parts
    - Grid lines

---

throughout the breast. The breast trabeculae and skin edge should be sharp. Blurring may cause subtle calcifications to be missed or cause incorrect characterization of calcification morphology. Images should have appropriate contrast and minimal noise. Mammograms should be free of artifacts, including motion, hair, skin folds, and antiperspirant, which may obscure or mimic pathology (Figs. 1.3–1.5).

APPROPRIATE POSITIONING

It is critical to assess if there is appropriate positioning with adequate breast tissue visualized on each view (Box 1.4) (Fig. 1.6). Appropriate positioning is important to ensure enough breast tissue is included in the mammogram to avoid potentially missing cancers. In fact, the majority of American College of Radiology (ACR) clinical image review and unit accreditation failures are due to poor positioning.

Positioning the nipple in profile helps to differentiate a nipple from a mass. As a practical approach in our practice, we will interpret a screening mammogram if the nipple is in profile on at least one view. Positioning the nipple in profile also helps identify nipple inversion or retraction that may be associated with an underlying mass. If the nipple does not naturally fall into profile, repositioning should not be performed at the expense of excluding breast tissue from the view. If the technologists cannot include both the nipple in profile and the appropriate amount of breast tissue in one view, an additional limited view can be obtained to demonstrate the nipple in profile.

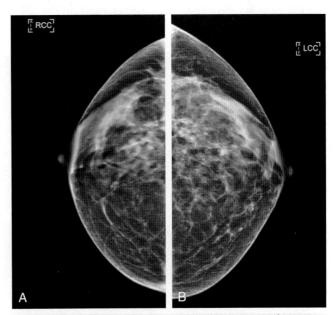

Fig. 1.3 Motion artifact. Craniocaudal (CC) views from a screening mammogram. Note the marked blurring due to motion artifact in the outer right breast (A), which could limit detection of subtle cancers. Compare this to the left breast (B), where the breast trabeculae and skin edge appear sharp with no blurring.

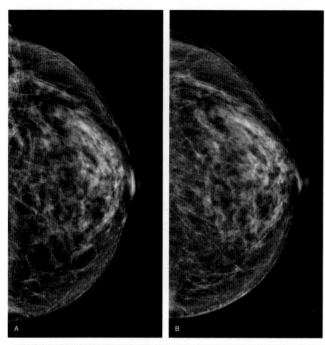

Fig. 1.4 Hair artifact. (A) Craniocaudal (CC) view of the left breast shows artifact from the patient's hair obscuring the outer posterior breast. (B) The patient was brought back for a repeat CC view, which shows resolution of the hair artifact.

The pectoralis muscle is an important landmark for evaluation of appropriate positioning. The posterior nipple line (PNL) is an imaginary line extending posteriorly and perpendicularly from the nipple to the pectoralis muscle. When the pectoralis muscle is not visible on the CC view, the PNL can be measured from the posterior nipple to the edge of the film. The length of the PNL on the CC and MLO views should be within 1 cm of each other. If the PNL length on the CC view is more than 1 cm shorter than on the MLO

view, it suggests that there is insufficient posterior breast tissue included on the CC view. It is important to clearly visualize the posterior medial breast on the CC view because it is often not well visualized on the MLO view.

On the MLO view, the visualized pectoralis muscle should extend inferior to the PNL. The pectoralis muscle should ideally demonstrate a convex anterior border and should be wider superiorly and gradually narrow inferiorly. The MLO view should attempt to show an open inframammary fold. If an open inframammary fold is not present, the breast should be pulled upward and outward as far as possible before compression is applied to reduce breast "sag" and overlapping tissue.

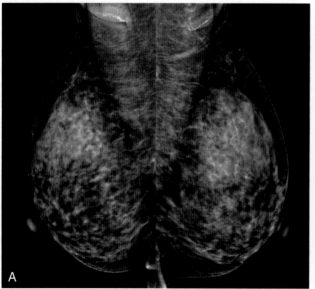
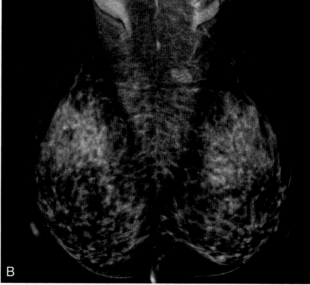

Fig. 1.5 Deodorant artifact. (A) Mediolateral oblique (MLO) views of the bilateral breasts shows radiopaque material over the bilateral axillae. (B) The patient was brought back for a repeat MLO views after wiping the bilateral axillae, which shows resolution of the artifact.

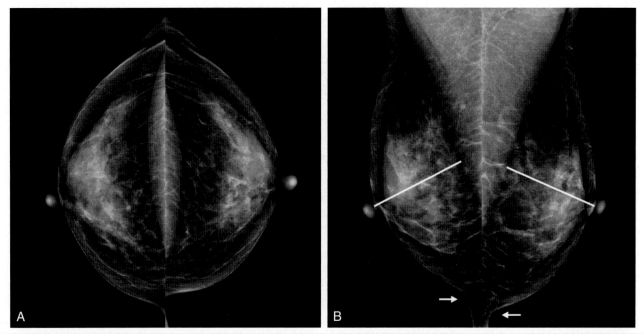

Fig. 1.6 Example of proper positioning for a bilateral screening mammogram. On the mediolateral oblique (MLO) view, note the pectoralis muscle extends inferior to the posterior nipple line (*line*) and the inframammary fold is open (*arrow*). The retroglandular fat is included and the nipple is in profile.

Special Views and Additional Views

SPOT COMPRESSION VIEW

Spot compression views can be obtained for further evaluation of a region of interest. A small spot compression paddle applies pressure to a smaller area of tissue (Fig. 1.7). This increases compression on the region of interest, improving tissue separation and visualization of the area. Spot compression can help discriminate a real lesion, such as a mass or architectural distortion, from summation artifact. A real lesion will typically persist on spot compression view, retaining its shape and density, whereas a summation artifact will disperse. When a mass is adjacent to fibroglandular tissue of similar density, the margins of a mass may be at least partially obscured. By dispersing the adjacent fibroglandular tissue, spot compression can help bring out the mass margins, allowing for more complete assessment of lesion morphology. Spot compression may be performed in conjunction with magnification when using 2D imaging, as described in the subsequent section on magnification view. Spot compression may also be used with tomosynthesis images, as described further in the tomosynthesis chapter.

MAGNIFICATION VIEW

Magnification views, in conjunction with spot compression, can be obtained to further evaluate microcalcifications and mass margins. The magnification stand positions the breast closer to the x-ray source (decreasing the source-to-object distance) and farther from the image receptor, allowing for 1.5 to 2 times magnification of the region of interest

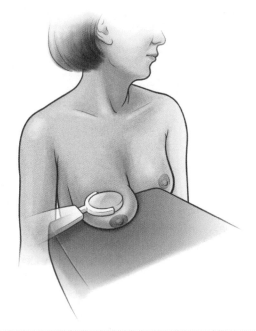

Fig. 1.7 Spot compression craniocaudal view.

(Fig. 1.8). Whereas geometric magnification alone typically reduces spatial resolution, the use of a smaller focal spot and increased compression allows for higher spatial resolution. Magnification views can help enhance visualization and characterization of calcification morphology and can help reveal calcifications not seen on nonmagnified images. Magnification views can also improve visualization of mass shapes and margins not discernible on full-field nonmagnified images.

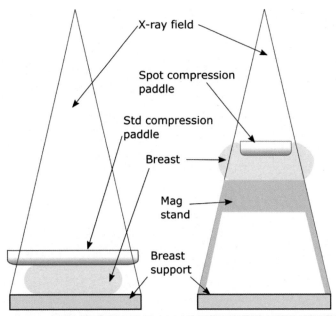

Fig. 1.8 Standard (Std) view (*left*) versus spot compression magnification view (*right*). Note that on the magnification view, the breast is placed on a magnification stand so the imaged tissue is closer to the x-ray source and farther from the image receptor, allowing for magnification of the region of interest (Image courtesy of James Mainprize).

Table 1.1 Additional Mammographic Views

Area of Interest	View	Abbreviation
Retroareolar	Spot compression with nipple in profile	–
Outer breast	Laterally exaggerated craniocaudal	XCCL
Inner breast	Medially exaggerated craniocaudal	XCCM
	Cleavage	CV
Upper breast	Craniocaudal (CC) from below	CCFB
Upper inner breast, lower outer breast	Superior-inferior oblique	SIO

ADDITIONAL VIEWS

When a portion of the breast is incompletely characterized, additional views can be obtained for further targeted evaluation (Table 1.1). These views include laterally exaggerated craniocaudal (XCCL), medially exaggerated craniocaudal (XCCM), cleavage view (CV), superior-inferior oblique (SIO), and CC from below. Use of additional views in diagnostic imaging is further discussed in Chapter 13 (Organized Approach to Diagnostic Imaging).

The Normal Mammogram

ANATOMY

The breast is composed of overlying skin, adipose tissue, and breast parenchymal tissue, which includes glandular tissue and stroma. The breast glandular tissue is divided into 15 to 20 lobes, each drained by a lactiferous duct. The lobes contain series of branching ducts that end in terminal ductal lobular units (TDLUs), which represent the functional units of the breast. TDLU is the origin of most breast carcinomas (e.g., ductal carcinoma in situ, invasive ductal carcinoma, and invasive lobular carcinoma). Each TDLU contains acini, ductules, and terminal ducts (Fig. 1.9). During lactation, breast milk is produced in the TDLUs and drain via the ductal system, which converge in the lactiferous sinus before opening into the nipple.

The breast is enveloped anteriorly by the superficial fascia just beneath the skin and posteriorly by the deep fascia just anterior to the pectoralis muscle. Cooper's ligaments are thin fibrous strands that connect the two fascial layers and support the breast (Fig. 1.10). Fibroglandular tissue is found in the mammary zone. There is fat anterior and posterior to the mammary zone, called premammary (or preglandular) and retromammary (or retroglandular) fat, respectively. Most of the glandular tissue are typically found in the upper outer quadrant of the breast near the axilla. Physiologic fatty involution occurs with aging and usually spares the upper outer breast until last.

RADIOLOGIC ANATOMY OF THE BREAST

The most anterior structure on a mammogram is the overlying skin, seen as a thin, 2- to 3-mm homogenous line against the radiolucent background of the premammary fat. Posterior to the premammary fat is the mammary zone, which appears as a radiodense (white) area with scalloped borders. The retromammary fat should be predominantly radiolucent without any glandular tissue. Any isolated asymmetry or mass in this area warrants further attention (Fig. 1.11).

The pectoralis muscle is seen at the most posterior aspect of the mammogram. On the lateral and MLO views, the pectoralis muscle is shaped like an upside-down triangle along the posterior, superior border of the images. On the CC

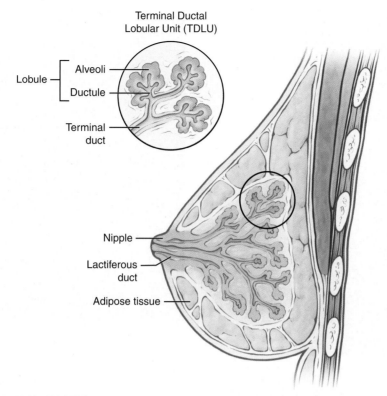

Fig. 1.9 Breast anatomy. The terminal ductal lobular unit (TDLU) is the origin of most breast carcinomas.

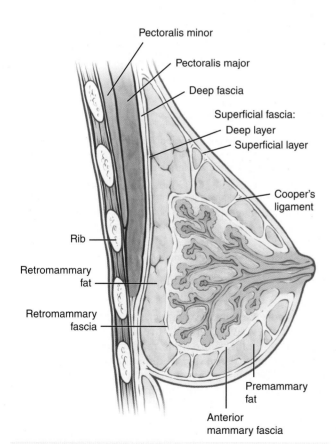

Fig. 1.10 Breast anatomy.

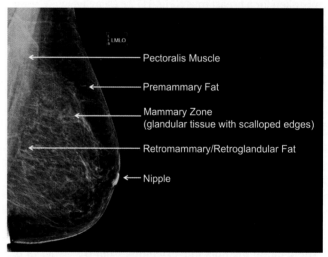

Fig. 1.11 Breast anatomy on a mammogram

view, the pectoralis usually appears crescent-shaped when visualized.

On the CC view, only fatty tissue should be seen in the far posterior medial breast. An exception is the sternalis muscle, a normal muscular variant of the anterior thoracic wall. It appears as a flame-shaped or small triangular soft tissue density in the inner breast on the CC view. Found in approximately 8% of the population, the sternalis muscle lies superficial and perpendicular to the pectoralis major muscle and parallel to the sternum. The sternalis muscle is most often unilateral, but can be bilateral. It should not be

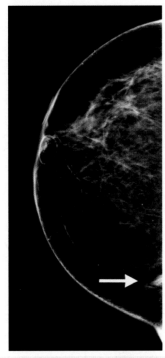

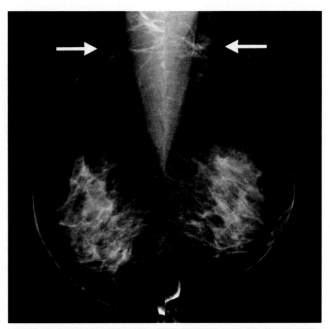

Fig. 1.13 Mediolateral oblique (MLO) views of the bilateral breasts show accessory breast tissue in the bilateral axillae (*arrows*). This is a normal variant of residual breast tissue persisting from embryologic development.

Fig. 1.12 The sternalis muscle is an anatomic variant of the chest wall musculature. The sternalis can appear as a triangular shaped asymmetry (*arrow*) in the inner breast at the posterior edge of the craniocaudal (CC) view.

Table 1.2   Image Contrast

Radiolucent (dark)	Fat
Intermediate density (white)	Fibroglandular tissue, muscle, lymph nodes, benign and malignant tumors, cysts
High density (whitest)	Calcifications, metals

mistaken for a breast mass (Fig. 1.12). Cleavage view, tomosynthesis, and/or target ultrasound could be obtained to verify as needed.

Normal axillary lymph nodes appear as circumscribed, oval, or reniform densities with radiolucent fatty hilum, typically overlying the pectoralis muscle on the MLO view. Normal lymph nodes can also be located within the breast parenchyma and are called intramammary lymph nodes. Intramammary lymph nodes are found most commonly in the lateral breast and seen in approximately 5% of all mammograms. If there is uncertainty regarding whether a lesion is a lymph node or mass, magnification views, tomosynthesis, and/or ultrasound can be obtained to better demonstrate the characteristic reniform shape and fatty hilum.

Accessory breast tissue is ectopic glandular parenchyma most commonly located in the axilla, but can be found anywhere along the milk line extending from the axilla to the abdomen. It is a normal, often bilateral variant (Fig. 1.13). Accessory breast tissue should demonstrate a similar radiographic appearance to normal glandular parenchyma. It is important to recognize the imaging appearance of accessory breast tissue to avoid mistaking the normal variant as a pathologic abnormality.

IMAGE CONTRAST

Mammography relies on the differences in x-ray attenuation between fat, fibroglandular tissue, and breast pathologies (Table 1.2). Fat is the least dense and appears radiolucent (dark) on mammography. Fibroglandular tissue, muscle, lymph nodes, neoplasms, and cysts are denser than fat and

---

Box 1.5   Breast Density

According to the Breast Imaging Reporting and Data System (BI-RADS) lexicon, mammographic density is assigned to indicate the relative possibility that a lesion could be obscured by normal tissue.

A. The breasts are almost entirely fatty

B. There are scattered areas of fibroglandular density

C. The breasts are heterogeneously dense, which may obscure small masses

D. The breasts are extremely dense, which lowers the sensitivity of mammography

appear more radiopaque (whiter). Calcifications and metals are the densest (whitest) structures on mammography.

Breast pathologies are more readily detected on a background of fatty tissue due to differences in tissue density. There can be overlap in tissue density between normal and pathologic tissues, and consequently 10% to 15% of breast cancers are mammographically occult. In these cases, a cancer is present in the absence of visible mammographic findings.

Breast density refers to the relative amount of radiopaque fibroglandular tissue to radiolucent fatty elements (Box 1.5). Relative proportions of fibrous and adipose tissue in breast

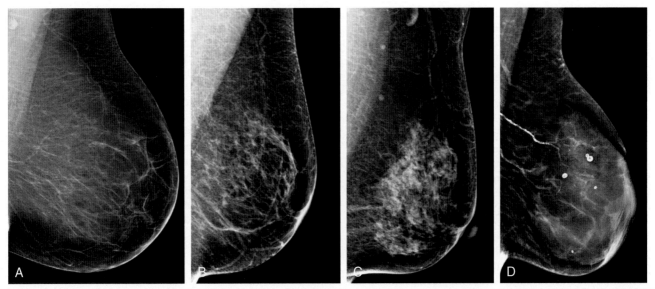

Fig. 1.14 Examples of the four breast density categories: (A) Almost entirely fatty, (B) scattered fibroglandular densities, (C) heterogeneously dense, and (D) extremely dense.

stroma vary by age and individual. Young, pregnant, and lactating women usually have a higher proportion of fibroglandular tissue. According to the Breast Imaging Reporting and Data System (BI-RADS) lexicon, mammographic density is assigned into one of four categories qualitatively indicating the relative possibility that a lesion could be obscured by normal tissue (Fig. 1.14). The categories from least to most dense are as follows: (1) The breasts are almost entirely fatty; (2) there are scattered areas of fibroglandular density; (3) the breasts are heterogeneously dense, which may obscure small masses; and (4) the breasts are extremely dense, which lowers the sensitivity of mammography. Dense fibroglandular tissue reduces the sensitivity of mammography by obscuring cancers. In addition, breast density has been shown to be an independent risk factor for developing breast cancer. Breast cancer risk and supplemental screening options are covered in detail in dedicated chapters.

Screening Versus Diagnostic Mammograms

Screening mammography is covered in detail in Chapter 12 (Organized Approach to Screening Mammography). Briefly, screening mammograms are performed in asymptomatic patients (Table 1.3). Screening mammograms are usually performed offline without a radiologist on site to guide the mammographic evaluation. After the standard CC and MLO views are obtained for each breast, patients typically leave the premises without receiving an immediate study result. The radiologist later interprets the screening mammograms in a batch and may decide to *recall* patients to return for additional imaging for suspicious findings requiring further workup. Patients may also be recalled for technical inadequacy (e.g., motion, positioning, artifact), referred to as a technical recall. Patients usually receive the mammogram

Table 1.3 Screening versus Diagnostic Mammograms

Screening	Diagnostic
Indications	Indications
■ Asymptomatic women of screening age	■ Suspicious breast signs or symptoms
	■ Abnormality detected on screening mammogram
	■ Short interval follow-up (e.g., for a Breast Imaging Reporting and Data System [BI-RADS] 3 "probably benign" lesion)
■ Patients usually leave the premises after the mammogram is obtained	■ Radiologist is actively guiding the evaluation while patients are present
■ Patients usually receive the mammogram result after leaving the premise	■ Images are interpreted at the time of examination and results communicated to patients before they leave the premises
■ Standard views: craniocaudal (CC) and mediolateral oblique (MLO) view of each breast	■ Diagnostic mammography views and/or ultrasound performed at the radiologist's discretion during the visit
■ Patients are recalled if additional imaging is needed	

results after leaving the premises, although some facilities may offer immediate interpretation.

Diagnostic mammograms are performed in patients with breast signs or symptoms and in those who need further evaluation of suspicious findings on screening mammograms. Diagnostic mammograms are also performed in patients requiring follow-up such as those who have recently received breast-conserving surgery or those with known BI-RADS 3 "probably benign" lesions. Diagnostic mammograms are performed while the radiologist is actively guiding the evaluation. Additional diagnostic imaging may include spot compression magnification views, other special views, and/or ultrasound. Diagnostic mammograms are interpreted in real time and results are communicated to patients before patients leave the facility. Diagnostic mammography is covered in detail in Chapter 13 (Organized Approach to Diagnostic Imaging).

- Breast compression reduces parenchymal superimposition and image blurring, decreases radiation dose, ensures adequate penetration, and improves spatial resolution and image contrast.
- Before interpreting a mammogram, assess the quality of the mammogram based on positioning, compression, exposure, contrast, sharpness, noise, and artifacts.
- The posterior nipple line (PNL) is an imaginary line from the posterior nipple perpendicular to the pectoralis muscle. The length of the posterior nipple line on craniocaudal (CC) and mediolateral oblique (MLO) views should be within 1 cm of each other.
- The CC view should demonstrate nipple in profile, well-visualized posterior medial breast, and fat posterior to the fibroglandular tissue.
- The MLO view should demonstrate an open inframammary fold, nipple in profile, pectoralis muscle extending inferior to the posterior nipple line, and convex anterior border of the pectoralis muscle.
- Spot compression views can provide better visualization of a region of interest, differentiating a real mass from summation artifact and bringing out mass margins.
- Magnification views allows for 1.5 to 2 times magnification of a region of interest and higher spatial resolution to aid in detection and evaluation of microcalcifications. This can be performed as spot compression with magnification (spot compression magnification view).
- Breast density categories from least to most dense are as follows: (1) almost entirely fatty, (2) scattered areas of fibroglandular density, (3) heterogeneously dense, and (4) extremely dense.
- Screening mammograms are performed in asymptomatic women of screening age. Only standard views are obtained without active, real time radiologist supervision. Most commonly, the study is interpreted and results communicated to patients after patients leave the premises.
- Diagnostic mammograms are performed in symptomatic women and those who need further evaluation of suspicious findings on screening mammograms. The radiologist is actively monitoring the diagnostic evaluation and deciding the specific mammography views to obtain. Studies are interpreted in real time and results communicated to patients before they leave the premises.

Suggested Readings

Boyd NF, Guo H, Martin LJ, et al. Mammographic density and the risk and detection of breast cancer. *NEJM.* 2007;356(3):227–238.

Broeders M, Moss S, Nyström L, et al. The impact of mammographic screening on breast cancer mortality in Europe: a review of observational studies. *J Med Screen.* 2012;19(Suppl 1):14–25.

Hendrick RE, Bassett LW, Botsco MA, et al. *Mammography quality control manual.* Reston, VA: American College of Radiology; 1999.

Logan WW, Janus J. Use of special mammographic views to maximize radiographic information. *Radiol Clin North Am.* 1987;25:953–959.

Mainiero MB, Moy L, Baron P, et al. "ACR Appropriateness Criteria Breast Cancer Screening." *J Am Coll Radiol.* 2017 Nov;14(11S):S383–S390.

Monsees BS. The Mammography Quality Standards Act. An overview of the regulations and guidance. *Radiol Clin North Am.* 2000;38:759–772.

Monticciolo DL, Newell MS, Hendrick RE, et al. Breast Cancer Screening for Average-Risk Women: Recommendations From the ACR Commission on Breast Imaging. *J Am Coll Radiol.* 2017 Sep;14(9):1137–1143.

Monticciolo DL, Newell MS, Moy L, et al. Breast Cancer Screening in Women at Higher-Than-Average Risk: Recommendations From the ACR. *J Am Coll Radiol.* 2018 Mar;15:408–414.

Park JM, Franken Jr EA. Triangulation of breast lesions: review and clinical applications. *Curr Probl Diagn Radiol.* 2008;37(1):1–14.

2 Why BI-RADS?: Overview of Breast Imaging Reporting and Data System (BI-RADS)

ANNE C. HOYT AND HANNAH S. MILCH

> **OVERVIEW** *This chapter summarizes the purpose and history of BI-RADS; introduces the BI-RADS lexicon, assessment categories, and standardized report; and answers frequently asked questions (FAQs) of using BI-RADS to communicate breast findings.*

Introduction

The Breast Imaging Reporting and Data System (BI-RADS) is a breast radiologist's second language. Spend 10 minutes in a breast radiology reading room and you will likely hear the word BI-RADS and its associated terminology uttered over a dozen times.

BI-RADS has three main goals:

1. Standardize breast imaging interpretation terminology (the BI-RADS lexicon), final assessments (the BI-RADS categories), and management recommendations.
2. Reduce confusion and optimize communication among radiologists, referring physicians, and patients.
3. Facilitate outcomes tracking and quality assurance.

Understanding BI-RADS will help you contextualize upcoming chapters on specific breast imaging findings and appropriate management steps.

HISTORY OF BI-RADS

The 1980s brought a sharp increase in mammography. In the early 1980s, only 15% to 20% of women had ever undergone a mammogram, and by the dawn of the 1990s, 65% had participated in mammography at least once.[1] This increase was largely due to favorable data showing effectiveness of screening mammography to reduce breast cancer mortality in multiple randomized controlled trials coupled with contemporaneous improvements in preoperative needle localization, making it easier to obtain a tissue diagnosis for suspicious lesions identified at mammography.[2] As mammography utilization grew in the United States during the 1980s, significant inconsistencies became apparent in mammography quality, radiation dose, radiologist interpretive skills, and result reporting. Due to the concerns raised by breast imaging specialists and the American Medical Association (AMA),[3–6] the American College of Radiology (ACR) convened two committees: the voluntary Mammography Accreditation Program (MAP) in 1987 and the Breast Imaging Reporting and Data System (BI-RADS) committee in 1988.[7] The BI-RADS committee was charged with developing guidelines for standardized mammography reporting and management recommendations.

Five years later, the ACR BI-RADS committee, composed of academic breast imagers and private practice radiologists and chaired by Dr. Carl J. D'Orsi, released the first edition of the BI-RADS lexicon in 1993.[7] This early BI-RADS document was robust and consisted of recommendations for (1) performance of screening and diagnostic mammography, (2) structure of the mammography report, (3) introduction of a mammography lexicon, and (4) final assessment categories with their respective management recommendations.[7] It should be noted that the authors fashioned BI-RADS with a clear understanding that it would be a malleable and adaptable reporting and data system with the ability to transform, improve, and expand as needed to incorporate the continuous new advances in breast imaging technology, research, and patient care.

After the successful release of the ACR MAP in 1987 and just before the 1993 ACR BI-RADS committee release of the first edition of BI-RADS, the 1992 Mammography Quality Standards Act (MQSA) became federal law and was enacted,[8] making breast imaging one of the most federally regulated medical specialties in the United States. By 1999, MQSA rules mandated, among other requirements, that every mammographic report include text for the final assessment category similar to that in the then-current 1998 third edition of BI-RADS. This new post-MQSA era in breast imaging marked a transition from inconsistent imaging quality and reporting to uniform mammography examination quality, interpretation, and reporting standards. MQSA regulations and accreditation requirements are covered in Chapter 20.

As envisioned, BI-RADS has undergone four revisions since its first edition in 1993 (1995, 1998, 2003, and 2013), with each carefully crafted to improve clarity, patient management, and quality assurance (Fig. 2.1). In 1998, the third edition included the first BI-RADS atlas with first-rate illustrations depicting each lexicon descriptor.

The fourth edition introduced many new lexicon descriptors such as the original asymmetry family (asymmetry, focal asymmetry, global asymmetry), division of suspicious calcifications into "intermediate risk" and "higher probability of malignancy," and the option to subclassify BI-RADS final assessment category 4 into subcategories (4 A, 4B, and 4 C) to better communicate the risk of malignancy to both the patient's health care provider and the pathologist interpreting a woman's biopsy tissue specimens. Furthermore, the fourth edition (2003) introduced the first BI-RADS ultrasound (US) and BI-RADS magnetic resonance imaging (MRI) lexicons. These new US and MRI lexicons were designed to mirror the same lexicon descriptors used in mammography whenever possible (e.g., mass, shape, and margin) but also allow for new modality-specific descriptors such as orientation and echo pattern in US or foci/focus and kinetic curve assessment in MRI. The current fifth edition (2013) further refines the lexicon using consistent terminology across mammography, US, and MRI sections with evidence-based justification and better quality images for all sections including mostly digital images for mammography. This edition also defines auditing rules that apply to all three sections and allows uncoupling of the final assessment category from its management recommendation as discussed in the section below.

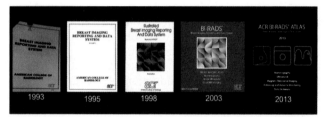

Fig. 2.1 Covers of the five editions of Breast Imaging Reporting and Data System (BI-RADS) beginning in 1993. (BI-RADS Atlas images obtained with permission from the American College of Radiology.)

THE BI-RADS LEXICON

The BI-RADS lexicon is a carefully constructed dictionary of descriptive terms for breast imaging findings, which has been published in numerous languages. It allows all radiologists to speak the same language and generate standard reports that are easily understood by referring providers and ancillary medical staff. The over 700-page BI-RADS Atlas provides detailed, annotated example images that illustrate the proper use of the lexicon terminology. Pathology of described findings is provided whenever possible. In addition to mammography, the most recent edition of the BI-RADS Atlas (2013) also includes comprehensive lexicons for breast US and MRI, plus a supplement with specific guidance for digital breast tomosynthesis (DBT).[9] Specifics of lexicon and lesion descriptors are described in the relevant modality-specific chapters to follow.

The BI-RADS lexicon is systematically organized in a uniform branching format for each imaging modality. The organization is first divided at the highest level by imaging modality (mammography, US, MRI) followed by breast tissue and findings. Breast tissue is classified by its *composition* on mammography and by the *amount of fibroglandular tissue* and *background parenchymal enhancement (BPE)* on MRI. Breast composition in mammography refers to a woman's individual admixture of dense fibroglandular tissue and fat within her breast (i.e., her breast density) and ranges from *almost entirely fatty* to *extremely dense* (Fig. 2.2). Similar terms are used to describe the amount of fibroglandular tissue on MRI. Sonographic tissue composition can also be described as *homogeneous* (fatty or fibroglandular) versus *heterogeneous* echotexture; however, these terms may only be used for screening and/or whole breast diagnostic US when the breast tissue can be assessed in its entirety. Further details on breast composition are outlined in the section titled

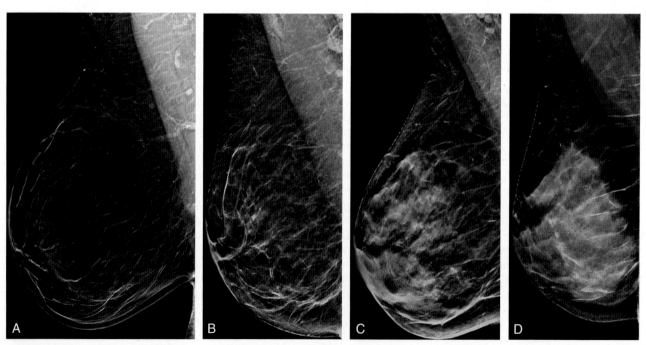

Fig. 2.2 Four synthetic mediolateral oblique mammograms depict the four Breast Imaging Reporting and Data System (BI-RADS) breast densities: (A) almost entirely fatty (type A); (B) scattered areas of fibroglandular density (type B); (C) heterogeneously dense, which may obscure small masses (type C); and (D) extremely dense, which lowers the sensitivity of mammography (type D).

"The Structured Breast Imaging Report" and subsequent chapters dedicated to specific imaging modalities.

Findings are divided by (1) type (i.e., mass), (2) features of each finding type, and (3) a list of descriptive terms. For example, a mass (a finding type) is characterized by three features: shape, margin, and density. Descriptive terms for the shape of a mass include oval, round, or irregular.

The lexicon has been developed such that selection of the correct descriptor leads to use of the appropriate final assessment category and management recommendation. This correlation applies across the full spectrum of breast imaging findings, ranging from completely benign to highly suspicious for breast cancer. If suspicious lexicon terminology is used, tissue diagnosis should be recommended. If benign lexicon terminology is used, routine annual follow-up should be recommended. For example, if calcifications are described as having a "fine-linear branching" morphology, they are suspicious and require a biopsy. If the calcifications are "popcorn-like," they are typically benign and can be left alone (Fig. 2.3). If calcifications are distributed in a "segmental" pattern, there is a high likelihood of breast cancer and tissue sampling is required. Combining a suspicious descriptor with a benign final assessment and routine annual follow-up recommendation is not advised. Improper use of BI-RADS causes confusion among other radiologists and referring health care providers and potentially leads to mismanagement of the patient.

Multiple lexicon descriptors may be used to describe a single breast finding, but the overall management assessment for that finding should match the most suspicious BI-RADS lexicon descriptor used. An example would be a mass seen on MRI that is *circumscribed* and T2-hyperintense but demonstrates a *heterogeneous internal enhancement* pattern. Circumscribed is a more benign descriptor, but heterogeneous internal enhancement is a suspicious descriptor, and therefore this mass should be biopsied (Fig. 2.4).

The BI-RADS lexicon is largely a data-driven document. For example, amorphous calcifications are considered moderately suspicious (BI-RADS 4B; Table 2.1) because studies have shown a 20% likelihood of association with malignancy. In some instances where supporting data is lacking,

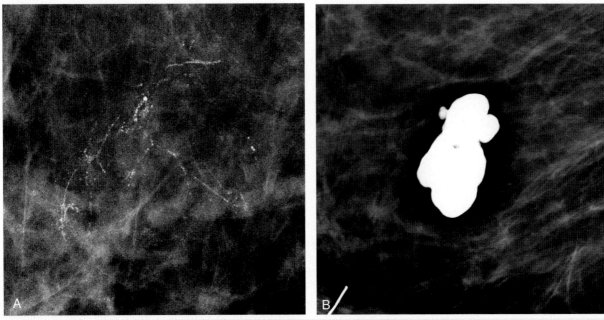

Fig. 2.3 Correct use of the lexicon descriptors lead to the lead the radiologist to the appropriate Breast Imaging Reporting and Data System (BI-RADS) final assessment category and management recommendation. (A) Fine-linear branching calcifications, a suspicious finding, are assigned BI-RADS category 4C, and tissue sampling is appropriate. (B) "Popcorn" calcification, a benign finding, is assigned BI-RADS category 2, with no further imaging or intervention needed.

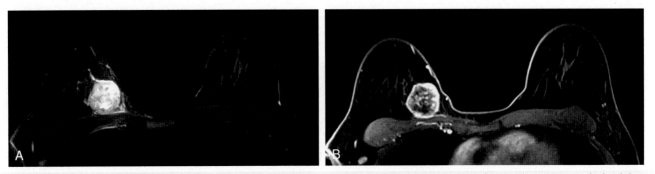

Fig. 2.4 The most suspicious descriptor guides management. (A) Magnetic resonance imaging (MRI) example of a mass that is *circumscribed* and short tau inversion recovery *(STIR) hyperintense*, two features that can be seen in more benign masses. (B) However, the mass demonstrates *heterogeneous internal enhancement* and therefore is suspicious and warrants biopsy. Final pathology was triple negative invasive ductal carcinoma.

guidance is derived from expert opinion by the BI-RADS committee in an effort to make the Atlas a practical and useful resource. Remember, BI-RADS is an ever-evolving document that is modified and updated as new knowledge is acquired.

Special Considerations for Other Imaging Modalities

Whenever possible the BI-RADS lexicon strives to use the same lexicon terminology across all three modalities to maximize consistency and facilitate learning. As such, some lexicon descriptors are universal for all modalities. For example, the shape of a mass is described by the descriptive terms *round*, *oval*, or *irregular* in all modalities. Likewise, the margin of a mass is either circumscribed or not circumscribed in all modalities. Some differences between the three

modalities are inevitable; for example, the BI-RADS language used to describe the margins of noncircumscribed masses (i.e., *angular* is specific to US, *obscured* is specific to mammography). The words used to describe the distribution (*diffuse*, *regional*, *linear*, *segmental*) of a non-mass finding are similar whether referring to calcifications on mammography or non-mass enhancement on MRI, with some small exceptions (i.e., *grouped* for calcifications and *focal* for non-mass enhancement).

Finally, some lexicon features are unique to a modality. For example, the shape of individual calcifications is only appreciable on mammography, and therefore *morphology* of calcifications is only described mammographically. The *orientation* of a mass is reserved for US imaging and refers to the orientation of the long axis of the mass relative to the skin line (*parallel* is more often benign, *not parallel* is suspicious; Fig. 2.5).

Specific guidance for DBT is included in a supplement to the mammography section of the ACR BI-RADS fifth edition. The mammography BI-RADS lexicon terminology is fully applicable to DBT. With DBT, multiple very low-dose projections are obtained in an arc, which allow reconstruction of those images into thin slices of breast tissue. These slices, when viewed like the pages of a book, sequentially remove overlying layers of fibroglandular breast tissue, occasionally exposing otherwise hidden or obscured breast cancers. Furthermore, many "asymmetries" on two-dimensional (2D) mammography are readily shown to be summation artifact (overlapping normal fibroglandular breast tissue at different depths within the breast) on DBT resulting in fewer patient recalls. In addition, the margins of masses are often better seen on DBT compared with 2D mammography, such that additional mammographic views may not always be necessary. In these situations, it is recommended that patients are still recalled—even if the mass is circumscribed—for additional evaluation with US to fully characterize the mass. DBT is covered in more detail in Chapter 6.

BI-RADS FINAL ASSESSMENT CATEGORIES

After using appropriate lexicon descriptive terms to describe findings in the body of the report, the next step is to assign a BI-RADS assessment category for the examination. If desired, separate BI-RADS assessments may be assigned to left and right breasts. The BI-RADS categories range

Table 2.1 Summary of BI-RADS Assessment Categories and Their Associated Management Recommendations and Likelihood of Malignancy

Assessment Category	Management Recommendation	Likelihood of Malignancy
BI-RADS 0: Incomplete	Recall for additional imaging and/or comparison with prior examination(s)	N/A
BI-RADS 1: Negative	Routine annual screening	Essentially 0%
BI-RADS 2: Benign	Routine annual screening	Essentially 0%
BI-RADS 3: Probably benign	Short-interval follow-up imaging or surveillance	>0% but ≤2%
BI-RADS 4: Suspicious	Tissue diagnosis	>2% but <95%
4A: Low suspicion		>2% to ≤10%
4B: Moderate suspicion		>10% to ≤50%
4C: High suspicion		>50% to <95%
BI-RADS 5: Highly suggestive of malignancy	Tissue diagnosis	≥95%
BI-RADS 6: Known biopsy/proven malignancy	Surgical excision when clinically appropriate	N/A

BI-RADS, Breast Imaging Reporting and Data System.
Adapted from D'Orsi CJ, Sickles EA, Mendelson EB, Morris EA, et al.; *ACR BI-RADS Atlas, Breast Imaging Reporting and Data System*. Reston, VA: American College of Radiology; 2013. Part I ACR BI-RADS Mammography, Appendix B, p. 175.

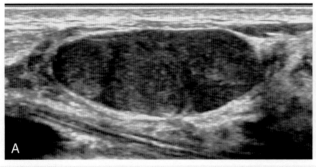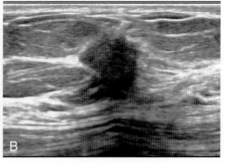

Fig. 2.5 Mass *orientation* on ultrasound. (A) A mass with *parallel* orientation, where the long axis is parallel to the skin surface, a benign feature commonly seen in fibroadenomas. (B) A mass with an irregular shape and a *not parallel* orientation, a suspicious feature worrisome for malignancy. This mass proved to be invasive ductal carcinoma.

from 0 to 6 and are divided into incomplete (category 0) and final assessments (categories 1–6). Each category is associated with a standardized management recommendation (see Table 2.1). In most cases, the management recommendation should match the assessment category; however, the fifth edition of the BI-RADS Atlas allows for uncoupling of the category and management under certain specific circumstances. Examples include women with appropriately categorized, probably benign findings (category 3) who desire biopsy for confirmation or a large painful cyst appropriately categorized as category 2 (benign) for which US-guided aspiration is recommended for symptomatic relief.

There are two types of breast imaging exams: screening and diagnostic. Screening mammography is an examination of an asymptomatic woman designed to detect clinically occult breast cancer. Diagnostic mammography is an examination of a symptomatic patient such as a woman with a breast lump or for a patient with a recent abnormal screening mammogram. The BI-RADS assessment categories are applicable to both of these imaging examination types; however, some assessment categories are more likely to be used in the setting of screening (BI-RADS 0) and some should be used only after a full diagnostic evaluation (BI-RADS 3, 4, 5, and 6). It is important to remember that a negative imaging evaluation can never guarantee that a woman does not have breast cancer, so any clinically suspicious lump or other breast symptom not explained by the diagnostic imaging evaluation should be referred to a surgeon to determine whether surgical biopsy is indicated in light of the negative imaging.

Box 2.1 summarizes key points for each of the seven assessment categories and their respective management recommendations. When the BI-RADS lexicon is followed, each assessment category is associated with a specific, rigorously proven likelihood of malignancy. The success of the BI-RADS lexicon and its final assessment categories is evident by its international adoption as the breast imaging reporting standard.

THE STRUCTURED BREAST IMAGING REPORT

The BI-RADS lexicon and assessment categories described above are incorporated into the structured breast imaging report. The exact division and order of sections will vary, but the following information should be included in every report:

- ***Examination modality/modalities:*** Mammography, DBT, US, MRI (can be more than one modality in a single report).
- ***Indication:*** Screening, callback from screening, palpable lump, breast pain, new breast cancer diagnosis, etc.
- ***Technique:*** A description of the type of imaging performed.
  - Mammography: Include technology full-field digital mammography (FFDM), DBT, views (mediolateral oblique [MLO], craniocaudal [CC]), and a statement regarding computer-aided detection (CAD) use if appropriate.
  - US: Include sonographic technique (targeted versus whole breast).
  - MRI: Include sequences performed and use of gadolinium.
- ***Comparison:*** Careful comparison to prior studies is a key component of breast imaging interpretation, which is one reason why baseline screening exams have higher recall rates.[9] If this section is not included in the report, it should be assumed that no comparison has been made.
- ***Overall breast composition/tissue density:*** Reporting overall breast composition is an important way to communicate the sensitivity of the examination to the referring health care provider. For example, the sensitivity of mammography is limited in a woman with extremely dense breasts (see Fig. 2.2). Providing information about breast density in a mammography report is required by law and may affect decision-making by the patient and health care provider, such as requesting DBT for future screening examinations or choosing to undergo supplemental screening US. The limitations of extremely dense breast tissue on mammogram is analogous to marked BPE limiting the sensitivity of MRI. Reporting US breast composition is optional as its effect on examination sensitivity requires further study.
- ***Clear description of important findings:*** Describing the appearance and location of each relevant finding is at the core of a good breast imaging report. Each finding is described using the BI-RADS lexicon without embellishment and without providing definitions of lexicon terms. The location of the finding refers to clockface and/or breast quadrant, as well as distance from the nipple and/or depth (anterior, middle, posterior third of breast tissue; Fig. 2.6). If a finding is seen best on DBT images, providing the slice number or range of slice numbers is recommended. A good rule of thumb when describing a finding is the following: Could someone accurately visualize what the finding looks like and where they are in the breast without looking at the images? If the answer is "yes," you have successfully described the finding.
- ***Assessment:*** The U.S. Food and Drug Administration (FDA) requires by law that the text corresponding to a single overall assessment category be included at the end of the report: negative, benign, probably benign, suspicious, etc. Although not required by the FDA, the ACR encourages use of a numeric code (0–6) along with the assessment category text. Certain practices may provide a BI-RADS assessment category for each breast and/or each finding; however this is optional. The overall final assessment must correlate with the most actionable finding. For example, if the right breast has benign scattered calcifications (BI-RADS 2) and the left breast has a suspicious mass (BI-RADS 4), the final overall assessment is "BI-RADS category 4: suspicious" because tissue diagnosis of the suspicious mass is the critical management step. The hierarchy of BI-RADS final assessment categories for findings of increasing clinical concern requiring action are as follows: category 1, 2, 3, 6, 0, 4, 5.
- ***Management recommendation:*** The specific management recommendation must be clearly stated at the end of the report. The use of a simple coded assessment and its coupled management recommendation (see Table 2.1) allows facile communication of both routine and higher priority next steps among the patient and members of the health care team—breast surgeons, referring physicians, nurses,

Box 2.1   Key Points for Each Breast Imaging Reporting and Data System (BI-RADS) Assessment Category

BI-RADS 0: Incomplete

- Intended for screening examinations ("callbacks")
- Can be used in the setting of a diagnostic examination when the study is incomplete
  - Examples: requesting prior imaging, patient unable to stay for full diagnostic workup, or ultrasound cannot be performed at time of diagnostic mammography

BI-RADS 1: Negative

- Intended for screening or diagnostic examinations
- No breast imaging findings described in report; normal examination

BI-RADS 2: Benign

- Intended for screening or diagnostic examinations
- Interpreting physician chooses to describe a benign finding in the report
  - Examples: scattered calcifications, bilateral circumscribed masses, postsurgical changes, breast implants, multiple simple cysts (ultrasound)

BI-RADS 3: Probably Benign

- Intended for diagnostic examinations; strongly discouraged for screening mammography examinations.
- The likelihood of malignancy is ≤2%.
- Management: 6-month follow-up imaging over the course of 1 year followed by annual surveillance until 2 years of stability is demonstrated, at which point the finding can be downgraded to BI-RADS 2. Some practices may choose to follow for 3 years before assessing as benign.
- Evidence supports the need for biopsy rather than continued follow-up if findings increase in size.
- Considered "positive" if assigned to a screening examination and "negative" if assigned to a diagnostic examination for MQSA/audit purposes.
- Reserved for findings where scientific evidence shows 2% or less likelihood of malignancy. Not to be used as an "indeterminate" assessment between categories 2 and 4. If unsure of benignity, then category 4 assessment with tissue sampling is appropriate.
  - Examples: Solitary group of round calcifications, focal asymmetry with no sonographic correlate parallel oval hypoechoic circumscribed mass, all at baseline imaging.

BI-RADS 4: Suspicious

- The level of suspicion (4A, 4B, 4C) communicates the likelihood of malignancy to referring provider, pathologist, and radiologist performing the biopsy and should correlate with PPV of imaging descriptors used.
- Intended for diagnostic examinations; strongly discouraged for screening examinations.
  - Examples: Fine linear branching calcifications have a PPV of 53%–81% and should be assigned a BI-RADS 4C (50%–95% likelihood of malignancy). Oval partially circumscribed hypoechoic mass suggestive of a fibroadenoma, and probable abscess should be assigned a BI-RADS 4A (2%–10% likelihood of malignancy).

BI-RADS 5: Highly Suspicious of Malignancy

- Historically, this category was included at the request of the American College of Surgeons to allow women in underserved communities who lack access to image-guided breast biopsy to proceed directly to open surgical biopsy and fresh frozen section confirmation of malignancy. It can also be useful to expedite surgical referral for a patient without waiting for biopsy results.
- If core needle biopsy is benign, then radiology-pathology correlation is considered *discordant* and surgical excision should be recommended.
- Intended for diagnostic examinations; strongly discouraged for screening examinations.

BI-RADS 6: Known Biopsy-Proven Malignancy

- Findings with a prior malignant tissue diagnosis that are reidentified on imaging.
- Continued surgical and oncologic management is recommended.
  - Examples: diagnostic MRI performed for extent of disease in a patient with known breast cancer, imaging follow-up of finding(s) in a patient undergoing neoadjuvant chemotherapy, older adult women with breast cancer and multiple medical comorbidities precluding lumpectomy whose breast cancer is managed with endocrine (tamoxifen) therapy only.

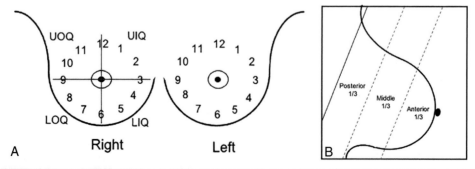

Fig. 2.6 The location of a finding on mammography is described by (A) the clockface with distance from nipple in centimeters or the quadrant and (B) the depth relative to the nipple. *UOQ*, upper outer quadrant; *UIQ*, upper inner quadrant; *LOQ*, lower outer quadrant; *LIQ*, lower inner quadrant.

Box 2.2 **Example of a standardized screening mammography report using appropriate report organization and BI-RADS terminology.**

Example Screening Report

May 30, 20XX

Bilateral Screening Digital Breast Tomosynthesis

Indication: Screening.

Comparison: None. Baseline examination.

Technique: The following digital breast tomosynthesis with 2D composite views were obtained: bilateral craniocaudal with tomosynthesis and bilateral mediolateral oblique with tomosynthesis.
Computer-aided detection was utilized by the radiologist in the interpretation of this examination.

Mammogram:
The breast tissue is heterogeneously dense, which may obscure small masses (density C).
There is a obscured oval mass in the left breast at 2:00, 5 cm from the nipple.
There is no suspicious mass, calcifications, or architectural distortion seen in the right breast.

Impression:
Left breast mass requires additional evaluation.

BI-RADS 0: Incomplete. Recommend additional mammographic views and, if indicated, targeted left breast ultrasound.

Box 2.3 **Example of a standardized diagnostic combined mammography and ultrasound report using appropriate report organization and BI-RADS terminology.**

Example Diagnostic Report

April 20, 20XX

Left Breast Diagnostic Digital Breast Tomosynthesis

Left Breast Diagnostic Ultrasound

Indication: Callback from screening

Comparison: Screening mammogram from April 12, 2021

Technique: The following digital breast tomosynthesis with 2D composite views were obtained: Left mediolateral with tomosynthesis, left mediolateral oblique spot compression with tomosynthesis, left craniocaudal spot compression with tomosynthesis.
Computer-aided detection was utilized by the radiologist in the interpretation of this examination.

Mammogram:
The breast tissue is heterogeneously dense, which may obscure small masses (density C).
Additional evaluation was performed for the partially obscured oval mass seen on prior mammogram. On the current examination, there is a circumscribed oval mass measuring 12 mm in the left breast upper outer quadrant at 2:00, 5 cm from the nipple.

Ultrasound:
Targeted left breast ultrasound was performed in the upper outer quadrant.
There is an oval circumscribed anechoic mass measuring $12 \times 6 \times 8$ mm in the left breast at 2:00, 5 cm from the nipple, demonstrating posterior enhancement. The finding corresponds to the mass seen on mammogram and is consistent with a simple cyst.

Impression:
Left breast simple cyst is benign. No mammographic evidence of malignancy.
Findings and recommendations were discussed with the patient by the radiologist Dr. Smith at the conclusion of the examination.

BI-RADS 2: Benign. Routine annual mammography recommended.

administrative office staff, schedulers, and radiologists—to help direct and guide the patient's care (Boxes 2.2 and 2.3).

BI-RADS FAQS

1. Why is using BI-RADS 3 "probably benign" on a screening examination discouraged?
   A screening examination should never replace a diagnostic workup. Additional imaging is required to optimally evaluate if a finding is benign, has subtle malignant features requiring biopsy, or should be classified as probably benign requiring short-interval follow-up. For example, calcifications that seem probably benign on a screening examination may layer on magnification views indicating milk of calcium, which requires no further follow-up (BI-RADS 2). Diagnostic imaging also affords the patient an opportunity to be informed about her breast imaging findings, ask questions, and weigh in on any decisions if appropriate. Assigning short-interval follow-up to a screening mammogram is not without risks; it can lead to unnecessary imaging cost, radiation exposure, patient anxiety, and delayed diagnosis of breast cancer. Performing diagnostic imaging of a screen-identified indeterminate finding leads to safer, more efficient, and cost-effective breast imaging.

2. If a screening mammogram is negative but you want to recommend MRI for high-risk screening, do you give it a BI-RADS 0 because you are recommending additional imaging?
   No. Never give a negative imaging examination a BI-RADS 0. Remember that the BI-RADS assessment category is specific to the imaging findings for the examination being interpreted in the report. If there are no significant imaging findings, the examination should be given BI-RADS 1 or 2. If you are recommending MRI for high-risk screening, add a sentence at the end of the report with the MRI recommendation.

3. If a patient has a known breast cancer (i.e., found on MRI) but the mammogram is negative, what BI-RADS should be given to the mammogram?
   BI-RADS 1 "negative" should be assigned because the mammogram did not show the malignancy. This is a false-negative mammogram, which does not reflect on the interpreting radiologist's skill unless the mammographic finding was overlooked or the radiologist interpreted a technically unacceptable mammogram.

4. If an MRI has a known cancer (BI-RADS 6) and an additional suspicious finding (BI-RADS 4), what is the overall BI-RADS?
   BI-RADS 4. The hierarchy of BI-RADS final assessment categories for findings of increasing clinical concern requiring action are as follows: category 1, 2, 3, 6, 0, 4, 5; hence a category 4 supersedes a category 6.

5. If a patient has axillary lymphadenopathy and no suspicious finding in the breasts, what is the BI-RADS?

The answer to this question depends on whether the adenopathy is unilateral or bilateral and if the patient has a known underlying malignancy or infectious, inflammatory, rheumatologic, or other condition that explains the adenopathy. Unilateral axillary lymphadenopathy is suspicious for occult breast cancer. Less common malignant causes include metastatic cancer (ovarian and melanoma, among others) or lymphoma. Benign causes may include inflammation or infection of the ipsilateral breast, axilla, or upper extremity. If a benign cause such as an infected nail bed is identified, then BI-RADS category 2 should be assigned. In the absence of a benign etiology, BI-RADS category 4 should be assigned. Bilateral axillary lymphadenopathy may be malignant or benign. BI-RADS category 2 "benign" is appropriate in cases of known infectious, reactive, or inflammatory etiologies such as human immunodeficiency virus (HIV), tuberculosis, sarcoid, rheumatoid arthritis, and psoriasis (Fig. 2.7). Suspicious causes of bilateral axillary adenopathy include lymphoma or leukemia and, in the absence of a known diagnosis of either condition, should be assigned a BI-RADS category 4. If a patient has known lymphoma or leukemia, a BI-RADS category 2 may be appropriate with an added phase "with bilateral axillary adenopathy presumed due to known lymphoma." If in the same patient the adenopathy suddenly increases after being mammographically stable or having resolved, then a BI-RADS category 4 is assigned to assess for potential disease recurrence. See Chapter 17: Lymph Node Evaluation in Breast Imaging for guidance on lymph node evaluation.

6. If an otherwise negative diagnostic mammogram and US are suggestive of implant rupture and MRI is recommended to evaluate for rupture, what is the appropriate BI-RADS assessment for the mammogram?

BI-RADS 2 because implant rupture is a benign finding and the mammogram is otherwise negative. A sentence should be added at the end of the report to recommend MRI evaluation for implant rupture as clinically appropriate.

7. If a biopsy is recommended for a low-suspicion breast mass (BI-RADS 4 A), but the patient opts for 6-month follow-up mammogram instead of biopsy, what is the BI-RADS assessment assuming stability at 6-month follow-up examination?

BI-RADS 4A. If a patient elects to follow a finding for which biopsy has been recommended, the assessment should continue to match the imaging finding and should not be changed to a category 3 to reflect the patient's wishes. Likewise, if a patient elects biopsy of a category 3 finding, the final assessment should not be changed to category 4 A. Simply add a sentence to the

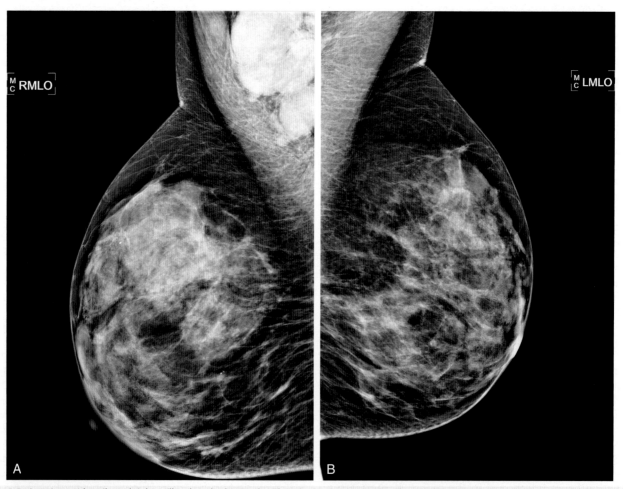

Fig. 2.7 A patient with unilateral right axillary lymphadenopathy. There is no mammographic abnormality in the breasts. This patient had known old tuberculosis. Breast Imaging Reporting and Data System (BI-RADS) category 2 "benign."

report stating that the patient prefers biopsy rather than follow-up imaging.

8. If an MRI is done to assess response to neoadjuvant chemotherapy in a patient with known breast cancer, and there is a complete imaging response to therapy such that the MRI is now negative, what is the BI-RADS assessment category?

BI-RADS 6. This is an exception to the statement in question #2 stating that the BI-RADS should match the imaging, because in the case of neoadjuvant chemotherapy, the definitive surgical management of the malignancy is delayed until chemotherapy has concluded. Hence, the patient's cancer has not yet been surgically removed and it is unknown if residual MRI-occult breast cancer remains.

9. An MRI is assessed as BI-RADS 4 for a suspicious finding with recommendation to obtain a targeted ("second-look") US for possible US biopsy in lieu of MRI biopsy. What BI-RADS assessment should be assigned to the MR-targeted US if there is no sonographic correlate?

An MRI-targeted diagnostic US performed for a suspicious (category 4) finding on MRI that does not show a sonographic correlate should be assessed as BI-RADS 1 "negative" because the US imaging is negative. A sentence should be added at the end of the US report restating the previous MRI recommendation for tissue diagnosis. An MRI-targeted diagnostic US that demonstrates a suspicious sonographic correlate for the MRI finding should receive a BI-RADS 4 final assessment and a sentence should be added at the end of the report stating that US-guided biopsy can be performed in lieu of an MRI biopsy for the suspicious MRI finding.

QUALITY ASSURANCE TOOL

A successful breast cancer detection program should (1) discover a high proportion of breast cancers that exist in a screened population, (2) minimize morbidity and cost, and (3) detect cancers that are more likely to be cured (minimal, node negative, stage 0 and 1). In order to evaluate the success of a breast cancer detection program, a mammography medical outcomes audit of each facility's mammography performance is required annually by the FDA in addition to the ACR's added requirement for annual individual radiologist audits. The audits should follow-up positive mammographic assessments and correlate pathology results with the interpreting physician's findings.[10] What at first sounds like a less-than-desirable task actually turns out to be a straightforward, powerful tool that provides valuable insight about a practice group's and its individual radiologist's interpretative performance. The success of the long-required MQSA mammography medical audit has led to the establishment of similarly structured auditing procedures for breast US and breast MRI, which are outside the scope of this chapter and can be found in the fifth edition of the BI-RADS Atlas.

Understanding and achieving desirable benchmark metrics is critical to the delivery of high-quality patient care and is actively becoming part of the equation used to calculate practice and individual clinical quality metrics for determining payment in this time of value-based medicine. Outcome monitoring also validates quality practice performance, facilitates research activities,

flags deficiencies, and allows identification of their root cause(s) so corrective action plans can be undertaken. The most valuable audit insights are gained by comparing all audit parameters to benchmark data as a measure of a group's or individual radiologist's breast imaging interpretative performance. Limiting comparison to only one or two audit metrics may be misleading and not reflect the true practice or radiologist's performance. For example, a recall rate within an acceptable range is of no value if the same reader's cancer detection rate is too low.[11] Comparing an individual or group's audit metrics over time allows for trend analysis and is a valuable quality assurance exercise. Average screening mammography audit metrics from the Breast Cancer Surveillance Consortium (BCSC) and the National Mammography Database (NMD), both large established screening mammography registries in the United States, are shown in Table 2.2. The last column in Table 2.2 lists acceptable screening mammography performance benchmarks as published in the BI-RADS Atlas 5th edition. (Table 2.2). It is important to compare any audit outcome to the most appropriate benchmark. The best benchmark with which an audit should be compared is the benchmark that was derived from a practice-type that most closely matches the practice-type of the group of radiologists being audited.[12]

The BCSC performance metrics are from practices selected to represent the many different mammography practice types in the United States. However, it is important to understand that the BCSC data is linked to cancer registries resulting in a very complete database, especially with regard to cancer staging data and inclusion of outcomes on near all-positive mammography examinations.[13] The NMD performance metrics are self-reported from a large number of everyday practices in the United States, most of which are not linked to cancer registries; hence the database is larger but less complete than the BCSC, since it has fewer known outcomes for positive examinations and less complete and accurate staging data.[14] The BI-RADS Atlas performance benchmarks were developed by a panel of expert breast imaging interpreting physicians after critical analysis of peer-reviewed literature, BCSC data, and personal experience.[10]

Breast imaging audits should be performed separately for both screening and diagnostic patient populations following either a "basic" or "more complete" analysis. "The basic clinically relevant audit" for screening will be the focus of this section. Additional information on "more complete" screening mammography, diagnostic mammography, and US or MRI audits can be found in the fifth edition BI-RADS Atlas. Box 2.4 details the data to be collected for the basic clinically relevant audit.

Understanding basic definitions (Box 2.5) allows one to more easily and accurately characterize an examination as positive or negative. A *positive screening examination* results in a recommendation for another imaging examination prior to the woman's next scheduled screening examination. A *negative screening examination* does not. *Cancer* is defined as ductal carcinoma in situ (DCIS) or primary breast cancer. The mammogram of a woman showing metastatic cancer to the breast is not counted as a detected cancer. The time interval used to assess whether an examination is a true or false positive or negative should match the screening interval used by the practice. For example, if a practice screens annually, then a negative screening examination is considered a true negative

Table 2.2 Screening Mammography Performance (BCSC, NMD) and BI-RADS Acceptable Benchmarks

	BCSC[a]	NMD[b]	BI-RADS[c]
Years	2007–2013	2017–2018	
Number of examinations	1,682,504	6,171,960	
Cancer detection rate per 1000 examinations	5.1	4.1	>2.5
Recall rate	11.6	9.9	5–12
PPV1 (abnormal interpretation)	4.4	3.8	3–8
PPV2 (recommendation for biopsy)	25.6	21.4	20–40
PPV3 (biopsy performed)	28.6	28.5	n/i
Cancer stage 0 or 1	76.9	71.8	n/i
Sensitivity	86.9	n/m	≥75%
Specificity	88.9	n/m	88%–95%
Cancer histology:			
DCIS	31.0	23.7	
Invasive cancer	69.0	76.3	
Lymph node status:			
Negative	79.4	88.2[d]	
Positive	20.6	11.8[d]	
Invasive cancer size:			
1–5 mm	12.7[e]	15.4[f]	
6–10 mm	25.6[e]	31.9[f]	
11–15 mm	25.5[e]	25.2[f]	
16–20 mm	14.7[e]	10.4[f]	
>20 mm	21.5[e]	17.1[f]	

Values are percentages (%) except for years, number of examinations, and cancer detection rate.
Table 2.2 lists three mammography medical audit benchmarks from the Breast Cancer Surveillance Consortium (BCSC) registry, the National Mammography Database (NMD) registry and the Breast Imaging Reporting and Data System (BI-RADS) Atlas. An individual practice's audit data should be compared with an audit benchmark derived from the same practice type.
[a]Breast Cancer Surveillance Consortium registry.
[b]National Mammography Database (Data obtained with permission).
[c]BI-RADS Atlas fifth edition acceptable benchmarks derived by a panel of expert breast imagers.
[d]Derived from 6926 invasive tumors with known nodal status of 19,215 reported invasive tumors.
[e]Derived from 5885 known invasive tumor sizes
[f]Derived from 7610 invasive tumors with known tumor size of 11,340 reported invasive tumors.
DCIS, Ductal carcinoma in situ; *n/i*, Not included in BI-RADS Atlas benchmark; *n/m*, not measurable since data set is not linked to tumor registries and is inherently less complete; *PPV*, positive predictive value.

if a breast cancer is not diagnosed within 1 year of the negative screening examination and a false negative if a breast cancer is diagnosed in less than 1 year. If a screening examination is assigned a category 3 (which is strongly discouraged), then it is considered a positive examination for screening audit purposes because the patient will undergo an imaging examination (short-interval follow-up) prior to what would have been her next annual screening examination. In the diagnostic setting the final assessment of category 3 is determined after a careful diagnostic workup. Hence the proper use of this category is associated with a 2% or less chance for malignancy and thus is considered a negative examination in the diagnostic audit. MQSA requires that when a facility becomes aware of a patient imaged at that facility but diagnosed with breast cancer after biopsy at an outside facility, the facility must attempt to obtain the outside pathology report and then review their facility's previously performed mammograms in order to identify any false negative examinations.

After collecting the data in Box 2.4, calculate the audit metrics listed in Box 2.5. Once complete, monitor your mammography performance metrics in comparison to recommended benchmarks (Table 2.2) to gain valuable insight about your practice group's and its individual radiologist's interpretative performance.

BI-RADS AND BEYOND/CONCLUSION

Implications for Research

Type "BI-RADS" into PubMed and the myriad of results provide a snapshot of breast imaging clinical research. One might think that a system with so many rules would hamper innovation, but in reality, the opposite is true. In fact, one of the fundamental roles of the BI-RADS system is to facilitate research. BI-RADS provides a framework to compare data among breast imaging practices and address areas requiring further study. BI-RADS has been adopted in nearly all parts of the world, affording an even greater opportunity to study the epidemiology and imaging characteristics of breast disease.

Beyond BI-RADS

Imitation is the greatest form of flattery, and BI-RADS has been used as the template for other ACR-endorsed reporting and data systems (RADS), including ovarian-adnexal (O-RADS), colon cancer (C-RADS), liver cancer (LI-RADS),

Box 2.4　Components of the Basic Clinically Relevant Audit

Box 2.4 lists the data to be collected for the basic clinically relevant audit.

1. Imaging modality
2. Beginning and end dates of audit
3. Total number of examinations performed in audit timeframe
4. Total number of screening examinations and total number of diagnostic examinations
5. Number of recommendations for additional imaging evaluation (category 0)
6. Number of recommendations for short-interval follow-up (category 3)
7. Number of recommendations for tissue diagnosis (category 4 and 5)
8. Tissue diagnosis results (positive or negative) for all category 0, 3, 4, and 5
9. Cancer histologic type, invasive cancer size, nodal status, and tumor grade
10. Analysis of any known false-negative mammography examination by attempting to obtain surgical and/or pathology results and by review of any negative mammography examinations (MQSA final rule)

Adapted from Sickles EA, D'Orsi CJ; ACR BI-RADS follow-up and outcome monitoring. In: ACRBI-RADS, ed. Breast Imaging Reporting and Data System. Reston, VA: American College of Radiology; 2013. Part IV ACR BI-RADS Follow-up and Outcome Monitoring, p. 23-24.

Box 2.5　Audit Metric Definitions

Audit metric equations and definitions to be calculated for a mammography medical outcomes audit.

Total number of examinations=TP+FP+TN+FN

True-positive (TP): Diagnosis of breast cancer within 1 year of a positive examination[a,b]

True-negative (TN): No diagnosis of breast cancer within 1 year of a negative examination[c,d]

False-negative (FN): Diagnosis of breast cancer within 1 year of a negative examination[c,d]

False-positive (FP): There are three false-positive audit calculations

　FP1: No known diagnosis of breast cancer within 1 year of a positive screening examination

　FP2: No known diagnosis of breast cancer within 1 year after a recommendation for biopsy

　FP3: No known diagnosis of breast cancer within 1 year after a recommended biopsy[e] is performed

Positive predictive value (PPV): There are three PPV audit calculations

　PPV[1]: Percentage of all positive screening examinations[a] that result in a diagnosis of breast cancer within 1 year. Metric is intended to evaluate screening[f] imaging studies.

　PPV[2]: Percentage of examinations[g] recommended for biopsy that result in a diagnosis of breast cancer within 1 year. Metric is intended to evaluate diagnostic imaging studies.

　PPV[3]: Percentage of examinations[g] recommended for biopsy where biopsy is performed and results in a diagnosis of breast cancer. Metric is intended to evaluate diagnostic imaging studies.

Sensitivity (sens): Sens=TP/(TP+FN)

Specificity (spec): Spec=TN/(TN+FP)

Cancer detection rate (CDR): Number of cancers detected per 1000 women screened. CDR is meaningful when calculated for screening populations. However, it may be calculated separately for prevalent and incident screening populations or for diagnostic populations.

Recall rate (RR): The percentage of screening examinations recalled for additional imaging (category 0)

Abnormal interpretation rate (AIR): Percentage of examinations interpreted as positive. This is intended to include category 0 exams in a screening audit and therefore should equal the recall rate; however the inclusion of the (not recommended) screening examination categories 3, 4, 5 will result in an AIR rate greater than the recall rate. If screening examinations are assigned to the (not recommended) categories 3, 4, and 5, then the AIR is a more meaningful metric than recall rate. For a diagnostic audit, AIR is intended to include categories 4 and 5.

[a]Category 0, 3, 4, 5 for screening. [b]Category 4, 5 for diagnostic. [c]Category 1, 2 for screening. [d]Category 1, 2, 3 for diagnostic. [e]Category 4, 5 for diagnostic and rare (not recommended) screening examinations. [f]Intended to include screening category 0 examinations only but may include the rare (not recommended) screening category 3, 4, 5. [g]Intended to include diagnostic category 4, 5 exams only, but may include the rare (not recommended) screening category 4, 5. Adapted from Sickles EA, D'Orsi CJ; ACR BI-RADS follow-up and outcome monitoring. In: ACRBI-RADS, ed. Breast Imaging Reporting and Data System. Reston, VA: American College of Radiology; 2013. Part IV ACR BI-RADS Follow-up and Outcome Monitoring, p. 23-24.

lung cancer (Lung-RADS), prostate cancer (PI-RADS), thyroid cancer (TI-RADS), and coronary artery disease (CAD-RADS). Each RADS has its own set of standards and guidelines specific to the organ system and its imaging modalities. With the exception of O-RADS, all of the RADS use some kind of numerical scoring system to evaluate the degree of suspicion for a particular disease. The goals of these systems are the same across the board: reduce ambiguous reporting by using standardized terminology, improve data collection, and assess practice and individual radiologist's interpretative performance, thus optimizing patient care.

The Art of Breast Imaging

This chapter has outlined the many rules and guidelines that govern breast imaging. With so many rules telling us exactly what to do, one might ask: Where is the *art* in breast imaging? The art of breast imaging is reflected in the nuances of every case. Few cases fit into a perfect formula, and a skilled breast radiologist has to be able to identify and accurately evaluate suspicious findings while not getting distracted by the numerous incidental, insignificant benign findings. The BI-RADS "formula" (lexicon, assessment categories, and standardized report) helps maintain consistency and has transformed the practice of breast imaging over the past 30+ years, but it does not replace the radiologist's ability to perceive subtle signs of breast cancer, which can take a lifetime to master.

KEY POINTS

- Breast Imaging Reporting and Data System (BI-RADS) is a fundamental component of breast imaging with three main goals: standardization of interpretative terminology and final assessment categories, unambiguous communication, and quality assurance optimization.
- The BI-RADS Atlas was first born in 1993 and has since undergone four revisions, with the fifth and most recent edition published in 2013. BI-RADS is meant to be a malleable and adaptable reporting and data system with the ability to transform, improve, and expand as needed

to incorporate the continuous new advances in breast imaging technology, research, and patient care.

- The BI-RADS lexicon is a carefully crafted dictionary of descriptive terms for breast imaging findings, systematically organized for each of the three modalities: mammography (includes digital breast tomosynthesis [DBT]), ultrasound, and magnetic resonance imaging (MRI).
- Proper use of the BI-RADS lexicon requires that suspicious lexicon words are used for suspicious findings and benign lexicon words are used for benign findings. Using the correct lexicon descriptors will lead to the most appropriate final assessment and management recommendations.
- The BI-RADS assessment categories range from 0 to 6, and each category is associated with a standardized management recommendation and likelihood of malignancy (see Table 2.1). Some assessment categories are more likely to be used in the setting of screening (BI-RADS 0), and some should only be used after a full diagnostic evaluation (BI-RADS 3, 4, 5, and 6).
- The BI-RADS lexicon and assessment categories are woven into the structured breast imaging report to clearly and consistently communicate significant imaging findings to patients and all members of the health care team, including referring physicians, breast surgeons, nurses, administrative office staff, schedulers, and radiologists, to help direct and guide the patient's care.
- Additional information embedded in the standardized report has important implications. For example, reporting breast density in the body of the report is how we communicate the sensitivity of the examination to the patient and referring physician (i.e., dense breast tissue decreases sensitivity of mammography).
- The Mammography Quality Standards Act (MQSA) mammography medical audit of each facility's mammography performance is required annually. Completion of the audit provides valuable insight about a practice group and its individual radiologist's interpretive performance.
- Understanding and achieving desirable benchmark metrics is critical to the delivery of high-quality patient care. BI-RADS is a key component used to generate trackable data. It is therefore not surprising that BI-RADS has been adopted across the globe and American College of Radiology (ACR) standardized reporting and data systems (RADS) have become common practice in other areas of radiology (e.g., LI-RADS (Liver Reporting and Data System), Lung-RADS (Lung Reporting and Data System), TI-RADS (Thyroid Imaging Reporting and Data System)).

Suggested Readings

D'Orsi CJ, Sickles EA, Mendelson EB, Morris EA, et al. *ACR BI-RADS Atlas, Breast Imaging Reporting and Data System*. Reston, VA: American College of Radiology; 2013.

Burnside ES, Sickles EA, Bassett LW, et al. The ACR BI-RADS experience: learning from history. *J Am Coll Radiol*. 2009;6(12):851–860. https://doi.org/10.1016/j.jacr.2009.07.023.

Rao AA, Feneis J, Lalonde C, et al. A Pictorial Review of Changes in the BI-RADS Fifth Edition. *Radiographics*. 2016 May–Jun;36(3):623–639.

References

1. Annual. Rev. Publ. Health. 1993. 14:605-33 Copyright 1993 by Annual Reviews Inc. All rights reserved. MAMMOGRAPHY UTILIZATION, PUBLIC HEALTH IMPACT, AND COST-EFFECTIVENESS IN THE UNITED STATES Emily White, Nicole Urban, and Victoria Taylor Cancer Prevention Research Program, Fred Hutchinson Cancer Research Center, Seattle, Washington 98104.
2. Joe BN, Sickles EA: The evolution of breast imaging: past to present, *Radiology*. 273(2 Suppl):S23–44, 2014 Nov. https://doi.org/10.1148/radiol.14141233. PMID: 25340437
3. McLelland R: Mammography 1984: challenge to radiology, *AJR Am J Roentgenol*. 143(1):1–4, 1984. https://doi.org/10.2214/ajr.143.1.
4. Galkin BM, Feig SA, Muir HD: The technical quality of mammography in centers participating in a regional breast cancer awareness program, *Radiographics* 8(1):133–145, 1988. https://doi.org/10.1148/radiographics.8.1.3353530.
5. Scott WC: *"Establishing mammographic criteria for recommending surgical biopsy."*. In *Report of the Council on Scientific Affairs*, Chicago, IL, 1989, *American Medical Association*.
6. Burnside ES, Sickles EA, Bassett LW, et al: The ACR BI-RADS experience: learning from history, *J Am Coll Radiol*. 6(12):851–860, 2009. https://doi.org/10.1016/j.jacr.2009.07.023.
7. Personal correspondence (e-mail) with Carl J. D'Orsi to validate historical elements. (April 30, 2020 - July 24, 2020).
8. 21 CFR Part 900: Mammography Quality Standards: Final Rule. Federal Register, Washington, DC: Government Printing Office, vol. 62: No. 208: pp. 55852-55994, October 28, 1997.
9. D'Orsi CJ, Sickles EA, Mendelson EB, Morris EA, et al: *ACR BI-RADS Atlas, Breast Imaging Reporting and Data System*, Reston, VA, 2013, American College of Radiology.
10. Sickles EA, D'Orsi CJ: ACR BI-RADS Follow-up and Outcome Monitoring. In Atlas ACRBI-RADS, editor: *Breast Imaging Reporting and Data System*, Reston, VA, 2013, American College of Radiology.
11. Schell MJ, Yankaskas BC, Ballard-Barbash R, et al: Evidence-based target recall rates for screening mammography, *Radiology* 243:681–689, 2007.
12. D'Orsi CJ, Sickles EA: 2017 Breast Cancer Surveillance Consortium Reports on Interpretive Performance at Screening and Diagnostic Mammography: Welcome New Data, But Not as Benchmarks for Practice, *Radiology* 283(1):7–9, 2017. https://doi.org/10.1148/radiol.2017170181.
13. Lehman CD, Arao RF, Sprague BL, et al: National Performance Benchmarks for Modern Screening Digital Mammography: Update from the Breast Cancer Surveillance Consortium, *Radiology* 283(1):49–58, 2017. https://doi.org/10.1148/radiol.2016161174.
14. American College of Radiology National Radiology Data Registry: National Mammography Database. January 2017-December 2018 data statistics as of 2/22/2019. Received with permission on 8/7/2020.

3 Mammographic Masses, Asymmetries, and Distortion

SHADI AMINOLOLAMA-SHAKERI AND RAMAN MUHAR

OVERVIEW *This chapter discusses the mammographic evaluation of breast masses, asymmetries, and architectural distortion. We will introduce the Breast Imaging Reporting and Data System (BI-RADS) descriptors as a tool to categorize these noncalcified lesions within the breast along with suggested management.*

Breast Masses

A mass occupies three-dimensional space with partially or completely convex borders, which bulges into the surrounding tissues. A mass should be identifiable on two orthogonal projections unless obscured by adjacent dense tissue. The radiologist's goal is to distinguish benign from malignant masses in order to appropriately manage the patient. Masses may be recognized at time of screening or may present as a palpable finding by the patient or referring provider in the diagnostic setting.

Once a mass has been identified, Breast Imaging Reporting and Data System (BI-RADS) lexicon descriptors are used for lesion characterization. Reporting also includes mass location by determining the laterality, quadrant or clockface, depth, and distance from the nipple to the mass. BI-RADS mammography descriptors for mass lesions are summarized in Table 3.1 and are illustrated with diagrams and image examples in Figs. 3.1–3.3 for mass shape, margin, and density. Adhering to BI-RADS terminology allows appropriate characterization of masses, which guides the next step in management. For example, a benign breast mass is assessed as BI-RADS 2 with a recommendation to return to annual screening. A suspicious breast mass is assessed as BI-RADS 4 with a recommendation for tissue diagnosis, usually using image-guided biopsy. Occasionally, a mass is assessed as BI-RADS 3 "probably benign" (with less than 2% probability of malignancy), and recommendation is for short-term imaging surveillance instead of immediate tissue sampling. When multiple suspicious mammographic findings are present suggesting a greater than 95% probability of malignancy (Box 3.1; Fig. 3.4) a BI-RADS 5 "highly suggestive of malignancy" assessment is appropriate.

BREAST MASS DESCRIPTORS SPECIFIC TO ULTRASOUND

Ultrasound is frequently performed in conjunction with mammography for further characterization of masses. Breast ultrasound is covered in more detail in Chapter 5: Breast Ultrasound Indications and Interpretation. Similar to mammography, mass shape on ultrasound is described as oval, round, and irregular. Ultrasound terminology for mass margin includes all of the mammographic descriptors, with the exception of "obscured" and an additional term specific to ultrasound: angular (Fig. 3.5). An angular margin indicates an area of a mass margin, which is sharply demarcated away from the mass. Other ultrasound specific descriptors include mass orientation, echo pattern, and posterior features (Fig. 3.6). Table 3.2 summarizes the ACR BI-RADS ultrasound descriptors.

Orientation is an ultrasound-specific descriptor. An antiparallel (older term: taller than wide) orientation refers to a mass with its long axis perpendicular to the skin line (or chest wall), indicating it may be growing against tissue planes, which is a suspicious feature.

Posterior features is an ultrasound-specific term that refers to the sound wave attenuation by tissue. This attribute of a mass may be characterized as having no posterior features, posterior enhancement, shadowing, or a combined appearance. The presence of shadowing is suspicious. Note, however, that not all cancers shadow. Highly cellular tumors such as mucinous, medullary, papillary, or cancers with necrosis can have increased through transmission.

Sonography is useful for distinguishing benign solid masses from indeterminate and malignant solid masses. In a prospective study of 750 sonographically identified breast masses, a negative predictive value of 99.5% was reached. Table 3.3 summarizes the individual sonographic characteristics used in this study. By excluding any mass with at least one malignant feature, sensitivity for cancer was 98.4%.[1]

When imaging a patient, the American College of Radiology requires specific labeling of saved ultrasound

Table 3.1 American College of Radiology (ACR) Breast Imaging Reporting and Data System (BI-RADS) Mammography Lexicon Descriptors

Shape	Margin	Density
Oval	Circumscribed	Fat containing
Round	Obscured	Low
Irregular	Microlobulated	Equal
	Indistinct	High
	Spiculated	

Mass Shape

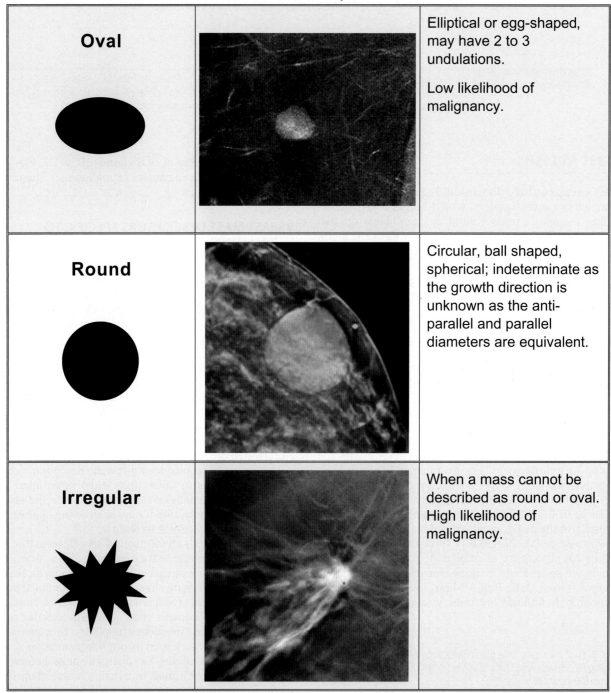

Oval		Elliptical or egg-shaped, may have 2 to 3 undulations. Low likelihood of malignancy.
Round		Circular, ball shaped, spherical; indeterminate as the growth direction is unknown as the anti-parallel and parallel diameters are equivalent.
Irregular		When a mass cannot be described as round or oval. High likelihood of malignancy.

Fig. 3.1 Diagrams and image examples illustrating mass shapes.

Mass Margin

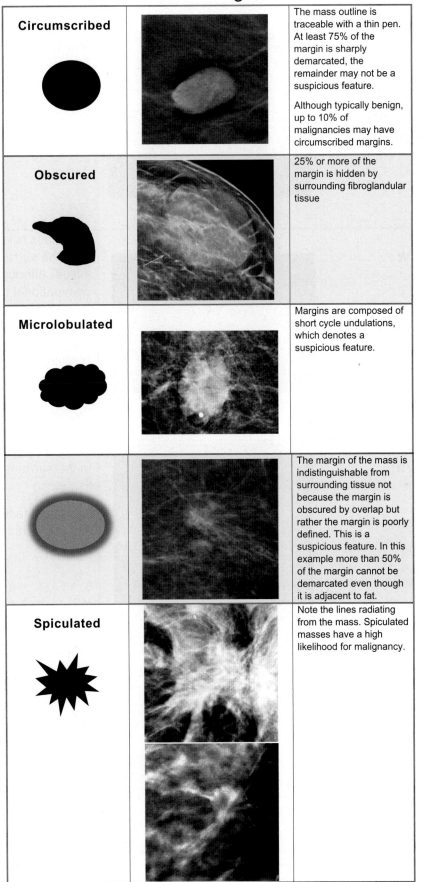

		The mass outline is traceable with a thin pen. At least 75% of the margin is sharply demarcated, the remainder may not be a suspicious feature. Although typically benign, up to 10% of malignancies may have circumscribed margins.
Circumscribed		
Obscured		25% or more of the margin is hidden by surrounding fibroglandular tissue
Microlobulated		Margins are composed of short cycle undulations, which denotes a suspicious feature.
		The margin of the mass is indistinguishable from surrounding tissue not because the margin is obscured by overlap but rather the margin is poorly defined. This is a suspicious feature. In this example more than 50% of the margin cannot be demarcated even though it is adjacent to fat.
Spiculated		Note the lines radiating from the mass. Spiculated masses have a high likelihood for malignancy.

Fig. 3.2 Diagrams and image examples illustrating mass margins

Mass Density

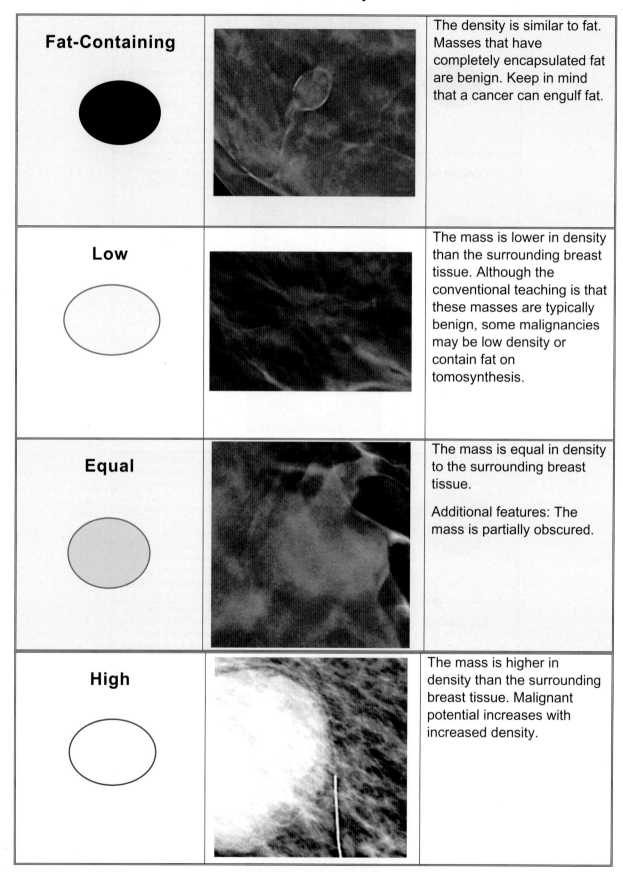

Fat-Containing		The density is similar to fat. Masses that have completely encapsulated fat are benign. Keep in mind that a cancer can engulf fat.
Low		The mass is lower in density than the surrounding breast tissue. Although the conventional teaching is that these masses are typically benign, some malignancies may be low density or contain fat on tomosynthesis.
Equal		The mass is equal in density to the surrounding breast tissue. Additional features: The mass is partially obscured.
High		The mass is higher in density than the surrounding breast tissue. Malignant potential increases with increased density.

Fig. 3.3 Diagrams and image examples illustrating mass density.

imaging. Breast ultrasound is covered in detail in Chapter 5: Breast Ultrasound Indications and Interpretation.

Specific pathologic entities presenting as breast masses are covered in detail in Chapter 9: Breast Pathology and Radiologic-Pathologic Correlation. Briefly, in addition to breast cancers, masses on imaging may result from a wide variety of pathologies, including fibroadenoma, hamartoma, pseudoangiomatous hyperplasia, papilloma, and phyllodes tumor. Please refer to Chapter 9 for an overview of the characteristic appearance and management of these lesions.

Asymmetries

An asymmetry is a noncalcified finding seen on one breast and not the other when comparing right and left mammograms. There are four types of asymmetries detailed further below: asymmetry, global asymmetry, focal asymmetry, and developing asymmetry. Asymmetries do not conform to the mammographic definition of a mass and may have the appearance of normal fibroglandular tissue. Slight differences between the two breasts are normal and may be best detected by examining the bilateral breasts back to back to look for differences in symmetry. Asymmetry is a term used

only in mammography and is not in the ultrasound or magnetic resonance imaging (MRI) BI-RADS lexicon.

The category of asymmetries refers to a space-occupying lesion that is discernible from the surrounding parenchyma with concave outward borders and usually interspersed with fat. It may be visualized on one or both orthogonal projections, which determines its subcategorization. In some cases, what initially appears as an asymmetry is revealed to be a mass on further workup. In such cases the mass may have been apparent on only one view and obscured by dense tissue on the orthogonal projection and categorized as an asymmetry until its three dimensionality is confirmed.

The next few sections will review the four types of asymmetries in the BI-RADS lexicon (see Box 3.2), their imaging evaluation and management including expected outcomes.

ASYMMETRY

This term is used to describe a discrete area of fibroglandular tissue visible on one 2D projection only. Although this single-view finding may potentially be a mass seen in only one projection, usually it represents superimposition of normal breast structures resulting in a summation artifact (Fig. 3.7). Asymmetry is a term used primarily at screening given that on further diagnostic workup it will be determined either not to be a true lesion or to represent a focal asymmetry or mass. Over 80% of asymmetries are due to summation of normal tissues.[2]

Discovery of an asymmetry on a screening mammogram therefore warrants further diagnostic workup to establish if it represents a true lesion (see Chapter 13: Organized Approach to Diagnostic Imaging). It is important to consider that a lesion that initially appears as an asymmetry, if demonstrated to represent a true finding, may be a focal asymmetry, mass, or architectural distortion. Workup and management should be based on a lesion's most suspicious feature.

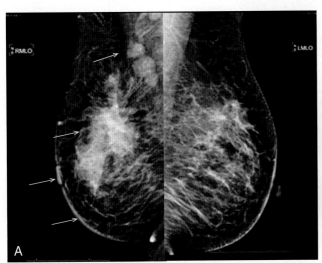
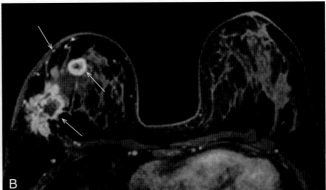

Fig. 3.4 (A–B) A 30-year-old woman presented with right upper outer quadrant breast tenderness and skin dimpling during pregnancy. On diagnostic mammogram (A) large, irregular, dense mass, skin thickening, nipple retraction, and lymphadenopathy are noted in the right breast (*arrows*). Post-contrast T1 fat-saturated magnetic resonance imaging (MRI) sequence (B) shows multifocal irregular enhancing mass with central necrosis, adjacent rim-enhancing mass along with skin thickening (*arrows*). Biopsy demonstrated invasive ductal carcinoma, estrogen receptor (ER), progestrone receptor (PR) positive, and human epidermal growth factor receptor (HER2) negative.

Ultrasound Mass Margin

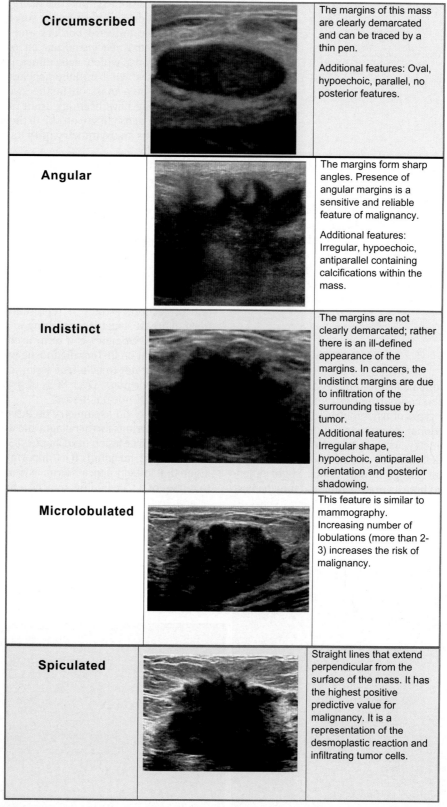

Circumscribed		The margins of this mass are clearly demarcated and can be traced by a thin pen. Additional features: Oval, hypoechoic, parallel, no posterior features.
Angular		The margins form sharp angles. Presence of angular margins is a sensitive and reliable feature of malignancy. Additional features: Irregular, hypoechoic, antiparallel containing calcifications within the mass.
Indistinct		The margins are not clearly demarcated; rather there is an ill-defined appearance of the margins. In cancers, the indistinct margins are due to infiltration of the surrounding tissue by tumor. Additional features: Irregular shape, hypoechoic, antiparallel orientation and posterior shadowing.
Microlobulated		This feature is similar to mammography. Increasing number of lobulations (more than 2-3) increases the risk of malignancy.
Spiculated		Straight lines that extend perpendicular from the surface of the mass. It has the highest positive predictive value for malignancy. It is a representation of the desmoplastic reaction and infiltrating tumor cells.

Fig. 3.5 Image examples illustrating mass margins at breast ultrasound.

Ultrasound Mass Echopatterns

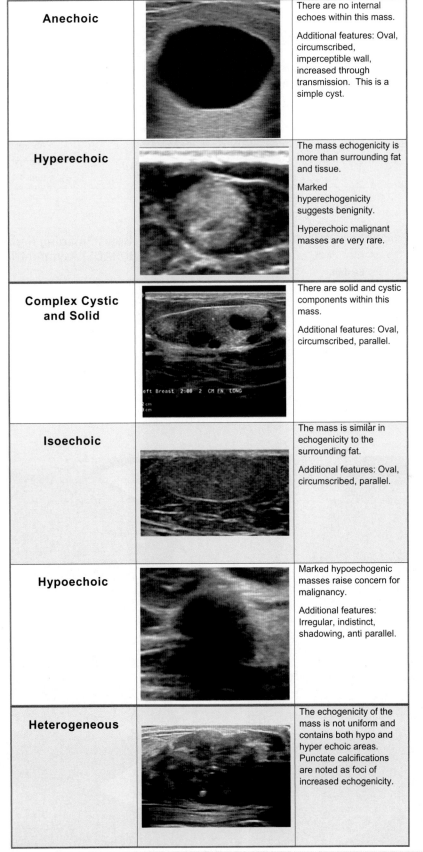

Anechoic		There are no internal echoes within this mass. Additional features: Oval, circumscribed, imperceptible wall, increased through transmission. This is a simple cyst.
Hyperechoic		The mass echogenicity is more than surrounding fat and tissue. Marked hyperechogenicity suggests benignity. Hyperechoic malignant masses are very rare.
Complex Cystic and Solid		There are solid and cystic components within this mass. Additional features: Oval, circumscribed, parallel.
Isoechoic		The mass is similar in echogenicity to the surrounding fat. Additional features: Oval, circumscribed, parallel.
Hypoechoic		Marked hypoechogenic masses raise concern for malignancy. Additional features: Irregular, indistinct, shadowing, anti parallel.
Heterogeneous		The echogenicity of the mass is not uniform and contains both hypo and hyper echoic areas. Punctate calcifications are noted as foci of increased echogenicity.

Fig. 3.6 Image examples illustrating mass echopatterns at breast ultrasound

Table 3.2   American College of Radiology (ACR) Breast Imaging Reporting and Data System (BI-RADS) Ultrasound Lexicon Descriptors

Shape	Margins	Echo Pattern	Posterior Acoustic Features	Orientation	Associated Features	Calcifications
▪ Oval	▪ Circumscribed	▪ Anechoic	▪ None	▪ Parallel	▪ Architectural distortion	▪ Inside of mass
▪ Round	▪ Not circumscribed:	▪ Hyperechoic	▪ Enhancement	▪ Not parallel	▪ Duct changes	▪ Outside of mass
▪ Irregular	▪ Angular	▪ Complex cystic and solid	▪ Shadowing		▪ Skin changes	▪ Intraductal
	▪ Indistinct	▪ Isoechoic	▪ Combined		▪ Edema	
	▪ Microlobulated	▪ Hypoechoic			▪ Vascularity:	
	▪ Spiculated				▪ Absent	
					▪ Internal	
					▪ Rim	

Table 3.3   Sonographic Appearance of Malignant and Benign Masses

Malignant	Benign
Margin	Absent malignant findings
Indistinct	Intense hyperechogenicity
Microlobulated	Ellipsoid shape
Angular	With no more than 2–3 gentle lobulations
Spiculated	
Marked hypoechogenicity	Thin capsule
Shadowing	
Ductal extension	

Box 3.2   Breast Imaging Reporting and Data System (BI-RADS) Asymmetries

1. Asymmetry (single-view finding)
2. Global asymmetry
3. Focal asymmetry
4. Developing asymmetry

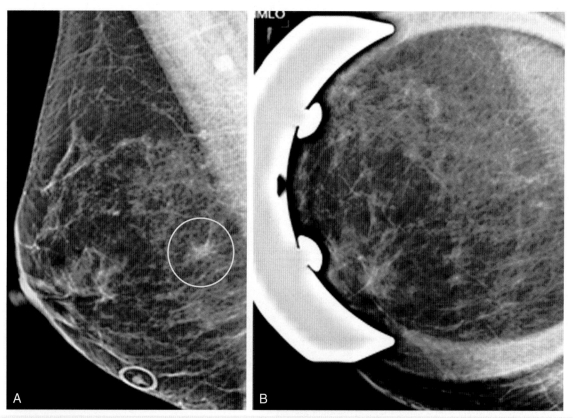

Fig. 3.7 Asymmetry. (A) Mediolateral oblique (MLO) view showing an asymmetry (*circle*), which was not seen on craniocaudal (CC) view (not shown), which effaces on MLO spot compression view (B).

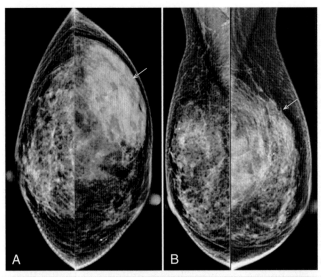

Fig. 3.8 Global asymmetry. (A–B): Two-dimensional (2D) craniocaudal (CC) and mediolateral oblique (MLO) views: There is a large global asymmetry involving the upper outer quadrant of the left breast (*arrows*). The area has remained stable for several years.

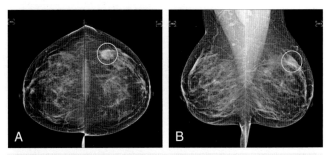

Fig. 3.9 Focal asymmetry. (A) Craniocaudal and (B) mediolateral oblique views show a left focal asymmetry (*circles*) compared with the contralateral breast.

Box 3.4   Workup of Focal Asymmetry

Probably benign unless new from prior or underlying:

- Solid mass or masses
- Architectural distortion
- Grouped microcalcifications

Benign if stable for ≥2–3 years

Box 3.3   Workup of Global Asymmetry

Benign unless at imaging see underlying:

- Solid mass or masses
- Architectural distortion
- Grouped microcalcifications

Be aware of the "shrinking breast sign" these are advanced cancers that actually scar the breast without forming a discrete mass.

GLOBAL ASYMMETRY

Global asymmetry is a large area of fibroglandular tissue density that is asymmetric with the analogous area in the contralateral breast (Fig. 3.8). Global asymmetry is seen in two different projections and involves at least one quadrant of the breast. It appears as a space-occupying lesion, with concave outward contours usually with interspersed fat. Global asymmetry usually represents a normal variant of tissues but may be significant when it corresponds to a palpable abnormality. There should not be any associated mass, architectural distortion, or microcalcifications. Be aware of the "shrinking breast sign," as these are advanced cancers that actually scar the breast without forming a discrete mass (Box 3.3).

FOCAL ASYMMETRY

Focal asymmetry is a relatively small area of fibroglandular tissue density involving less than a quadrant of the breast and seen in two different projections. Like global asymmetry, focal asymmetry is a space-occupying lesion with concave-outward contours, usually with interspersed fat. In contrast, a mass exhibits convex-outward contours. Recognizing a focal asymmetry requires comparison with the analogous area of the contralateral breast (Fig. 3.9).

Often, a focal asymmetry at screening mammography is determined to actually represent a mass after diagnostic evaluation. The workup of a focal asymmetry is summarized in Box 3.4.

DEVELOPING ASYMMETRY

A developing asymmetry is a focal asymmetry that is either new or increased in size or conspicuity compared with a previous examination (Fig. 3.10). Comparison with multiple prior examinations is recommended, as developing asymmetries can present as a subtle increasing density over time. A developing asymmetry requires further workup as the change from prior examinations is concerning (Box 3.5). Developing asymmetries are malignant in approximately 15% of cases at screening mammography and approximately 27% of cases at diagnostic mammography. Thus a developing asymmetry confirmed at diagnostic mammography should be assessed as BI-RADS 4 (suspicious) and tissue sampling should be performed (Box 3.6).

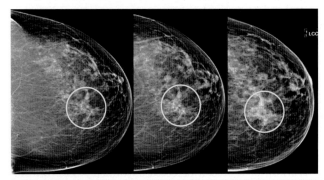

Fig. 3.10 Developing asymmetry. Craniocaudal view from 3 consecutive years (latest is the rightmost panel) of screening demonstrates increasing density of an asymmetry (*circled*) prompting recall for diagnostic workup.

ASSESSMENT OF ASYMMETRY AT SCREENING MAMMOGRAPHY

A review of the patient's provided medical history may be helpful in this evaluation. For example, a woman may have had an excisional biopsy in the intervening period since her prior examination with loss of asymmetry between the two breasts. Therefore asymmetric findings due to removal of tissue is benign. Comparison to any available prior examinations is essential when evaluating an asymmetry. Diligent comparison with prior examinations, at least two including the most recent, is critical. Comparison to multiple priors is helpful for recognition of change indicating the presence of a developing asymmetry.

A diagnosis of summation artifact is possible at screening. If an asymmetry is seen on one view and not the other, the depth of included tissue on the two views needs to be evaluated. If the finding on one view is in the deepest third of the breast that is not included on the other view, the patient needs to be recalled for visualization of deeper tissue fully. If the depth of the views match, and there is enough dense tissue that the asymmetry may be obscured on the other view, then the patient needs to be recalled for further diagnostic workup. Tomosynthesis has been found particularly useful for the evaluation of asymmetries and decreases recall rates from screening.[3,4]

ASSESSMENT OF ASYMMETRY AT DIAGNOSTIC MAMMOGRAPHY

Diagnostic workup of a focal asymmetry or developing asymmetry, seen on two projections at screening mammography, is similar to the evaluation of a mammographic mass. If the lesion is not due to summation of tissues, ultrasound should be performed targeted to the location of the lesion.

Workup of a screen detected asymmetry seen on only one view can be more challenging. At diagnostic mammography, the view on which the asymmetry was originally identified may be repeated. If the finding resolves on the repeat projection on which it was originally seen, then it may be concluded that the asymmetry was due to summation of tissues. Similarly, slightly varying the view in which the asymmetry was originally seen by changing the beam obliquity by a few degrees allows tissues to spread apart to diminish superimposition. By changing the beam obliquity only very slightly, if the asymmetry is a real lesion, its position won't change enough for it to be obscured in adjacent dense tissue. Spot compression and magnification techniques can also be used to spread tissues apart.

If the asymmetry persists on the repeat views and on spot compression and magnification views, its location on the orthogonal projection may be determined by using triangulation, rolled views, step oblique views, or tomosynthesis. If the asymmetry is recalled from tomosynthesis, the next step in the diagnostic workup may be targeted ultrasound. Utilizing the position bar on the tomosynthesis view where the asymmetry is seen is helpful for estimating the location of the finding (see also Chapter 6: Basics of Digital Breast Tomosynthesis). When tomosynthesis is not utilized, triangulation is useful to search for the location of an asymmetry that is identified only on the mediolateral oblique (MLO) view or only on the craniocaudal (CC) view. A 90-degree projection may be obtained at the time of diagnostic workup. The CC, MLO, and 90-degree view should be placed in order of decreasing projection angle (90, 45, 0 degrees) with an invisible horizontal line used to align the nipple on the three projections. A line drawn through the asymmetry on the lateral and continued through the MLO will then determine whether the finding is lateral or medial when the line is extrapolated to the CC (Fig. 3.11). Similarly, obtaining step oblique views will allow an asymmetry seen on the MLO projection to be identified on the CC projection. This may be accomplished by obtaining a series of projections at incremental decreases in angle, for example by 15 degrees starting from 45 degrees (MLO) to 0 degrees (CC) (Fig. 3.12) (see Chapter 13: Organized Approach to Diagnostic Imaging).

Rolled views can also be performed to roughly localize the position of an asymmetry seen only on the CC view. In this technique, the breast is positioned on the image receptor in

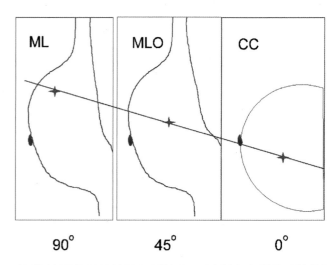

Fig. 3.11 Triangulation.

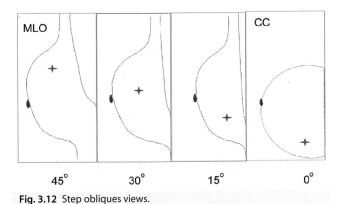

Fig. 3.12 Step obliques views.

the CC position, then the upper breast is "rolled" medially or laterally relative to the nipple. The direction of shift of the asymmetry on the rolled images allows a rough estimation of where the lesion is located. However, shifting breast tissue in rolled views is more difficult to control and less precise than triangulation.

Once the location of an asymmetry has been established in the breast and is identified in more than one view, it may be categorized as a mass, a focal asymmetry, or developing asymmetry, and ultrasound may be utilized for further characterization and biopsy planning. If no sonographic correlate to a focal asymmetry is identified, management depends on whether it was called back from a baseline screening mammogram. If called back from a baseline screening mammogram, the focal asymmetry with no sonographic correlate may be assessed as BI-RADS 3 (probably benign). If the finding is new or increased compared with prior mammograms, the lesion should be assessed as BI-RADS 4 (suspicious) and stereotactic or tomosynthesis-guided biopsy would be warranted (Fig. 3.13).

Architectural Distortion

Architectural distortion is a distortion of the breast parenchyma, which appears as straight lines radiating from a central point without a visible mass. Architectural distortion is the third most common presentation of breast cancer[5]

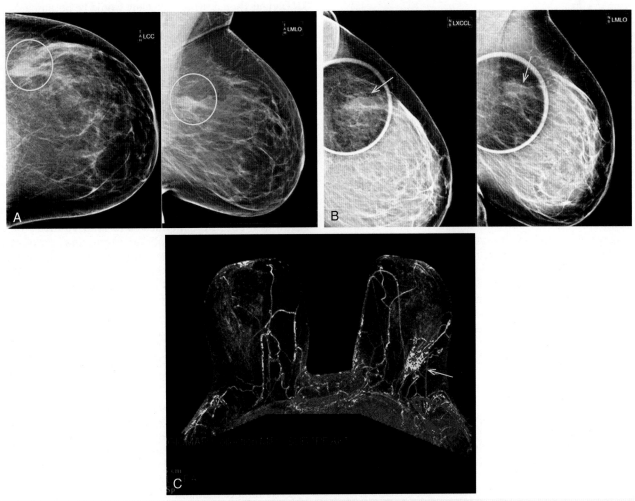

Fig. 3.13 A 43-year-old woman. (A) Focal asymmetry (*circles*) seen on left craniocaudal (CC) and mediolateral oblique (MLO) views, increased compared with examination 6 months prior. (B) Spot compression views show persistence of focal asymmetry (*arrows*) without underlying mass. Targeted ultrasound (not shown) did not show a correlate to the mammographic focal asymmetry. (C) Diagnostic magnetic resonance imaging (MRI) revealed a heterogeneously enhancing area of nonmass enhancement (*arrow*) in the upper outer quadrant corresponding to the mammographic focal asymmetry. Stereotactic biopsy demonstrated invasive lobular carcinoma.

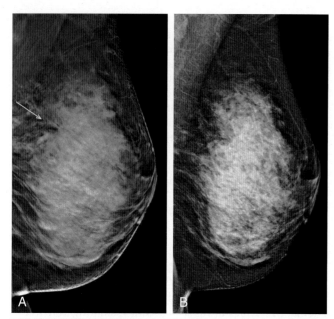

Fig. 3.14 (A) Architectural distortion (*arrow*) only visible on digital breast tomosynthesis (DBT) mediolateral oblique (MLO) view and not seen on the conventional mammogram (B). Biopsy showed radial scar.

on mammograms following mass and calcifications and may be associated with microcalcifications or asymmetry. Architectural distortion is also the most commonly missed imaging presentation of cancer at mammography.[6–8] Digital breast tomosynthesis (DBT) improves detection of architectural distortion in comparison to digital mammography (DM) by increasing sensitivity (Fig. 3.14). Of architectural distortion findings detected only by tomosynthesis, 10% to 47% were found to be due to cancer.[9–12]

Benign causes of architectural distortion include postsurgical scar, sclerosing adenosis, radial scar, and complex sclerosing lesion. Radial scar or complex sclerosing lesion is a benign, proliferative process of the breast and not related to prior surgery or trauma. There is an association with atypical ductal hyperplasia, lobular carcinoma in situ, and tubular carcinoma; therefore surgical excision is typically recommended, although the management of radial scars is controversial (see Chapter 9: Breast Pathology and Radiologic-Pathologic Correlation). Although radial scars can be palpable, more commonly they are initially diagnosed on mammography. Architectural distortion of a radial scar appears as a "black star," or a central dark area lacking a central mass with long, thin dense lines radiating outward. It has an appearance similar to carcinoma, but the center has been described as low density in comparison to carcinomas, which are high density. Note, however, that this is not a reliable feature to avoid biopsy. On ultrasound, radial scars appear similar to carcinoma as an irregular, spiculated, ill-defined hypoechoic mass with posterior shadowing. Secondary signs to suggest carcinoma such as skin thickening and retraction should not be present. As with architectural distortion at mammography, biopsy is needed to exclude malignancy. MRI features are similar. Radial scars that enhance may contain a malignant component. Box 3.7 summarizes the differential diagnosis for architectural distortion.

ASSESSMENT OF ARCHITECTURAL DISTORTION ON DIAGNOSTIC MAMMOGRAPHY WORKUP

In the absence of DBT, the diagnostic evaluation of architectural distortion at mammography follows the same principles as described in Chapter 13: Organized Approach to Diagnostic Imaging. Architectural distortion found on 2D digital mammography may be further assessed using spot compression views. In cases in which the architectural distortion was only seen on one view at screening mammography, additional views may be performed in the same projection as that in which it was originally seen but also at a different angulation to verify finding is real and for localization. For example, if architectural distortion is found on MLO view, then a 90-degree view would be obtained. Some malignant architectural distortion is only seen on DBT. Due to variability of tumor visualization with 5% to 9% of cancers seen on craniocaudal view only and 1% to 2% on MLO view only, two-view tomosynthesis diagnostic exam should be performed.[13]

Once the location of the architectural distortion has been established in the breast, ultrasound may be utilized for further characterization and biopsy planning. When architectural distortion is detected on DBT, the next diagnostic step should be ultrasound. Further 2D imaging with spot compression views generally does not provide additional information to avoid biopsy. Lesions with an ultrasound correlate have a higher likelihood of being malignant.[14] Of malignant architectural distortion on DBT, 50% were occult and 20% were manifested as an asymmetry on 2D mammography. Invasive lobular carcinomas account for 20% of malignant architectural distortion detected on DBT. When ultrasound is negative and architectural distortion is only seen on 2D digital mammography or DBT, biopsy must be performed using stereotactic 2D or DBT core biopsy.

KEY POINTS

1. Mammographic lesions that are not calcifications include masses, asymmetries, and distortion.
2. A mass is three-dimensional, seen on at least two mammographic projections, and demonstrates at least partial convex outward borders.
3. There are four types of asymmetries: Asymmetry (seen on only one view), global asymmetry (large area of asymmetric tissue density, >1 quadrant), focal asymmetry (small area of asymmetric tissue density seen on more than one view, lacking the conspicuity and convex margins of a mass), and developing asymmetry (a focal asymmetry that is new or increasing in size).

4. A circumscribed mass or a focal asymmetry identified on a baseline screening mammogram with no sonographic correlate on diagnostic imaging may be assessed as BI-RADS 3 (probably benign). This rule only holds true for lesions identified from baseline imaging, not for new or growing findings.

5. Architectural distortion appears as lines radiating from a central point without a visible mass.

6. Architectural distortion has a high predictive value for malignancy but is often subtle and missed on two-dimensional mammography. Tomosynthesis increases sensitivity for malignancies presenting as architectural distortion.

7. Nonmalignant causes of architectural distortion include surgical scar, sclerosing adenosis, and radial scar or complex sclerosing lesion.

References

1. Stavros AT, Thickman D, Rapp CL, Dennis MA, Parker SH, Sisney GA. Solid breast nodules: use of sonography to distinguish between benign and malignant lesions. *Radiology*. 1995;196:123–134.
2. Sickles EA. Findings at mammographic screening on only one standard projection: outcomes analysis. *Radiology*. 1998;208:471–475.
3. Durand MA, Haas BM, Yao X, et al. Early clinical experience with digital breast tomosynthesis for screening mammography. *Radiology*. 2015;274:85–92.
4. Price ER, Joe BN, Sickles EA. The developing asymmetry: revisiting a perceptual and diagnostic challenge. *Radiology*. 2015;274:642–651.
5. Burrell HC, Pinder SE, Wilson AR, et al. The positive predictive value of mammographic signs: a review of 425 non-palpable breast lesions. *Clin Radiol*. 1996;51:277–281.
6. Burrell HC, Evans AJ, Wilson AR, Pinder SE. False-negative breast screening assessment: what lessons can we learn? *Clin Radiol*. 2001;56:385–388.
7. Huynh PT, Jarolimek AM, Daye S. The false-negative mammogram. *Radiographics*. 1998;18:1137–1154. quiz 243-4.
8. Suleiman WI, McEntee MF, Lewis SJ, et al. In the digital era, architectural distortion remains a challenging radiological task. *Clin Radiol*. 2016;71:e35–e40.
9. Partyka L, Lourenco AP, Mainiero MB. Detection of mammographically occult architectural distortion on digital breast tomosynthesis screening: initial clinical experience. *AJR Am J Roentgenol*. 2014;203:216–222.
10. Freer PE, Niell B, Rafferty EA. Preoperative Tomosynthesis-guided Needle Localization of Mammographically and Sonographically Occult Breast Lesions. *Radiology*. 2015;275:377–383.
11. Alshafeiy TI, Nguyen JV, Rochman CM, Nicholson BT, Patrie JT, Harvey JA. Outcome of Architectural Distortion Detected Only at Breast Tomosynthesis versus 2D Mammography. *Radiology*. 2018;288:38–46.
12. Patel BK, Covington M, Pizzitola VJ, et al. Initial experience of tomosynthesis-guided vacuum-assisted biopsies of tomosynthesis-detected (2D mammography and ultrasound occult) architectural distortions. *AJR Am J Roentgenol*. 2018;210:1395–1400.
13. Korhonen KE, Weinstein SP, McDonald ES, Conant EF. Strategies to increase cancer detection: review of true-positive and false-negative results at digital breast tomosynthesis screening. *Radiographics*. 2016;36:1954–1965.
14. Vijapura C, Yang L, Xiong J, Fajardo LL. Imaging features of nonmalignant and malignant architectural distortion detected by tomosynthesis. *AJR Am J Roentgenol*. 2018;211:1397–1404.

Suggested Readings

Cohen EO, Tso HH, Leung JWT. Multiple bilateral circumscribed breast masses detected at imaging: review of evidence for management recommendations. *AJR Am J Roentgenol*. 2020;214:276–281.

D'Orsi C, Sickles EA, Mendelson EB, Morris EA, et al. *ACR BI-RADS Atlas, Breast Imaging Reporting and Data System*. Reston, VA: American College of Radiology; 2013.

Durand MA, Wang S, Hooley RJ, Raghu M, Philpotts LE. Tomosynthesis-detected architectural distortion: management algorithm with radiologic-pathologic correlation. *Radiographics*. 2016;36:311–321.

Friedewald SM, Rafferty EA, Rose SL, et al. Breast cancer screening using tomosynthesis in combination with digital mammography. *JAMA*. 2014;311:2499–2507.

Gaur S, Dialani V, Slanetz PJ, Eisenberg RL. Architectural distortion of the breast. *AJR Am J Roentgenol*. 2013;201:W662–W670.

Korhonen KE, Weinstein SP, McDonald ES, Conant EF. Strategies to increase cancer detection: review of true-positive and false-negative results at digital breast tomosynthesis screening. *Radiographics*. 2016;36:1954–1965.

Pearson KL, Sickles EA, Frankel SD, Leung JW. Efficacy of step-oblique mammography for confirmation and localization of densities seen on only one standard mammographic view. *AJR Am J Roentgenol*. 2000;174:745–752.

Price ER, Joe BN, Sickles EA. The developing asymmetry: revisiting a perceptual and diagnostic challenge. *Radiology*. 2015;274:642–651.

Sickles EA. Findings at mammographic screening on only one standard projection: outcomes analysis. *Radiology*. 1998;208:471–475.

Stavros AT, Thickman D, Rapp CL, Dennis MA, Parker SH, Sisney GA. Solid breast nodules: use of sonography to distinguish between benign and malignant lesions. *Radiology*. 1995;196:123–134.

4 *Mammographic Analysis of Breast Calcifications*

HEATHER I. GREENWOOD

OVERVIEW *This chapter covers mammographic appearance of benign, probably benign, and malignant breast calcifications. It reviews the list of typically benign breast calcifications. Analysis of breast calcifications using Breast Imaging Reporting and Data System (BI-RADS) morphology and distribution to determine appropriate assessment, and management recommendations are also covered.*

Breast calcifications are a common mammographic finding. The majority of calcifications in the breast are related to benign causes. However, not all calcifications are benign, and some calcifications are caused by malignant lesions in the breast. In addition, calcifications are the most common mammographic presentation of nonpalpable breast cancer. High-risk breast lesions may also present with calcifications on imaging.

The vast majority of calcifications in the breast can be readily identified as typically benign (BI-RADS 2). Benign calcifications tend to be larger in size, more regular, and easier to detect than suspicious calcifications, which tend to be smaller in size. The calcifications that are not typically benign on mammography can be analyzed by evaluating the Breast Imaging Reporting and Data System (BI-RADS) morphology and distribution descriptors to determine an appropriate BI-RADS assessment. Some may be assessed as probably benign (BI-RADS 3) or suspicious for malignancy (BI-RADS 4 or 5). Suspicious calcifications should be biopsied.

Pathogenesis

Calcifications are neither benign or malignant; rather, they represent mineral deposition within the breast that results from various physiologic processes including secretory, inflammatory, senescence, traumatic injury, and necrosis. Necrosis may be related to benign or malignant processes. Calcifications may occur anywhere in the breast, such as in the ducts, lobules, vessels, and skin. Most breast calcifications form either within the terminal ducts (intraductal) or within the acini (lobular), which together compose the terminal ductal lobular unit (TDLU).

There are two types of calcifications that occur within the breast. Calcium phosphate, usually in the form of hydroxyapatite, is the more common form, which is associated with both benign and malignant processes. Benign processes include fibrocystic changes such as cysts, usual ductal hyperplasia, adenosis and sclerosing adenosis, and fibroadenomas. Malignant processes include both in situ and invasive carcinomas. Calcium phosphate stain blue or dark purple on hematoxylin and eosin (H&E) stains. Calcium oxalate is less common and is always associated with benign processes. Calcium oxalate is colorless on H&E staining, and the pathologist may need to look at these under polarized light to see. Unfortunately, mammography cannot distinguish between the two types.

Screening and Diagnostic Assessment

If calcifications cannot be definitively assessed as typically benign at screening mammography, then they should be recalled as a BI-RADS 0 (needs additional imaging), and diagnostic views including magnification mammography are necessary for further evaluation. Calcifications are the smallest structures identified on mammography and are best visualized when there is no patient motion on images and by using high-resolution techniques. Magnification views provide more precise information on the morphology and number of calcifications than standard full-field views. The vast majority of calcifications are not visualized on ultrasound. Occasionally calcifications, particularly larger ones, may be seen on ultrasound. It is important to note that while ultrasound may visualize calcifications, it does not adequately characterize them.

Occasionally artifacts may be confused for calcifications in the breast. Radiopaque material on the skin as can be seen in the setting of deodorant and some skin powders/lotions that contain metals such as zinc oxide, magnesium, aluminum, or iodine. In the setting of possible deodorant artifact, the patient may wipe off/wash the skin of the axilla, and the artifact should be removed on repeat imaging.

Typically Benign Calcifications

In the current BI-RADS fifth edition for mammography, calcifications are separated into two categories: typically benign and suspicious morphology. There are several types of breast calcifications that can be classified as benign based on a characteristic mammographic appearance. The first step in interpreting breast calcifications is to identify those that are characteristically benign. If calcifications can be classified as typically benign, they may be dismissed at screening as a BI-RADS 2 (benign) finding (Box 4.1). Sometimes further evaluation may be needed, and diagnostic mammography and spot magnification views may be necessary to characterize calcifications as typically benign (BI-RADS 2).

SKIN CALCIFICATIONS

Skin calcifications are located in the sebaceous glands of the breast and tend to be tightly grouped together and have lucent centers. They appear in typical locations such as the areola, axilla, inframammary fold, and cleavage (Fig. 4.1). A sign that has been described as suggestive of a dermal origin is the "tattoo" sign. The tattoo sign refers to calcifications that maintain a fixed relationship to each other in different mammographic projections and are suggestive of a dermal location. Digital breast tomosynthesis (DBT) may also be helpful in showing dermal location of calcifications. On DBT, the skin often appears on the first and last few images of the DBT sequence. However, when parts of the skin are not touching the detector or compression paddle, the calcifications may not appear on these first and last few images. This is more frequently the case in areas of the breast that are thinner, such as anteriorly. If needed, additional views such as tangential views can be performed to confirm whether calcifications localize to the skin. To perform a tangential view, the skin calcifications are localized with an alphanumeric grid, a radiopaque BB marker is placed directly over the calcifications, and an image is taken with the radiopaque BB marker in tangent to the beam. Skin calcifications will project within the skin on the tangential view (Fig. 4.2).

VASCULAR

Vascular breast calcifications are a very common finding on mammography. These represent calcifications within

Box 4.1	Benign Breast Calcifications
Skin	
Vascular	
Coarse "popcorn-like"	
Large rod-like	
Rim	
Dystrophic	
Milk of calcium	
Suture	
Round	

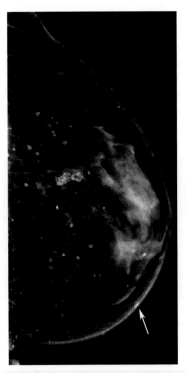

Fig. 4.1 Diffuse skin calcifications, note some project within skin itself (*arrow*).

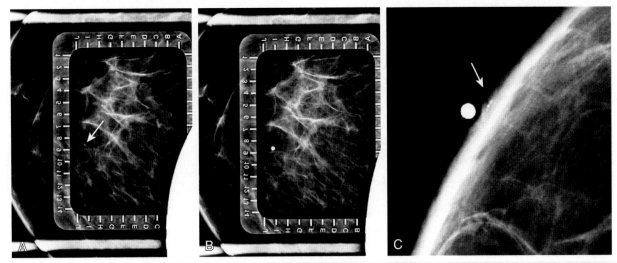

Fig. 4.2 Tangential views. Calcifications (*arrow*) placed in an alphanumeric grid (A), a radiopaque BB marker is placed directly over the calcifications (B), view performed tangential to the radiopaque BB marker shows the calcifications within the skin (*arrows*) (C) confirming the dermal location.

the medial layer of the vessel. These are usually bilateral but may be unilateral or more prominent on one side. A classic appearance on mammography includes a tram-track configuration of calcifications paralleling the wall of the vessel (Fig. 4.3). Often the soft tissue of the tubular vessel will also be apparent. They tend to have a serpentine course rather than a branching ductal pattern. If not definitively vascular on screening, as may occur in the case of smaller vessels, spot magnification or DBT views may be helpful to determine a vascular etiology. The parallel orientation of the calcifications or the tubular vessel may be easier to see on DBT.

COARSE "POPCORN-LIKE"

Coarse "popcorn-like" calcifications are produced by involuting fibroadenomas. These are large, dense calcifications, greater than 2 to 3 mm in diameter. Often an associated soft tissue mass may be seen. The calcifications tend to be at the periphery of the soft tissue mass, and these fibroadenomas may calcify to varying degrees (Fig. 4.4). Over time the calcifications may coalesce. In some cases, the entire soft tissue mass is calcified and only a large calcification may be seen.

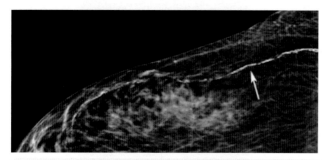

Fig. 4.3 Vascular calcifications (*arrow*) in the breast with classic parallel "tram-track" calcifications paralleling the vessel wall.

LARGE ROD-LIKE

Large rod-like calcifications are benign calcifications in the ducts, related to benign duct ectasia. These are calcifications of inspissated secretions in or immediately adjacent to dilated benign ducts. These have a cigar-shape appearance, with a smooth thick rod shape, >0.5 mm diameter. Given the ductal location, there may be a diffuse linear branching distribution pattern. A less common appearance of this type of calcification has a lucent center. This occurs when the calcifications are periductal, or along the wall of the duct in location (Fig. 4.5). These tend to occur in women who are 60 years of age or older. They are most commonly bilateral, but when they first begin to develop, they may be unilateral. These can most often be distinguished from the suspicious linear calcifications of ductal carcinoma in situ (DCIS) by the thickness and smoothness of these calcifications versus the calcifications of DCIS, which appear more irregular in appearance.

RIM

Rim calcifications are thin benign calcifications that appear to coat the surface of a sphere. They may be round or oval and have smooth surfaces with lucent centers (Fig. 4.6). These calcifications represent areas of fat necrosis or calcifications in the walls of oil cysts. In the most recent BI-RADS fifth edition, the old terms *egg-shell* and *lucent centered* were combined into the single new term *rim*. These may occur anywhere in the breast and often may be seen in a superficial location.

DYSTROPHIC

Dystrophic calcifications form in the breast following various types of trauma, commonly after radiation or surgery. These may also form in patients following trauma such as

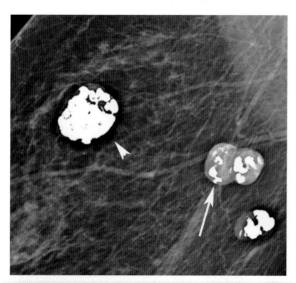

Fig. 4.4 Coarse or "popcorn-like" calcifications. Note varying degree of calcified masses with completely calcified mass (*arrowhead*) and partially calcified mass (*arrow*).

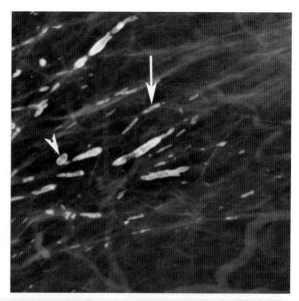

Fig. 4.5 Large rod-like calcifications with smooth margins with classic cigar shape appearance (*arrow*) and less commonly with lucent center (*arrowhead*).

seat belt injuries during motor vehicle collisions. These are coarse, thick calcifications that are often irregular in shape and usually greater than 1 mm in size (Fig. 4.7). These are often seen associated with scars in the breast. Over time these calcifications tend to coalesce and may become very large and readily palpable (Fig. 4.8).

MILK OF CALCIUM

Milk of calcium represents sedimented or layering calcifications that occur in macro- or microcysts in the breast. This process has a characteristic appearance on mammography. On a mediolateral (ML) or lateromedial (LM) projection, layering calcifications within cysts appear as linear, curvilinear, crescent, or "tea cup" shaped. (Fig. 4.9A). On the craniocaudal (CC) view, these layering calcifications are much less evident, appearing as indistinct, smudgy, or amorphous deposits (Fig. 4.9B). The particles must change shape on different projections (CC and LM or ML) in order to be characterized as benign milk of calcium. This concept is illustrated in the diagram shown in Fig. 4.9C.

SUTURE

Sutural calcifications have a typical tubular or linear appearance and sometimes knots may be present (Fig. 4.10).

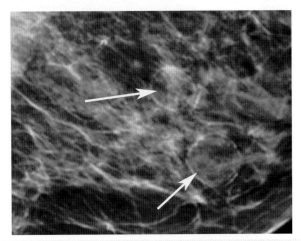

Fig. 4.6 Multiple rim calcifications, note the peripheral calcifications that appear to coat the surface of a sphere with a lucent center (*arrows*).

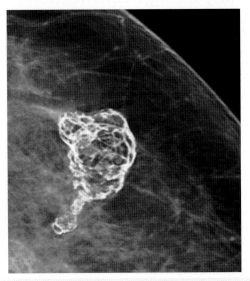

Fig. 4.7 Dystrophic calcifications at a site of prior surgery (*arrow*).

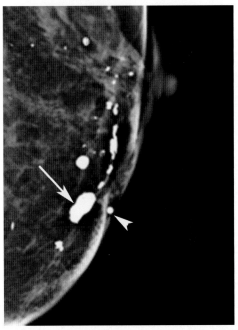

Fig. 4.8 Multiple large dystrophic calcifications. Note the radiopaque BB marker (*arrowhead*) marking the site of palpable lump corresponding to large dystrophic calcification (*arrow*).

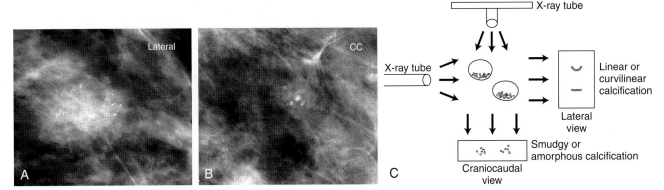

Fig. 4.9 Milk of calcium. Calcifications layering in cysts appear linear and crescentic on lateral view (A) and appear as smudgy, amorphous deposits on craniocaudal (CC) view (B). Diagram illustrates the concept behind different appearances of milk of calcium on CC and lateral views (C).

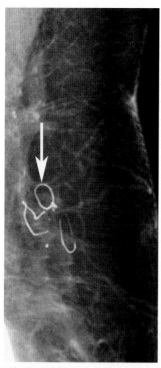

Fig. 4.10 Sutural calcifications (*arrow*) with typical curvilinear appearance.

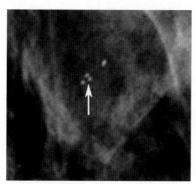

Fig. 4.11 Round calcifications (*arrow*).

Sutural calcifications are most often seen in the surgical bed of an irradiated breast.

ROUND

In the current BI-RADS fifth edition, the term *round* encompasses both round and punctate. These are round calcifications of varying sizes (Fig. 4.11). The assessment and management of round calcifications depend on the distribution as well as whether they are stable, new, and/or increasing. When they are diffuse, they may be dismissed as benign. Assessment and management of other distributions of round calcifications will be discussed later in this chapter.

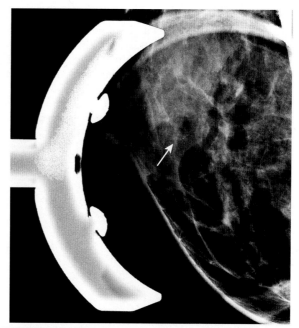

Fig. 4.12 Grouped round and punctate calcifications (*arrow*).

Probably Benign Calcifications (BI-RADS 3) and Their Management

Grouped round and/or punctate calcifications (Fig. 4.12) on baseline mammogram—whether the patient's first mammogram or no priors are available—warrant a BI-RADS 3 "probably benign" assessment with recommendation for short-interval imaging surveillance. Of note, the calcifications must be fully evaluated with diagnostic imaging, including magnification views, before making a BI-RADS 3 assessment. Once stability is documented for a period of at least 2 years, a BI-RADS 2 benign assessment may be made. During follow-up, if there is an increase in the number of calcifications not consistent with an evolving benign cause or a change in the morphology that appears more suspicious, then a recommendation for biopsy should be made.

Suspicious Calcifications

When evaluating all other calcifications in the breast—those that cannot be classified as typically benign or probably benign—it is important to use both the BI-RADS distribution and the BI-RADS morphology (shape) to determine the appropriate BI-RADS assessment category and the need for biopsy. Suspicious calcifications tend to be smaller and more irregular than benign calcifications.

Distribution

The BI-RADS lexicon defines various distribution patterns for breast calcifications (Fig. 4.13A–D). The different distributions are listed in Table 4.1 in order of most benign to

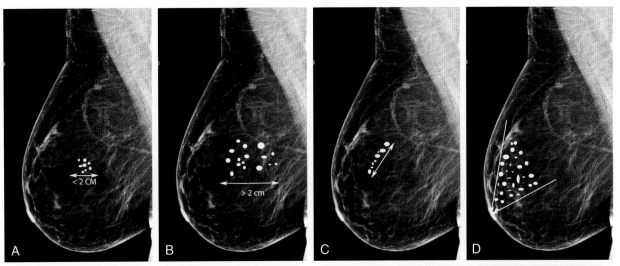

Fig. 4.13 Distributions of calcifications, grouped calcifications (A), regional calcifications (B), linear calcifications (C), and segmental calcifications (D).

Table 4.1 Distribution Patterns and Likelihood of Malignancy

Distribution	Likelihood of Malignancy
Diffuse	0%
Regional	26%
Grouped	31%
Linear	60%
Segmental	62%

Adapted from: Sickles et al., 2013.

most suspicious. Distribution assists with the assessment of breast calcifications and must always be considered with morphology.

DIFFUSE

A diffuse distribution is defined as randomly scattered throughout the breast (Fig. 4.14). This was previously known as "scattered." This does not mean that the calcifications are distributed evenly, as the tendency of calcifications is to group together. The key is that no area is more suspicious than any other area in the breast. This pattern suggests a benign process, especially when bilateral. For example, punctate and amorphous calcifications in a diffuse distribution are almost always benign, particularly if they are in both breasts. Diffuse punctate and amorphous calcifications are often associated with benign fibrocystic change.

REGIONAL

A regional distribution is defined as numerous calcifications that occupy over 2 cm of breast tissue in greatest dimension that is not in a ductal distribution (Fig. 4.15). This distribution pattern is suggestive of a benign process, but morphology must also be considered. Often calcifications related to sclerosing adenosis or fibrocystic change may present with a regional distribution pattern.

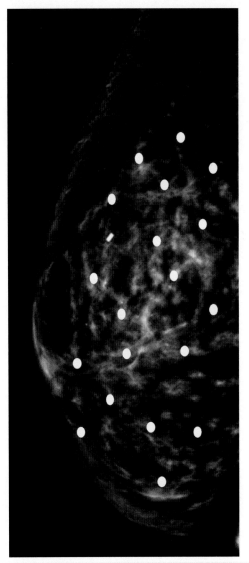

Fig. 4.14 Diffuse distribution of calcifications in a patient with a clip from a prior benign breast biopsy.

GROUPED

A group (previously "clustered") is defined as five calcifications or more in 1 cm of breast tissue spanning up to 2 cm of breast tissue (Fig. 4.16). This distribution pattern is of intermediate concern, and assessment will depend on the morphology of the calcifications. Of note, if calcifications appear grouped only in one projection, it may not be a true group and rather be related to overlapping calcifications. To confirm a group, calcifications should appear grouped in two different projections (CC, MLO, and/or true lateral). Differential diagnoses for grouped calcifications are listed in Table 4.2.

LINEAR

A linear distribution is defined as calcifications in a line (Fig. 4.17). This is a suspicious distribution pattern for all morphologies of calcifications, as this suggests deposits in a duct. Note this excludes those calcifications on the typically benign list, such as vascular and large rod-like calcifications.

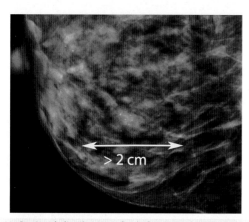

Fig. 4.15 Regional distribution of calcifications occupy over 2 cm of breast tissue in greatest dimension.

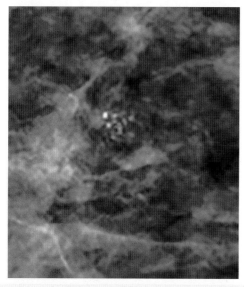

Fig. 4.16 Grouped calcifications: There are greater than five calcifications and these span less than 2 cm of breast tissue.

Differential diagnoses for grouped calcifications are listed in Table 4.3.

SEGMENTAL

A segmental distribution pattern is defined as a wedge-shaped area with the apex of the wedge pointing toward the nipple (Fig. 4.18). This is the most suspicious pattern and suggests calcification deposits along a ductal distribution.

Morphology

There are four morphologies of calcifications that usually warrant a biopsy recommendation. The suspicious

Table 4.2 Differential Diagnosis Grouped Breast Calcifications

Benign	Malignant
Skin	DCIS
Fibrocystic change/milk of calcium	Invasive carcinoma
Fibroadenoma	
Fat necrosis	
Sclerosing adenosis	
Papilloma	
Atypia (ADH, ALH, LCIS)	

ADH, Atypical ductal hyperplasia; *ALH*, atypical lobular hyperplasia; *LCIS*, lobular carcinoma in situ
Adapted from: Sickles et al., 2013.

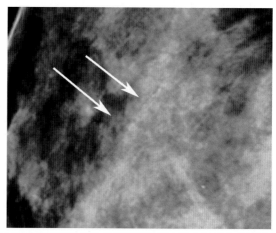

Fig. 4.17 Linear calcifications in a linear distribution (*arrows*).

Table 4.3 Differential Diagnosis Linear Breast Calcifications

Benign	Malignant
Vascular	DCIS
Large rod-like	Invasive ductal carcinoma
Sutural	

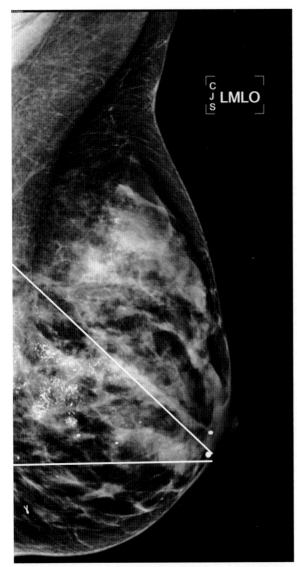

Fig. 4.18 Calcifications in a segmental distribution, wedge-shaped with apex pointing toward the nipple.

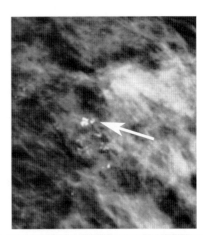

Fig. 4.19 Coarse heterogeneous calcifications in a grouped distribution (*arrow*).

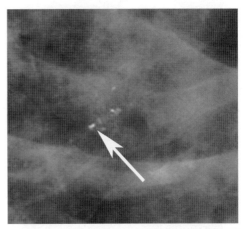

Fig. 4.20 Amorphous calcifications in a grouped distribution pattern (*arrow*).

Table 4.4 Suspicious Morphology Calcifications and Likelihood of Malignancy

Morphology	Likelihood of Malignancy
Coarse heterogeneous	13%
Amorphous	21%
Fine pleomorphic	29%
Fine-linear or fine-linear branching	70%

Adapted from: Sickles et al., 2013.

morphologies and corresponding likelihood for malignancy are listed in Table 4.4, in order of least to most suspicious.

COARSE HETEROGENEOUS

Coarse heterogeneous calcifications are irregular, conspicuous calcifications that are larger than 0.5 mm (Fig. 4.19). They are usually between 0.5 and 1.0 mm and have a tendency to coalesce. These calcifications are larger than fine pleomorphic calcifications and smaller than dystrophic calcifications. This shape is of intermediate concern. The majority of these calcifications represent a benign etiology such as a fibroadenoma, trauma, or fibrosis; however, malignancy is in the differential diagnosis, particularly DCIS. Per BI-RADS, "numerous bilateral groups of coarse heterogeneous calcifications may be dismissed as benign, although baseline magnification views may be helpful." Otherwise, coarse heterogeneous calcifications warrant a BI-RADS 4 assessment and should undergo sampling.

AMORPHOUS

Amorphous calcifications are small and have hazy borders. These calcifications are so small and or indistinct that it is hard to define an exact size or shape (Fig. 4.20). This morphology is of intermediate concern. The positive predictive value (PPV) for malignancy has been shown to be approximately 21% (BI-RADS). The distribution of these calcifications determines the assessment. If amorphous calcifications are diffuse and bilateral, they may be dismissed as benign (BI-RADS 2). Amorphous calcifications that are in a grouped, linear, or segmental distribution warrant a BI-RADS 4 (suspicious) assessment and stereotactic core biopsy should be recommended.

FINE PLEOMORPHIC

Fine pleomorphic calcifications are small, less than 0.5 cm, that are variable in size and shape (Fig. 4.21). These are smaller than coarse heterogeneous calcifications These have a higher probability of malignancy and are suspicious in any distribution pattern, warranting tissue sampling.

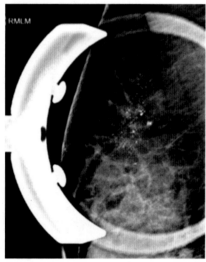

Fig. 4.21 Spot magnification view showing fine pleomorphic calcifications.

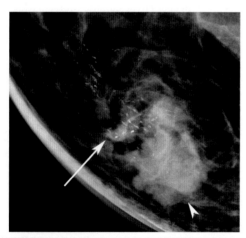

Fig. 4.22 Fine linear/linear branching calcifications (*arrow*) extending anteriorly from a mass (*arrowhead*)

FINE LINEAR/LINEAR BRANCHING

Fine linear/linear branching calcifications are thin, linear, curvilinear, or irregular in shape. They tend to be small, less than 0.5 mm (Fig. 4.22). These often have irregular edges. These have the highest PPV of malignancy of all the suspicious morphologies and are suspicious in any distribution pattern, warranting tissue sampling.

Management of Suspicious Calcifications

Suspicious calcifications assessed as a BI-RADS 4 or 5 most commonly undergo percutaneous sampling via stereotactic core biopsy. If stereotactic core biopsy is not feasible, for example in the setting of thin breasts, far posterior lesions, or any other reason, surgical excisional biopsy can be performed for tissue diagnosis. Rarely, one may see a correlate to calcifications on ultrasound, and in those cases ultrasound-guided biopsy could be performed with specimen radiography to confirm presence of calcifications in the biopsy sample.

Summary

In summary, breast calcifications may be classified as benign, probably benign, or suspicious for malignancy. The majority of calcifications in the breast can be recognized as typically benign. Those that are not typically benign can be assessed using BI-RADS distribution and morphology terminology to determine appropriate management recommendations. Suspicious calcifications should undergo sampling, most commonly stereotactic core biopsy.

KEY POINTS

Most calcifications in the breast can be characterized as typically benign (BI-RADS 2).

Calcifications that are not typically benign can be assessed by their Breast Imaging Reporting and Data System (BI-RADS) morphology and distribution.

A group of round punctate calcifications on a baseline mammogram meets criteria for a probably benign assessment, BI-RADS 3, with a recommendation for short-imaging surveillance.

Calcifications that cannot be classified as probably benign or typically benign are suspicious, and these should be sampled.

Stereotactic core biopsy is the most common sampling method for suspicious calcifications.

Suggested Reading

Demetri-Lewis A, Slanetz PJ, Eisenberg RL. Breast calcifications: the focal group. *AJR.* 2012;198:W325–W343.

Horvat JV, Keating DM, Rodrigues-Duarte H, Morris EA, Mango VL. Calcifications at digital breast tomosynthesis: imaging features and biopsy techniques. Radiographics 2019;39:307–318.

Lai KC, Slanetz PJ, Eisenberg RL. Linear breast calcifications. *AJR*. 2012;199:W151–W157.

Park GE, Kim SH, Lee JM, et al. Comparison of positive predictive values of categorization of suspicious calcifications using the 4th and 5th Editions of BI-RADS. *AJR*. 2019;213:710–715.

Sickles EA, D'Orsi CJ, Bassett LW, et al. *ACR-BIRADS® Mammography*. In: *ACR-BIRADS® Atlas, Breat Imaging Reporting and Data System*. Reston, VA: American College of Radiology; 2013.

Sickles EA. Breast calcifications: mammographic evaluation. *Radiology*. 1986;160:289–293.

5 *Breast Ultrasound Indications and Interpretation*

JOCELYN RAPELYEA

OVERVIEW *This chapter covers screening and diagnostic indications for breast ultrasound and Breast Imaging Reporting and Data System (BI-RADS) interpretation. Additional topics covered include ultrasound technique for optimizing image quality, basic ultrasound physics, and artifacts.*

Indications

Breast ultrasound can be used for both screening and diagnostic indications (Table 5.1). Ultrasound evaluates breast tissue without the use of ionizing radiation or the injection of contrast material and is affordable, readily available, and well tolerated by patients. The following sections will review some common applications of breast ultrasound.

SUPPLEMENTAL SCREENING IN ADDITION TO MAMMOGRAPHY

Even with the advancements in breast cancer screening, such as full-field digital mammography (FFDM) and digital breast tomosynthesis (DBT), breast ultrasound continues to be essential in breast cancer detection. Historically, the principal function of ultrasound was to discover if a mammographic mass was solid or cystic. Yet in recent years, the recognition of mammography's diminished accuracy

Table 5.1 Appropriate Indications for Breast Ultrasound

1. Evaluation and characterization of palpable masses and other breast-related signs and/or symptoms

2. Evaluation of suspected or apparent abnormalities detected on mammography (with or without digital breast tomosynthesis), breast magnetic resonance imaging (MRI), or other imaging modalities

3. Initial imaging evaluation of palpable breast masses in patients under 30 years of age who are not at high risk for development of breast cancer and in lactating and pregnant women

4. Evaluation of problems associated with breast implants

5. Guidance for breast biopsy and other interventional procedures

6. Treatment planning for radiation therapy

7. As a supplement to mammography, screening for occult cancers in certain populations, including of women with heterogeneously or extremely dense breasts who are determined to be at elevated risk of breast cancer or with newly suspected breast cancer, who are not candidates for MRI or have no easy access to MRI

8. Identification of and biopsy guidance for abnormal axillary lymph node(s), for example, in patients with newly diagnosed or recurrent breast cancer or with findings highly suggestive of malignancy or other significant pathology

American College of Radiology: *ACR practice parameter for the performance of a breast ultrasound examination*, Reston, 2016, American College of Radiology.

in women with dense breast tissue has changed the use of ultrasound from a fundamental diagnostic examination to a hybrid tool of screening and diagnosis.

Many single and multi-institutional screening studies, including the American College of Radiology Imaging Network (ACRIN) 6666 trial, confirm the utility of supplemental screening using ultrasound or magnetic resonance imaging (MRI) in women at elevated risk. The American College of Radiology (ACR) Appropriateness Criteria Practice Parameters and guidelines recommend bilateral whole breast ultrasound for women at elevated risk who qualify but are unable to undergo breast MRI or for women at increased risk solely due to breast density. (Breast MRI is discussed in Chapter 8: Breast MRI Indications, Interpretation, Interventions.)

Compared with screening mammography alone, supplemental screening breast ultrasound detects an additional three to four cancers per 1000 women screened (Table 5.2). Most of these cancers are invasive and without evidence of lymph node involvement.

The added benefit of supplemental screening with breast ultrasound is balanced against an increase in false-positive findings relative to mammography. The ACRIN 6666 trial found an initial 8.1% false-positive rate for ultrasound compared with 4.4% for mammography. False positive biopsy rate for ultrasound screening decreased to ~5% on subsequent incidence screening rounds with only 7.4% of those biopsies positive for cancer.[2] Many single and multicenter studies evaluating a whole breast ultrasound screening program in their practice show a decline of false-positive findings on subsequent screening rounds. The recommendation to perform an independent audit may change practice habits and improve outcomes.

Technique

Screening breast ultrasound may be performed manually by a technician or physician using a handheld device or by using an automated breast ultrasound system (ABUS). Each method has distinct advantages and disadvantages. The manual handheld technique relies on the individual's experience acquiring the ultrasound images and directly corresponds to the study's quality and diagnostic accuracy. Following the ACR practice parameter for performance

Table 5.2 Single and multi-institutional screening breast ultrasound publications.

Author (Year)	Center	Type	Examinations	Ultrasound-Only Cancers	Yield per 1000
Lee et al. (2019)	Multi	HHUS	6,081	33	5.4
Ohuchi et al. (2016)	Multi	HHUS	36,859	61	3.3
Brem et al. (2014)	Multi	ABUS	15,318	30	1.96
Berg et al. (2012)	Multi	HHUS	4,814	32	4.28
Hooley et al. (2012)	Single	HHUS	935	3	3.21
Kelly et al. (2010)	Multi	AWBUS	6,425	23	3.58
Corsetti et al. (2008)	Multi	HHUS	9,157	37	4.04
Crystal et al. (2003)	Single	HHUS	1,517	7	4.61
Leconte et al. (2003)	Single	HHUS	4,236	16	3.78
Kolb et al. (2002)	Single	HHUS	13,547	37	2.73

HHUS, Hand held ultrasound. *ABUS*, Automated breast ultrasound. *AWBUS*, Automated whole breast ultrasound.
Modified from Butler RS, Hooley RJ: Screening breast ultrasound: update after 10 years of breast density notification laws, *American Journal of Roentgenology* 214(6), 1424–1435, 2020. https://doi.org/10.2214/AJR.19.22275.

of whole breast ultrasound, standard examination documentation for a negative examination consists of a single representative image of each quadrant plus an image of the retroareolar region. If an abnormality is missed by the technician or the physician during real-time scanning, this information is not available for interpretation or later review and could result in a false-negative examination.

Automated breast ultrasound systems resolve the operator dependence of the handheld technique and have the capacity to record the entire ultrasound examination using cine capability. The recording of the whole study decouples the experience and expertise of the individual acquiring the images from the physician's diagnostic interpretation. Moreover, some automated systems use a large 15-cm transducer to obtain an extended field of view with axial/transverse images, which are immediately available for reconstruction into multiple planes (coronal and sagittal). The cross-sectional (three-dimensional) data facilitates understanding of the patient's breast anatomy, including potential pathologic findings that may identify more extensive disease from adjacent normal tissue. The reconstructed coronal view is especially useful in detecting areas of architectural distortion that are not as conspicuous on the transverse (axial) images (Fig. 5.1). Although the use of panoramic software found in a conventional ultrasound machine can achieve a similar transverse extended field of view image, multiplanar reconstruction is unattainable. The long transverse or panoramic view can improve visualization and distinguish abnormal findings from the surrounding tissue; however, this technique is conducted only on a focused portion of the breast that displays the abnormality (Fig. 5.2).

Screening ultrasound, like screening mammography, can have a final Breast Imaging Reporting and Data System (BI-RADS) assessment code of 0. Because there are fixed images of the screening examination, any further evaluation would be consistent with a diagnostic study. An incomplete assessment code is not appropriate for a diagnostic ultrasound scan, since the goal of the study is to explain an abnormal finding, even if the second ultrasound examination takes place on the same day or later.

DIAGNOSTIC EVALUATION

Besides screening in dense breast tissue, breast ultrasound is the initial examination performed in women younger than 30 years of age and pregnant or lactating women complaining of breast-related symptoms. According to ACR practice parameter guidelines for the performance of breast ultrasound examination, in women 40 years of

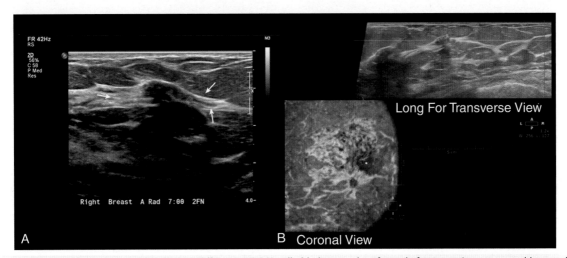

Fig. 5.1 Indications: screening ultrasound technique differences. (A) Handheld ultrasound performed after screening automated breast ultrasound examination demonstrates a hypoechoic irregular mass with posterior acoustic shadowing. There is associated architectural distortion (*arrows*), duct changes (*^*), and Cooper ligament straightening and thickening. (B) Reconstructed coronal view of the same breast during screening ultrasound demonstrates increase conspicuity of the mass with associated architectural distortion. Long field-of-view (FOV) transverse image demonstrates similar findings to handheld ultrasound.

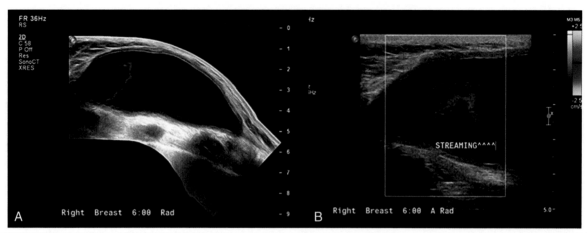

Fig. 5.2 Indications: postsurgical breast. A 68-year-old woman with recent mastectomy surgery. (A) Long field of view or panoramic view is useful for visualizing larger areas and for understanding the relationship to the surrounding tissue. The panoramic view demonstrates a 20-cm complex cystic and solid mass with posterior acoustic enhancement. This lesion with nondependent echoes and wall thickening would typically be categorized as BI-RADS 4: suspicious. However, in the setting of recent mastectomy, these ultrasound findings are consistent with a hematoma/seroma. (B) The handheld ultrasound transducer can image only 5 cm of the fluid collection. There is no vascularity associated with this lesion and active movement of the intracystic echogenic material was observed as "streaming" on color Doppler imaging suggestive of proteinaceous blood products and clot. Assessment is benign: BI-RADS 2.

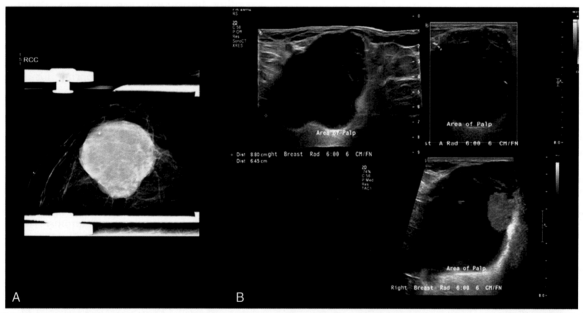

Fig. 5.3 Mass orientation: antiparallel. (A) Spot compression mammographic view of a palpable mass demonstrates a circumscribed dense mass. (B) Further characterization with ultrasound demonstrates that the mammographic finding is a complex cystic and solid mass with antiparallel orientation as its longest dimension is perpendicular to the skin. Pathology diagnosis intracystic papillary carcinoma.

age and older, mammography is recommended as the initial examination to evaluate a patient's symptoms (see Chapter 14: The Symptomatic Breast). Ultrasound provides a direct correlation between imaging and clinical findings. Its use gives a characterization of palpable lumps and breast-related symptoms such as focal noncyclical pain or nipple discharge (Fig. 5.3). The complaint of nipple discharge is concerning when it occurs from one orifice of one breast. Bilateral nipple discharge is usually secondary to hormonal effects or fibrocystic changes. Evaluation with ultrasound with the guidance of color or power Doppler can be performed to search for an intraductal mass when nipple discharge is unilateral. Papillary lesions are common intraductal masses and can be single or multiple. A single intraductal papilloma

within the milk duct can appear as an expansile hypoechoic mass or as a complex cystic and solid mass. Color Doppler imaging helps identify internal vascularity, which can differentiate a papillary lesion from an inflamed cyst. Papillary cystic neoplasms are more complex in appearance and may contain a mural nodule with or without a fibrovascular stalk and thick septations (see Fig. 5.3).

Diagnostic evaluation of palpable areas of concern is a common use of ultrasound. The two-finger technique, which surrounds the lump in question while using the ultrasound probe to scan in between will increase sensitivity. The sonographic appearance of the symptomatic area can differentiate between a dense island of tissue or an underlying abnormality and reassure the patient and clinician when

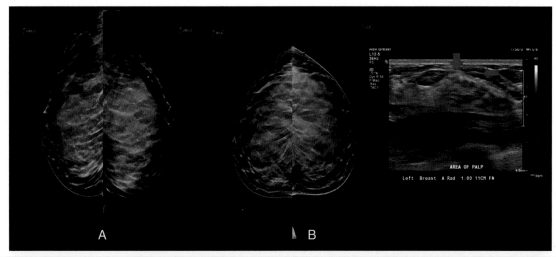

Fig. 5.4 Indications: diagnostic evaluation. Palpable lump. Bilateral mammogram and left breast ultrasound was performed to evaluate a palpable mass in a 42-year-old woman. (A) There is no discrete mass identified on the mammogram; however the sensitivity of mammography is limited by extremely dense breast tissue. The ultrasound examination is not impeded by breast density, and upon correlation with the physical examination demonstrates a normal ridge of dense glandular tissue (*arrows*). The negative predictive value of the combined mammogram and ultrasound examination exceeds 99%.

there is a negative examination (Fig. 5.4). Women who present for ultrasound examinations after a negative mammogram have an ultrasound finding that correlates 50% of the time, with most results categorized as benign, for example a cyst or ridge of dense glandular tissue. According to the ACR appropriateness criteria and best practices for palpable breast mass, it may be appropriate to perform an ultrasound examination as the initial test in symptomatic women with a recent mammogram in the previous 6 months. A repeat mammogram may be unnecessary, given that ultrasound is highly diagnostic in this setting.

Ultrasound Evaluation of Mammographic Finding

Breast ultrasound is the most common adjunct tool used in the evaluation of a mammographic abnormality. When correlating between the two modalities, careful consideration is made to lesion location, lesion size, and lesion shape with a clear understanding of the surrounding tissue. Lesion location is the most important feature, since an upper outer ultrasound mass does not correlate with a lower inner mammographic mass, even if the masses appear similar in shape and size. Interrogation of the correct area requires understanding how positioning and acquisition of the mammographic examination can affect differing appearances on the two modalities.

First, one must understand the varying degrees of obliquity and positioning when acquiring images for the two types of examinations. The interrogation of a mass in the radial (extending as rays from the nipple) and antiradial projections (perpendicular to the radial axis) on ultrasound will appear similar but not exact to the mediolateral oblique (MLO) and craniocaudal (CC) mammographic views. Second, a general awareness of lesion depth is useful, but it is critical to determine its related position to the mammary zone (anterior, middle, or posterior). A mammographic abnormality should resemble a similar positional depth on ultrasound with allowances for technique—mammographic compression pulls a lesion away from the chest wall, while the application of compression

during the ultrasound examination is toward the chest wall. Compression and positional differences may give the false impression that a lesion is closer to the pectoralis muscle on the ultrasound examination compared with mammography. In this latter case, a detailed understanding of the adjacent tissue density is essential to correlate findings accurately. A mass that is nearly surrounded by fat density on mammography bears no resemblance to a finding surrounded by dense fibroglandular changes on ultrasound. The third discrepancy between the two modalities affects the orientation of the mass. Depending on the degree of compression applied during the ultrasound examination, an obliquely oriented mass can change to a horizontal position, which may not correlate to the mammographic finding.

Besides location, the size of the lesion on mammography must resemble the findings identified on ultrasound. In more difficult cases, such as asymmetry, it may be hard to correlate between the mammographic and sonographic findings. Asymmetry on mammography can represent a summation of smaller sonographic structures. One must consider the surrounding tissue to account for the asymmetry identified on mammography confidently. Ultrasound dimensions obtained should include the longest measurements in two views with calipers spanning the outside edges of the lesion. If you measure the inside of the lesion, the ultrasound lesion may not correlate and will always be smaller than the mammographic finding.

Lastly, the lesion shape on mammography must correlate with the shape of the lesion seen on ultrasound. An irregular mass on mammography is suspected to be irregular on ultrasound. Differences that cannot be accounted for by the adjacent surrounding tissue suggest there is no correlative finding. The ultrasound section of the ACR BI-RADS lexicon gives a guide to ultrasound interpretation and aids in determining the level of suspicion (see Ultrasound BI-RADS and Interpretation section in this chapter). Examples of mammography and ultrasound correlation are shown in Figs. 5.5 and 5.6.

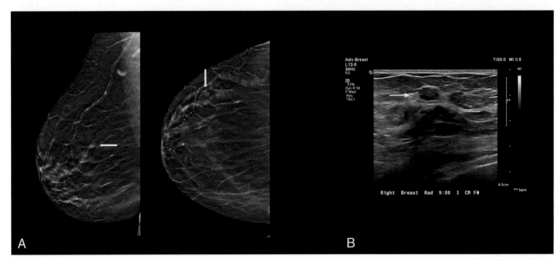

Fig. 5.5 Indications: diagnostic evaluation. Mammography and ultrasound correlation. (A) 56-year-old woman with abnormal screening mammogram demonstrates a 7-mm circumscribed mass (arrow) in the right upper outer breast. (B) Further evaluation with ultrasound shows corresponding finding with a similar size, shape, and location to the mammographic mass. The circumscribed oval mass (*arrow*) is located in the middle depth of the breast tissue immediately surrounded by fatty and glandular tissue.

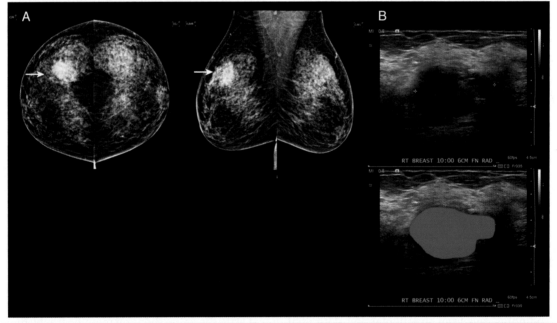

Fig. 5.6 Indication: diagnostic evaluation. Mammographic asymmetry and ultrasound correlation. (A) Bilateral mammogram demonstrates a focal asymmetry in the right upper outer breast (*arrows*). (B) The corresponding location (clockface, distance from the nipple), size, and shape on ultrasound agrees with the mammographic examination. (Ultrasound mass size and shape indicated by blue overlay.) The parallel-oriented (largest dimension is parallel to the skin) microlobulated hypoechoic mass found on ultrasound has posterior acoustic enhancement. Core needle biopsy confirmed a diagnosis of mucinous breast cancer.

Targeted Ultrasound After MRI and Other Imaging

Targeted ultrasound has the potential to identify a suspicious lesion recognized on physiologically based imaging such as breast magnetic resonance imaging (MRI), breast-specific gamma imaging (BSGI), positron emission mammography (PEM), and contrast-enhanced spectral mammography (CESM) with the intent to biopsy. Ultrasound plays a significant role in characterizing suspicious findings identified on most, if not all, breast imaging modalities. Implementation of ultrasound in this way is sometimes referred to as a "second look" since ultrasound evaluates a lesion initially identified with a different modality, which may or may not be visible on the second review with sonographic interrogation. Figs. 5.7 and 5.8 show examples of targeted second-look ultrasound for BSGI and MRI findings.

Lesions detected with physiologic-based imaging may not be readily apparent on ultrasound imaging that relies on anatomic variations. The efficiency of second-look ultrasound is best investigated for MRI. Reported ultrasound detection rates for MRI findings vary between 22.6% and 82.1%. Ultrasound correlates are more likely to be found for mass lesions than nonmass lesions and for malignant masses versus benign. Technical differences, software advancements, and reader experience contribute to the range of published results. When performing the ultrasound examination, there must be consideration of multiple factors, such as surrounding landmarks, size, and shape of lesion and location in the breast. If there is no ultrasound correlate, then a biopsy should be performed using the modality that demonstrates the lesion best.

Postsurgical Breast

The postsurgical breast includes a spectrum of findings related to fat necrosis. Fat necrosis evolves and has a variable presentation on all modalities of breast imaging. Ultrasound characteristics consist of skin thickening and edema (hyperechoic appearance) of the tissue surrounding the surgical site. Additional findings include hematoma/seroma that develops in the lumpectomy bed and can be present for years. The seroma takes the shape of the surgical cavity and can have an anechoic ultrasound appearance or one that is more heterogeneous with low-level echoes (see

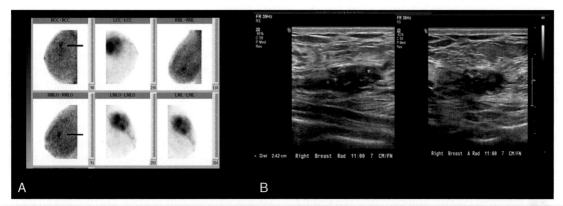

Fig. 5.7 Indications: diagnostic evaluation. Breast-specific gamma imaging (BSGI) targeted a 63-year-old woman with recent diagnosis of left breast cancer. (A) BSGI was performed for extent of disease. The examination demonstrates asymmetric uptake with large mass-like radiotracer uptake in the left upper outer breast with nonmass like extension toward the nipple. Additional focal mass like area was identified in the contralateral breast (*arrow*) in the craniocaudal (CC) and medial lateral oblique (MLO) projections. A targeted second-look ultrasound was performed. (B) Targeted ultrasound demonstrates a microlobulated heterogenous hypoechoic mass containing calcifications and no posterior acoustic features. An ultrasound-guided biopsy was performed demonstrating ductal carcinoma in situ (DCIS).

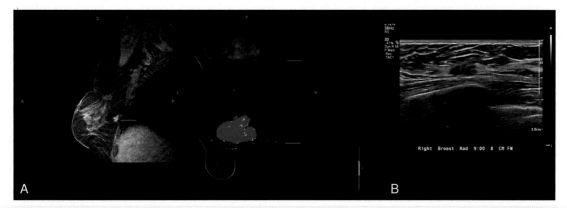

Fig. 5.8 Indications: diagnostic evaluation. Magnetic resonance imagining (MRI) surveillance and targeted ultrasound. A 65-year-old woman is status post–bilateral lumpectomy surgery for breast cancer. (A) MRI demonstrates stable postsurgical change and a new irregular enhancing mass in the upper outer right breast demonstrating suspicious kinetics (*arrow*). Targeted ultrasound was recommended with intent to biopsy. (B) Targeted ultrasound of the right breast demonstrates an irregular hypoechoic mass with similar shape and size identified on recent MRI. Pathology demonstrated recurrent invasive lobular breast cancer that was mammographically occult.

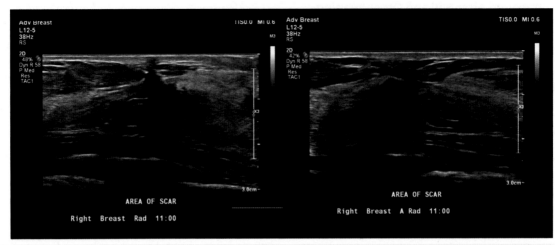

Fig. 5.9 Indication: postsurgical evaluation. Radial and antiradial projections of a lumpectomy scar demonstrate an irregular hypoechoic angular mass with posterior acoustic shadowing. Scar should connect with the surgical tract on one of the orthogonal views (*arrows*). Surgical scars can evolve over time and may show suspicious characteristics suggestive of malignancy. Correlation with mammography and clinical history will help in discerning benign from suspicious findings and whether tissue sampling is warranted.

Fig. 5.2). Both presentations are benign; however, a spontaneous increase in seroma size should raise suspicion. Any morphologic descriptor that describes the findings and is suspicious will also dictate an image-guided biopsy.

Over time, the fluid/debris within the surgical bed will get reabsorbed, and a fibrinous scar develops. Ultrasound characteristics of postoperative changes can mimic cancer and must be viewed in two orthogonal views to help differentiate disease from a scar. Scar tissue can usually be followed to the skin in an oblique line, whereas the orthogonal view may appear as a hypoechoic irregular mass with posterior acoustic shadowing (Fig. 5.9). Worrisome ultrasound findings for disease recurrence include a new mass adjacent to the excisional site, increased volume of the hypoechoic scar (that persists in two projections), and eccentric thickening or nodularity of the seroma cavity. Doppler may help determine whether there is internal vascularity, which would be more indicative of recurrent disease.

NEOADJUVANT TREATMENT

With the increasing use of neoadjuvant chemotherapy and localized brachytherapy, ultrasound has played a pivotal role in management and pretreatment decisions. Ultrasound evaluation can explore the potential for multifocal/multicentric disease, cancer involvement of the skin, and axillary lymph nodes, which are all-important prognostic indicators. Chest wall involvement is best identified with breast MRI, which has the advantage of discriminating the prepectoral fascial plane, chest wall musculature, and tumor margin. There are competing issues that may limit ultrasound visibility, such as shadowing from the mass and decreased penetration of the beam in deeper tissue that will make it less favorable in this evaluation.

The normal appearance of a lymph node, whether in the axilla or the breast, is a circumscribed hypoechoic oval (mostly reniform) mass containing an echogenic fatty hilum. Size is usually not taken into consideration, except for a new or enlarging lymph node. Benign reactive lymph nodes have morphologic characteristics that overlap with

more suspicious features such as enlargement or cortical thickening, albeit these characteristics are more uniform in appearance (Fig. 5.10). When such questionable overlapping features are present, evaluation of the contralateral axilla can be helpful. The discovery of bilaterally enlarged lymph nodes would suggest an underlying systemic process such as lymphoma, human immunodeficiency virus (HIV), sarcoid, or rheumatoid arthritis. Please also refer to Chapter 17: Lymph Node Evaluation in Breast Imaging.

Signs suspicious for metastatic involvement of a lymph node include eccentric cortical thickening >3 mm and hilar effacement or replacement. The underlying pathology coincides with imaging whereby metastatic cells are carried to the lymph node through the capsule and lodge in the cortical and subcapsular sinuses. This creates an eccentric thickening of the lymph node (Fig. 5.11). Perinodal spread of tumor beyond the capsule accounts for the loss of the outer capsule, presenting as cortical irregularity and a finding that warrants a biopsy to confirm a diagnosis.

According to the recent guidelines from the National Comprehensive Cancer Network, systemic treatment in the adjuvant or neoadjuvant setting is recommended for locally advanced cancer that measures more than 5 cm (stage IIB and III) with axillary lymph nodes demonstrating significant tumor burden, or cancer with direct extension and involvement of the chest musculature and skin (NCCN guidelines). The administration of preoperative (neoadjuvant) systemic treatment can improve the odds of breast-conserving surgery and reduce disease recurrence rates. Compared with physical examination or mammography alone, breast ultrasound is superior at assessing the extent of disease. Its use during the neoadjuvant setting can help tailor treatment based on tumor response. Favorable signs, such as decreased size and reduced vascularity of cancer while undergoing treatment, translates to improved outcomes. Breast MRI, which includes morphologic and physiologic information, is extremely sensitive in assessing tumor response in this setting but is more expensive (Fig. 5.12). After neoadjuvant treatment, the residual tumor surrounding the biopsy clip is removed through image-guided

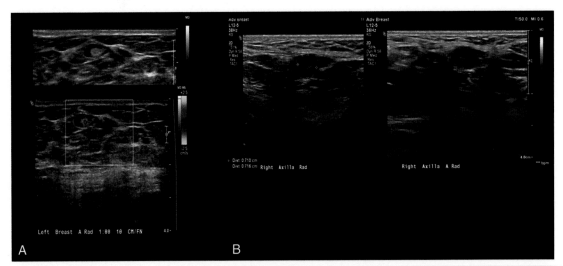

Fig. 5.10 Indications: neoadjuvant setting. Lymph nodes. (A) Normal lymph node demonstrates a circumscribed parallel oriented oval (reniform) hypoechoic mass. (B) Reactive lymph node can have characteristics that overlap with malignant features. Cortical thickening measures 3 mm and is circumferential. The absence of surrounding or cortical vascularity and no other abnormalities is characteristic of a benign reactive lymph node.

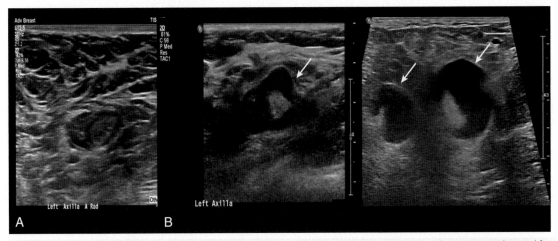

Fig. 5.11 Indications: neoadjuvant setting. Lymph node metastasis. (A) Normal lymph node with <3 mm hypoechoic cortex and central fatty hilum. (B) Two examples of metastatic involvement (*arrows*) of axillary lymph nodes. The presence of fat in the hilus does not exclude a diagnosis of malignancy. Cortical thickening or irregularity, eccentric thickening, or replacement of the fatty hilum are all suspicious findings at ultrasound.

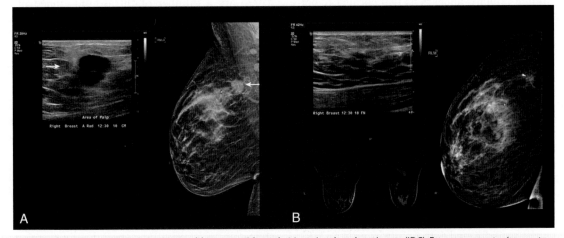

Fig. 5.12 Indications: neoadjuvant setting. A 32-year-old woman with grade 3 invasive ductal carcinoma (IDC), Estrogen receptor/progesterone receptor (ER/PR), and human epidermal growth factor receptor (HER2) negative. (A) Ultrasound and mammogram demonstrate a microlobulated antiparallel oriented mass (*arrows*) biopsy proven to represent IDC. (B) Postneoadjuvant images (ultrasound, axial T1 postcontrast magnetic resonance imaging [MRI], and postbiopsy mammogram) demonstrates presence of the clip and surrounding soft tissue. There is no abnormal enhancement suggesting fibrosis and not residual disease. Both ultrasound and mammography examinations are good at predicting the presence of disease; however, MRI is superior in determining pathologic complete response.

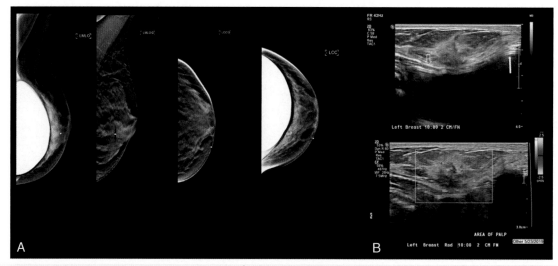

Fig. 5.13 Indications: breast implants. (A) Unilateral mammogram with push back (implant displaced) views demonstrates heterogeneously dense tissue and a retro pectoral silicone implant. Radiopaque BB marker overlies the upper inner left breast denoting area of concern. (B) Static ultrasound images of the palpable area demonstrates an irregular angular hypoechoic mass with an echogenic rim and no posterior acoustic features. Notice that the field of view and focal zone positioning in the second ultrasound image improves characterization of the mass. Diagnosis was invasive ductal carcinoma, grade 2. Fibrous capsule (open arrow) and implant shell (arrow) are also included in the field of view.

localization. If there is no longer a visible tumor on imaging, then the biopsy marker is removed along with the surrounding tissue. A complete pathologic response is an excellent prognostic indicator.

BREAST IMPLANTS

Although women with implants have similar breast complaints as women who do not, the use of ultrasound can improve visualization of the overlying breast tissue, axilla, and the anterior edge of the prosthesis. Both silicone and saline implants appear anechoic on ultrasound. The outer shell of the implant can have a variable appearance depending on the type of implant (double or single lumen), and shell surface (textured or smooth). The shell of a single lumen implant appears as two parallel hyperechoic lines separated by an anechoic intermediary layer. A third outer hyperechoic layer represents the fibrous capsule and can appear as one with the implant's outer shell (Fig. 5.13). In the subcapsular region, surrounding the implant is a small but variable amount of normal anechoic fluid. The disruption of this appearance and relationship of these layers can signify pathology and possible implant rupture.

Ultrasound is sensitive in evaluating implant integrity; however, limitations in beam focusing with increasing depth of the tissue can reduce sensitivity when evaluating intracapsular rupture. The rupture of saline implants is a clinical diagnosis without any need for imaging, yet the majority of silicone implant ruptures are clinically silent. In symptomatic patients, the investigation of implant integrity is performed with an ultrasound or MRI. MRI is more sensitive than ultrasound in this evaluation. The classic sonographic appearance of intracapsular rupture resembles a stepladder, with alternating hyperechoic and anechoic parallel lines. This finding corresponds to

the implant shell floating in the anechoic viscose fluid. Extracapsular silicone implant rupture refers to free silicone outside of the implant with deposition in the breast tissue. Extracapsular rupture appears as an indistinct hyperechoic mass with variable posterior acoustic shadowing, typical "snowstorm" appearance (Fig. 5.14). Recently an increasing number of breast implant–associated lymphocytic lymphoma cases has prompted evaluation and tissue sampling with ultrasound. Sonographic findings such as heterogeneity, asymmetry, or an enlarging peri-implant effusion are suspicious (see Chapter 18: The Augmented and Reconstructed Breast).

INTERVENTIONAL PROCEDURES

There are a number of ultrasound-guided percutaneous procedures, including fine-needle aspiration, core needle biopsy, and presurgical localization of nonpalpable masses. Using ultrasound assistance is preferred, since these procedures are less invasive, less expensive, and comparable in accuracy to surgical excision. The advantage of improved patient comfort with no contrast injection and no additional radiation makes it widely employed. The benefit of performing ultrasound procedures in real time makes it safer, since there is full control of the needle position. During the process, the intermittent use of color Doppler can identify and avoid complications and reduce bleeding risk. Optimal use of ultrasound-guided procedures improves access to lesions in difficult locations such as the axilla, lesions near the chest wall, or breast implants.

Procedural complications include hematomas, arteriovenous malformations, pseudoaneurysm, and abscess formation. The use of the ultrasound probe to apply compression and visualize improvement is one distinct advantage. Ultrasound is more than 95% accurate in diagnosing pseudoaneurysm (Fig. 5.15). For further information on

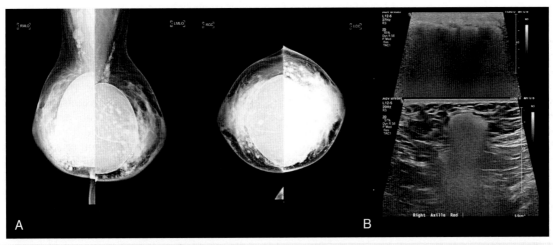

Fig. 5.14 Indications: breast implants. Silicone injections with saline implants. A 38-year-old transgender patient with new palpable mass in the left breast. (A) Bilateral mammogram demonstrates retro glandular saline implants with bilateral scattered circumscribed hyperdense masses with involvement of the right axillary lymph nodes. Ultrasound examination was performed to evaluate the new clinical symptoms. Although ultrasound sensitivity is reduced in the setting of silicone granulomas, its use is quick and easy to directly correlate clinical and imaging findings. (B) Trapezoidal ultrasound images of the palpable regions suggest the patient's symptoms are due to free silicone granulomas with the typical "snowstorm" appearance. Although this finding is due to injection of free silicone, similar ultrasound findings are appreciated in extracapsular silicone implant rupture.

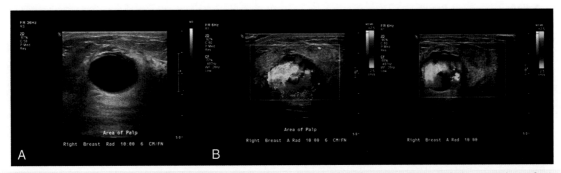

Fig. 5.15 Indications: interventional procedures. Pseudoaneurysm. A 47-year-old woman with recent stereotactic biopsy complains of pain and a new lump. (A) Ultrasound evaluation was performed and demonstrates a circumscribed anechoic mass with enhanced through transmission. Finding suggestive of a hematoma but color Doppler images will help determine blood flow. (B) Color Doppler images demonstrate blood flow inside of the cystic mass characteristic of a pseudoaneurysm (*swirl pattern*). This complication is the result of a puncture of the arterial wall with subsequent development of blood flowing into the adjacent tissue and communicating with the vessel.

image-guided procedures, see Chapter 7: Mammographic and Ultrasound-Guided Breast Biopsy Procedures.

Technical Parameters

Proper technique and optimal position are needed to maximize the quality of the ultrasound image. B mode ultrasound, or brightness mode, is used to construct the conventional two-dimensional (2D) grayscale image. The formation of an ultrasound image occurs after a spectrum of frequencies is emitted, and the resulting echoes received to the transducer. The brightness of the gray value of the ultrasound image corresponds to the energy of the returning echoes.

During the ultrasound examination, the patient is positioned supine and oblique on a wedge-shaped cushion with the arm raised above the head. This position allows for the reduction in breast thickness and helps maximize the ultrasound beam's penetration. Using this technique, the maximum penetration of the ultrasound beam is approximately

5 cm deep through a highly attenuating structure such as the breast. Gel or lotion is used as a medium to allow sound waves to propagate from the transducer into the tissue. Gentle transducer pressure is applied while scanning the patient to reduce artifactual shadowing from typical normal structures. Real-time ultrasound scanning allows the operator to change the transducer's angle to improve the overall quality of the examination and, thus, interpretation. Per the ACR appropriateness guidelines and practice parameters, a recorded ultrasound image should have a permanent identification that labels the facility name, patient name and ID (or date of birth), examination date, laterality of the breast, and sonographer's initials.

Image Quality

Image quality relies on three fundamental principles, transducer frequency, resolution, and contrast. The ACR practice parameter for the performance of breast ultrasound examination recommends a transducer with a broad bandwidth operating at a center frequency of at least 12 MHz and preferably higher.[1] A high-frequency ultrasound transducer provides superior contrast and spatial resolution. The penetration of breast tissue is inversely proportional to transducer frequency. Ultrasound beams are composed of a range of frequencies determined by the number of sound waves in a unit time. The width of the spectrum of frequencies transmitted defines the bandwidth. The more sound waves to interrogate a mass, such as in broad bandwidth, the better. The transducer with a higher frequency improves resolution but has less penetration, whereas lower frequency provides greater penetration and less resolution (Table 5.3). Thus, when evaluating deep tissue in patients or large breasts, it may be helpful to select lower frequency settings for the beam to penetrate deeper tissue and give better characterization.

The field of view must include visualization of the skin to the pectoralis muscle and is optimized to visualize an abnormality (Fig. 5.16). Image labeling requires annotation

describing the laterality (right or left breast), location of the lesion (clockface and distance from the nipple), and transducer orientation in relation to the breast. This information may also be designated using a breast pictogram. Documentation of the lesion's largest size in two orthogonal planes (radial/antiradial or transverse/longitudinal) can record its maximum dimensions. Ultrasound features are essential and give an accurate assessment of a breast mass, so images with and without caliper measurements are recommended. An additional set of images with and without color/power Doppler will help assess the presence or absence of vascularity.

ARTIFACTS

Artifacts are routinely encountered in breast ultrasound imaging (Table 5.4). Speckle (noise) artifact refers to the diffuse granular appearance of breast tissue on the ultrasound image. This common artifact occurs from the interference of acoustic soundwaves with scattered low-amplitude echoes originating from the many microstructural surfaces of the breast. This artifact reduces image contrast and

Table 5.3   Image Resolution

	Action	Result	
Transducer frequency	↑ Frequency	↑ Attenuation	Improves near field
	↓ Frequency	↓ Attenuation	Improved depth penetration
Compound imaging		↑ Mass margin interrogation	
Harmonics		↓ Artifactual internal echoes	
		↑ Real internal echoes	
Spatial resolution	↑ Transducer frequency	Axial resolution improves	
	↑ Number of focal zones and position of ultrasound beam	Lateral resolution improves	
	Use standoff gel/pad	Elevation resolution Improves	

Table 5.4   Breast Ultrasound Artifacts

Artifact Type	Description	Examples	Resolution
Reverberation	Occurs due to multiple reflections	Anechoic cyst	Add THI
Speckle artifact	Decreases image contrast and lesion characterization	↑ Noise of image	Add THI
Clutter	Decreases contrast resolution	↑ Noise of image	Add THI
Acoustic shadowing	Occurs behind a highly attenuating object creating a "shadow"	Solid mass	
Acoustic enhancement	Occurs behind a minimally attenuating object causing increased echo intensity	Cyst	

THI, Tissue harmonic imaging.
THI will reduce artifactual echoes.

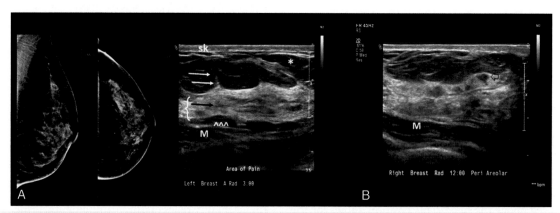

Fig. 5.16 Breast anatomy. (A) Unilateral left mammogram and sonogram of a patient complaining of breast pain demonstrates normal ultrasound anatomy. The skin (*sk*), subcutaneous fat (***) is the reference for sonographic findings, Cooper ligaments (*arrows*), glandular parenchymal tissue (*bracket*) containing branching ducts, retromammary fat (*^*), and chest wall musculature (*M*). Ultrasound image demonstrates normal branching ductule (*black arrow*). (B) A 23-year-old woman with complaint of focal breast pain with normal appearing lobular units (*open arrow*) and chest wall musculature (*M*).

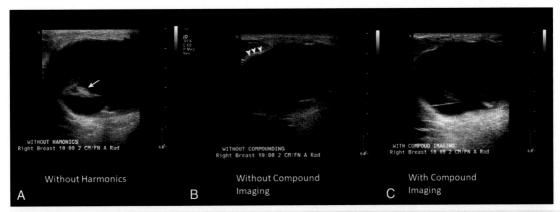

Fig. 5.17 Artifacts: image resolution (harmonics and compound imaging). There is an increase in artifactual echoes identified in images A and B. (A) Image obtained without tissue harmonic imaging (THI). THI will clear up artifactual echoes and enhance real echoes (*arrow*). (B) Image obtained without compound imaging. Notice the clutter artifact appreciated in this complex cystic solid mass (*arrowheads*) compared with the image with compound imaging. (C) Image obtained with compound imaging demonstrates improvement in lateral resolution and margin characterization. Notice that refraction artifact in A is no longer visible with the use of compound imaging. THI and compound imaging will enhance contrast and clear up low-level echoes in cystic structures. Harmonics imaging and compound imaging reduces artifactual echoes.

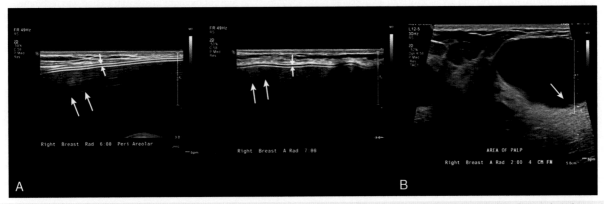

Fig. 5.18 Artifacts: reverberation artifact. (A) Multiple parallel hyperechoic lines in an anechoic structure (*arrows*). Hyperechoic/hypoechoic/hyperechoic lines of the inner and outer shell of the implant (*open arrows*). (B) The trapezoidal image of the fibrocystic changes is less pronounced with the use of tissue harmonic imaging. Clutter is still apparent in the far field of the cyst (*arrow*).

lesion characterization. Similarly, clutter is also considered a noise artifact that can degrade contrast resolution. Clutter is evident in anechoic or hypoechoic structures such as cysts presenting as artifactual echoes or "filling" in of cysts (Fig. 5.17). Harmonic imaging can help reduce this artifact. Refraction artifacts occur from a change in the direction of the ultrasound beam when it encounters a curved interface. The two different sound speeds lead to edge shadowing in circumscribed structures such as cysts or breast implants. Refraction can also occur at the interface of fat lobules and Cooper ligaments. In the latter, changing the transducer's angle or increasing transducer pressure can sometimes mitigate this artifact. Reverberation artifact is identified in anechoic structures and results from the ultrasound beam bouncing between two highly reflective parallel interfaces. It appears as multiple parallel hyperechoic (bright) lines in a cystic structure (Fig. 5.18).

While artifacts can degrade an image, common attenuation artifacts seen in breast ultrasound, such as acoustic shadowing and enhanced through transmission, help further characterize findings. Sound attenuation as it passes through a solid structure determines a solid mass from a cystic lesion. Shadowing occurs when there is a highly attenuating structure relative to the surrounding tissue. The low amplitude of the returning ultrasound beam distal to the highly attenuating structure causes a hypoechoic or dark band. In breast ultrasound, shadowing is indicative of a solid mass. However, it is essential to note that some masses can have enhanced through transmission. In this case further characterization with color Doppler imaging can aid in differentiating a solid lesion.

Image Optimization

Image optimization (see Table 5.3) can reduce artifacts, improve spatial resolution, and enhance diagnostic accuracy. Although a high-frequency transducer can improve axial and lateral resolution, technical parameters such as gain settings, focal zone selections, and field of view can enhance the image's integrity (Fig. 5.19).

IMAGE RESOLUTION

Contrast resolution, which is dependent on spatial resolution, improves the conspicuity of lesions from the

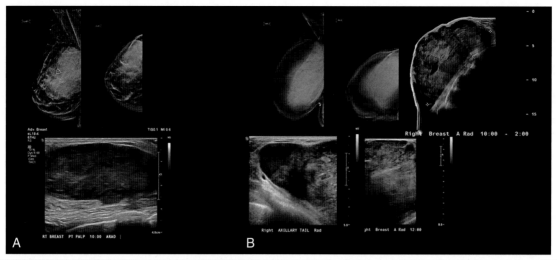

Fig. 5.19 Image optimization: field of view. (A) Unilateral right mammogram demonstrates a partially obscured mass in the upper outer breast correlating with the patient's palpable concern (*marked with a triangle*). A targeted ultrasound demonstrates an oval circumscribed hypoechoic mass not visible in its entirety. Percutaneous needle biopsy revealed a diagnosis of a phyllodes tumor. The patient declined surgery and returned 16 months later. (B) Unilateral mammogram demonstrates increasing asymmetry with an obscured mass encompassing most of the right breast. Ultrasound was recommended for further characterization and demonstrates a large circumscribed heterogenous mass. A panoramic view gives full characterization of the lesion and its relationship to the adjacent tissue. This mass measured 15 cm in diameter (*calipers*) and is incompletely visualized on the standard 5 cm field of view.

surrounding normal glandular tissue. The enhancement of spatial resolution depends on the number and location of focal zones and the grayscale gain. Proper positioning of a single focal zone is at the anterior to the middle third of a region of interest for maximum resolution. The ultrasound beam is the most narrow and intense at the focal zone. Because there is the attenuation of the ultrasound beam with depth, the time gain compensation or TGC curve should increase gradually with the evaluation of deeper tissue, thus keeping fat uniform at multiple depths. The gain should be adjusted so fat is gray to improve contrast resolution. Too much gain gives artifactual echoes and can make simple anechoic cysts appear solid, while too little gain can provide a false impression that solid masses appear cystic.

Three things determine spatial resolution: axial, lateral, and elevation resolution. The axial resolution is always superior to lateral resolution and allows one to delineate similar structures in the direction of the ultrasound wave (anterior and posterior to a lesion). Axial resolution is enhanced using a higher-frequency transducer with a shorter pulse length and an ultrasound beam with broader bandwidth. The discrimination of adjacent findings at the same depth and plane (side-by-side discrimination of a lesion) depends on the ultrasound beam width and is called *lateral resolution*. An increase in focal zone number and focal zone positioning at mulitple depths will narrow the beam's width and can improve resolution of two adjacent objects in a region of interest.

Elevation resolution is the last component of spatial resolution. It is related to the section thickness of the ultrasound-producing elements in the transducer—artifacts associated with elevation resolution present as low-level internal echoes in anechoic structures. Superficial lesions are susceptible to this artifact and can be corrected using a standoff pad or layer of gel to decrease averaging the structures within the section thickness and bring them closer to the focal zone (Fig. 5.20).

TISSUE HARMONICS

Tissue harmonics imaging (THI) improves the signal-to-noise ratio of the ultrasound beam and provides higher-quality images than those obtained with conventional ultrasound. The production of harmonic waves occurs in the native tissue from high-pressure waves delivered at the ultrasound beam's center through the tissue. Different signals will be generated at distinct anatomic sites with similar impedances, leading to higher-contrast resolution. The use of THI can help reduce artifacts such as sidelobe, near field, and reverberation artifacts. Speckle artifact, which appears as a granular appearance to the ultrasound image, can be reduced by THI and compound imaging and many postprocessing algorithms (see Fig. 5.17). Similarly, reverberation artifact is reduced with THI, at least in the near field.

COMPOUND IMAGING

Compound imaging improves contrast and spatial resolution. The conventional ultrasound beam examines a mass from one angle, whereas compound imaging combines information obtained from multiple angles (Fig. 5.21). Because there is averaging of data from numerous angles, lateral resolution is improved. For example, speckle artifact, which results from the interference of the ultrasound beam from acoustic scatterings made by small tissue reflectors, improves with the use of compound imaging (see Fig. 5.17). This inherent noise gives a grainy appearance of the ultrasound image and can be reduced using compound imaging as signal-to-noise is improved. One disadvantage of using compound imaging is reduced temporal resolution. With several frames of information averaged in one image, the frame rate decreases with real-time scanning. Given this obstacle, many ultrasound machines deliver postprocessing algorithms to automatically minimize speckle artifacts and lessen this random phenomenon's appearance.

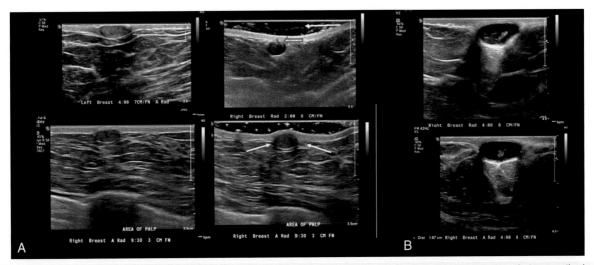

Fig. 5.20 Breast anatomy: sebaceous/epidermal inclusion cyst. (A) In all examples the ultrasound findings demonstrate an oval, circumscribed mass. A layer of gel (*arrow*) acts as a standoff pad to help improve characterization. Notice the layer of gel places the lesion deeper at the level of the focal zone. Careful attention to visualize a punctum-gland neck/hair follicle (*open arrow*) traversing the dermal layer gives confidence in the diagnosis of a benign assessment, BI-RADS 2. The amount of sebum and internal debris may dictate the posterior acoustic features. The transition angle between the skin and the edge of the lesion can help determine the location with reference to the dermis. An acute angle (where the skin wraps around the lesion) is referred to as the "claw" sign (*arrows*) and suggests a location within the dermal layer. (B) In this case a more heterogenous mixed echo pattern can help differentiate epidermal inclusion cysts from sebaceous cysts. Epidermal inclusion cysts will contain keratin that may layer or float freely within the sebum.

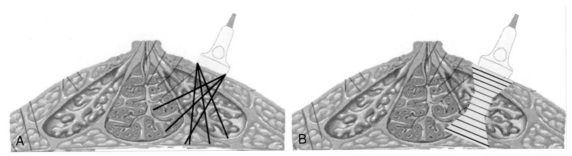

Fig. 5.21 (A) Compound imaging combines information obtained from multiple angles which improves lateral resolution. (B) Conventional beam examines a mass from one angle and has less spatial resolution compared with compound imaging.

DOPPLER IMAGING

Color Doppler imaging (CDI) evaluates the presence or absence of vascularity in tissue and can help distinguish solid masses from complicated cysts. The superimposition of blood flow on a 2D grayscale image allows the radiologist to simultaneously determine the characteristics of a lesion and vascular flow patterns (Fig. 5.22). The difference between the transmitted ultrasound frequency and the frequency reflected off an object determines movement. If the target moves relative to the transmitted ultrasound beam and a frequency change is detected, a color is assigned.

Power color Doppler is independent of flow direction or velocity and is three to five times more sensitive than color Doppler imaging (Fig. 5.23). The gain defines the amount of amplification of echoes from the receiver. The setting for color gain is calibrated so that it is visible only within the boundaries of a vascular structure. If the gain is set too high, there is the suppression of the color data. In both techniques, CDI and power Doppler, the application of too much pressure with the ultrasound probe can diminish the color reading.

Additional Ultrasound Techniques

There are additional qualitative and quantitative assessments that improve the specificity of the ultrasound examination. By differentiating the elasticity of soft, healthy breast tissue from the breast's stiff pathologic disorders, one can stratify lesions into benign and suspicious categories and enhance the ultrasound examination's diagnostic accuracy. Different elastography techniques are classified based on the compression force applied to a breast finding.

STRAIN ELASTOGRAPHY

The more common technique called strain elastography records the degree of tissue elasticity before and after mechanical compression. Strain elastography technique will allow a qualitative description of a lesion (soft, intermediate, and hard) relative to the surrounding tissue. Applied pressure with the ultrasound transducer is considered active compression, while passive compression is stress related to respiratory or cardiac motion. Cancers tend to

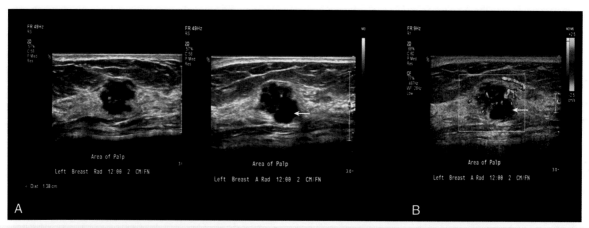

Fig. 5.22 Image resolution (with and without compound imaging). (A) Radial and antiradial sonographic evaluation of a microlobulated complex cystic and solid mass with posterior acoustic enhancement. Compound imaging improves characterization (calcifications within the mass), margin analysis and reduces speckle artifact (*arrow*) compared with color Doppler image. (B) Color Doppler image of the same mass without the use of compound imaging decreases visualization of the mass margin and increases speckle artifact (*arrow*) throughout the image (increase in image noise or graininess). Pathologic diagnosis was high-grade ductal carcinoma in situ (DCIS).

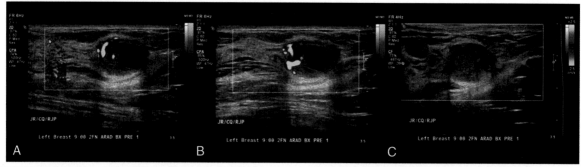

Fig. 5.23 Image resolution: power Doppler imaging in A and B is independent of flow direction or velocity and is three to five times more sensitive than color Doppler imaging. (C) Color Doppler imaging of the same mass. A 67-year-old woman with an indistinct complex cystic and solid mass on ultrasound. Findings demonstrate a heterogenous, mixed iso- to anechoic pattern with posterior acoustic enhancement. Increased vascularity is noted inside and surrounding the lesion (rim of vessels). Pathologic diagnosis was mucinous carcinoma.

be rigid and benign masses softer. The elastography image called an "elastogram" is a color image that overlays the conventional grayscale image and translates the degree of stiffness of the underlying tissue. When findings are considered benign, there is no significant difference in the size of the two images, whereas breast cancer's elastogram image tends to be larger compared with the B mode grayscale image. The increase in size is due to the desmoplastic inflammatory response surrounding the invasive tumor; the surrounding tissue associated with malignancy is stiff.

SHEAR WAVE ELASTOGRAPHY

Shear wave elastography (SWE) is the quantitative assessment of tissue stiffness measured from the speed of shear waves propagating through tissue. Shear waves are generated in the tissue by high-intensity focused ultrasound pulses. The speed of propagation through tissue renders an absolute stiffness value measured in kPa (kiloPascals) or m/s. Shear waves travel faster through stiff tissue and slower through softer tissue. Higher values are associated with malignancy, while lower numbers suggest tissue is soft and associated with benign disease. In a large multinational study, BE1 Multinational study, SWE significantly improved

the accuracy and specificity of the ultrasound examination more than BI-RADS characteristic features alone. The ACR BI-RADS lexicon emphasizes that ultrasound morphologic qualities, such as shape, margin, and orientation, are far more predictive of malignancy than hardness or softness.

Breast Anatomy

Arterial supply of the breast comes from the perforating branches of the lateral thoracic and thoracoacromial branches of the axillary and subclavian artery. The medial aspect of the breast is supplied by the perforating branches of the internal mammary artery. Beneath the nipple is the venous plexus, which drains into the intercostal, internal thoracic, and axillary veins. Ninety percent of lymphatic drainage goes into the ipsilateral axillary lymph nodes, and only a small percentage flows into the internal mammary chain. Ultrasound, like mammography, focuses on anatomic differences between normal tissue and abnormal findings and has the resolution to differentiate between the two. Understanding normal breast development and anatomy is essential for accurate interpretation of the pathologic findings. Because the development of the breast begins in

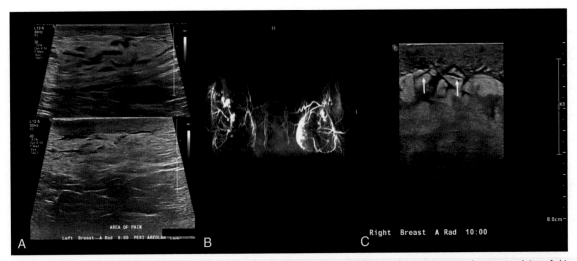

Fig. 5.24 Breast anatomy: skin edema/inflammation. A 46-year-old woman with an increased risk for breast cancer has a complaint of skin changes and pain in the medial and inferior left breast minimal erythema noted. (A) Ultrasound images demonstrate skin thickening with no other abnormality. (B) Breast magnetic resonance imaging (MRI) was performed and demonstrates skin thickening, edema, and enhancement with no parenchymal abnormality. Skin punch biopsy was performed and was negative for carcinoma. (C) Patient with enlarging right breast with increasing asymmetry and trabecular thickening on mammography. Ultrasound demonstrates skin thickening, prominent lymphatic channels (*arrows*), and edema. Hyperechoic underlying breast parenchyma is consistent with edema. Skin punch biopsy was positive suggesting a diagnosis of inflammatory breast carcinoma.

utero, some female and male newborns may have transient enlargement of the rudimentary breast bud due to circulating maternal hormones. This is normal and will resolve on its own. The female breast goes through many maturation phases, driven by hormonal changes, and will be discussed in the next section.

The female breast lies anterior to the thoracic wall musculature and extends from the second to the sixth rib. The breast tissue frequently extends into the axilla and is enclosed between two fascial layers. The superficial fascia abuts the undersurface of the dermis, while the deep fascial plane lies anterior to the pectoralis muscle. At the same time, Cooper ligaments act as suspensory ligaments that support and attach the breast glandular tissue to the subcutaneous and deep fascia.

The breast is composed of 8 to 20 lobes, each of which contains branching ductules that drain into larger lactiferous ducts. These ducts empty into their respective lactiferous sinus just beneath the nipple. Ultrasound has the resolution to interrogate findings inside of the lumen such as debris or a mass and helps improve diagnostic capability in a patient complaining of nipple discharge. The ductal system extends radially from the nipple and is anechoic (intraductal fluid) to isoechoic. Ultrasound has become a useful tool to recognize and assess intraluminal disease and the surrounding tissue. The use of color Doppler can improve specificity by demonstrating increased vascular flow in a lesion or a vascular pedicle and feeding vessels in a ductal mass.

The nipple-areolar complex is challenging to image without proper ultrasound technique. The shadowing observed posterior to the nipple can be reduced using a thick layer of gel or a standoff pad to improve resolution. The ultrasound transducer must be angled so that the beam is perpendicular to the milk duct's long axis to minimize acoustic shadowing. Color or power Doppler is instrumental when trying to distinguish intraluminal masses from debris. The presence of internal vascularity would suggest a mass. The ballottement technique is also useful. This maneuver applies intermittent compression on the milk duct and determines whether there is free movement of intraluminal debris. The intraluminal secretions' back-and-forth motion is accentuated with this technique and is consistent with a benign finding.

Ultrasound can reflect six distinct layers: skin, subcutaneous fat, glandular (mammary) tissue, retromammary fat, pectoralis musculature, and ribs (see Fig. 5.16). On ultrasound, fibrous and dense glandular tissue is white or hyperechoic, while fatty glandular tissue is gray and the frame of reference for other findings. Ultrasound visualization of superficial lesions warrants evaluation with a standoff acoustic pad or a thick layer of gel to improve resolution. The skin appears as a hyperechoic narrow band at the top of the ultrasound image and should be no more than 2 mm thick. Skin thickening is pathologic and could represent signs of edema (Congestive heart failure (CHF), renal failure), inflammation (cellulitis, inflamed sebaceous cyst, or epidermal inclusion cyst), or cancer involvement (inflammatory breast carcinoma, melanoma) (Fig. 5.24). The angle produced at the edge of a superficial lesion and the cutaneous layer can help differentiate origin. Acute angles imply a dermal location, whereas obtuse angles suggest the lesion is below the skin and present in the breast parenchyma. One caveat is the presence of a linear tract that extends from the superficial mass to the epidermis, which is consistent with a diagnosis of a benign epidermal or sebaceous cyst (see Fig. 5.20).

Female Hormonal Phases

The prepubertal breast has a limited number of ducts located in the retroareolar area. During adolescence, estrogen stimulates ductal proliferation and appears as a mound of tissue in the retroareolar region. In late adolescence, lobular proliferation is stimulated by progesterone. During pregnancy, the lobules increase in size and number

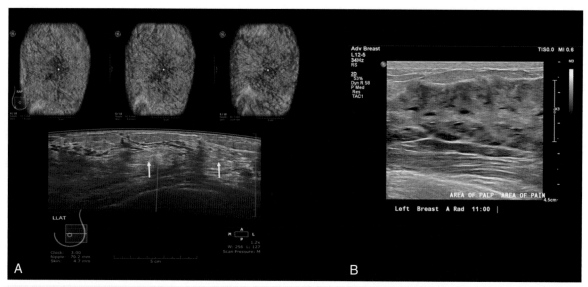

Fig. 5.25 Female hormonal phases: lactation changes. (A) Coronal and long field-of-view (FOV) transverse ultrasound images demonstrates increase echotexture of the breast parenchyma (*arrows*) as a result of the enlargement of the glandular tissue and proliferation of the milk ducts containing milk rich in fat. (B) Handheld ultrasound demonstrates ductal prominence and distention with intraluminal echoes.

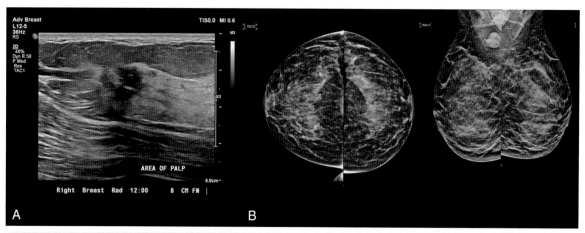

Fig. 5.26 Female hormonal phases: pregnancy-associated breast cancer (PABC) has similar imaging characteristics to nonpregnant women. Ultrasound is usually the first imaging performed. (A) Ultrasound of the right breast demonstrates an irregular hypoechoic mass with angular margins with combined posterior acoustic features. Part of the mass demonstrated posterior acoustic shadowing and part of the mass has no posterior features. An ultrasound-guided biopsy was performed of this lesion and an abnormal appearing axillary lymph node. (B) Postbiopsy mammogram was performed to evaluate extent of disease. Bilateral mammogram demonstrates right breast segmental pleomorphic calcifications extending toward the nipple for approximately 7 cm. Mammography has higher sensitivity for evaluating calcifications; however, ultrasound can help identify an invasive component. Pathologic diagnosis: high-grade invasive ductal carcinoma.

in preparation for lactation. This proliferation coexists with secretory modifications occurring in the breast's ductal and lobular components preparing for milk production. These lactation changes are visible by 12 weeks of gestation and progress up until delivery. On ultrasound, the mammary zone appears hypoechoic and is enlarged due to lobular proliferation and retained secretions in the lobular acinus (Fig. 5.25). As the hormonal influence continues, it causes breast-related changes that manifest as ductal prominence and distention with intraluminal echoes.

Breast ultrasound is the initial examination performed in a pregnant female, since there is no ionizing radiation, and it is not affected by breast density. Mammography can be performed after ultrasound evaluation of a highly

suspicious malignant lesion, mainly to evaluate disease extent. Diagnostic ultrasound evaluation in a pregnant patient who is symptomatic is near 100% sensitivity and has a 100% negative predictive value in evaluating pregnancy-associated breast cancer (Fig. 5.26).

During pregnancy and lactation, there are unique conditions diagnosed, such as galactocele, lactating adenoma, and pregnancy-associated breast cancer. Galactoceles are the most common lesion identified in women who have just completed and are currently breastfeeding. These masses are cysts containing fluid that resembles milk thought to occur from stagnation and ductal dilatation of milk products. The ultrasound appearance can be quite variable, resembling a complicated cyst with a look coinciding with

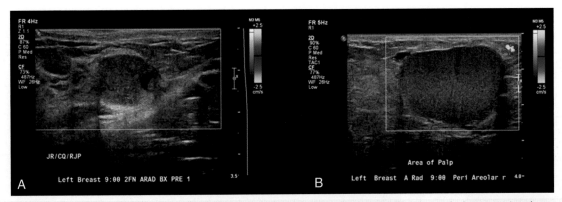

Fig. 5.27 Associated findings: vascularity. (A) Papillary carcinoma demonstrating internal vascularity. (B) Galactocele demonstrating absent vascularity. Both are circumscribed masses and have a similar echotexture. In the latter case, the patient was lactating with a new palpable mass. Galactoceles are focal collections of breast milk in the lobular structures of the breast. They can present as a palpable lump and have a variable appearance on ultrasound. Depending on the milk fat contents, galactoceles can appear as anechoic, hypoechoic, or a fluid-fluid level.

the amount of fat and water contents (Fig. 5.27). Another common mass that occurs during pregnancy is lactating adenomas. Both lactating adenoma and fibroadenoma appear similar on ultrasound as a homogenous hypoechoic oval mass with septa demonstrating posterior acoustic enhancement. Lactating adenomas are a common concern for pregnant and lactating women and can quickly enlarge. There is increase echogenicity due to the enlargement of the lobular tissue and the proliferation of the milk ducts containing milk rich in fat. Typical lactational changes seen are due to ductal prominence with distention containing intraluminal echoes (see Fig. 5.25B).

The diagnosis of pregnancy-associated breast cancer occurs during pregnancy or 1 year postpartum. This type of cancer is usually aggressive and has a poor prognosis. Approximately 80% are invasive ductal cancer, and the majority of women present with positive lymph nodes. Ultrasound can aid in diagnosis and biopsy guidance (see Fig. 5.26). Imaging in pregnancy and lactation is further discussed in Chapter 19: Special Populations in Breast Imaging.

Although mastitis is a clinical diagnosis in pregnant and nonpregnant patients, ultrasound can assess complications such as abscess formation. Most infections that arise during lactation come from the retrograde movement of bacteria (most *Staphylococcus* and *Streptococcus* bacteria) through a cracked nipple. The appearance of mastitis on ultrasound is similar to all inflammatory changes. Changes consist of edema (hyperechoic areas within the breast parenchyma) and skin thickening. Visualization of a focal hypoechoic mass with surrounding vascularity (ring of vessels) is concerning for focal inflammation and abscess formation. A more mature abscess appears as a thick-walled complex cystic and solid mass with increased adjacent vascularity and posterior acoustic enhancement. There should be no internal vascularity present, since the abscess contains pus and possible blood products and not a tumor. If there is internal vascularity, biopsy should be performed after a course of antibiotic treatment to rule out underlying breast cancer. Ultrasound can guide the aspiration of the fluid for diagnostic and therapeutic reasons. Breastfeeding should resume after the procedure to reduce milk stagnation. If a core biopsy is performed, the rare complication of

a milk fistula can occur. The continuation of breastfeeding decreases that risk.

Male Breast

High-resolution ultrasound is just as useful in evaluating the male breast as the female breast. Most pathologic findings in the male breast arise from the ducts and periductal stroma since male patients do not have fully developed lobules. The enlargement of the male breast is called gynecomastia and is often due to the hormonal imbalance of estrogen and androgen hormones. Gynecomastia can be physiologic or pathologic

The appearance of gynecomastia on ultrasound can be quite variable, and it may be helpful to scan both sides. Ducts and stroma in the retroareolar region may resemble a focal hypoechoic mass with associated vascularity. The hyperemia observed in this tissue may directly correlate to the amount of hyperplasia and proliferation of the ducts. Most gynecomastia cases have breast tissue that is triangular in appearance containing branching ducts that extend posterolateral from the nipple (Fig. 5.28). Although gynecomastia is not a risk for male breast cancer, it coexists with the diagnosis 50% of the time (Fig. 5.29). Imaging of the male breast is further discussed in Chapter 19: Special Populations in Breast Imaging.

Ultrasound BI-RADS and Interpretation

As with mammography, the ACR BI-RADS lexicon for ultrasound aides in the interpretation of findings. Descriptors outlined below help differentiate benign from malignant disease (Table 5.5). The presence or absence of vascularity along with elastography features can contribute to the analysis and assessment of a sonographic mass. There is no set number of descriptors required to describe an ultrasound finding, but in general, shape, orientation, and margin will lead to an appropriate final assessment code. For example, oval, parallel-oriented, and circumscribed margins suggest

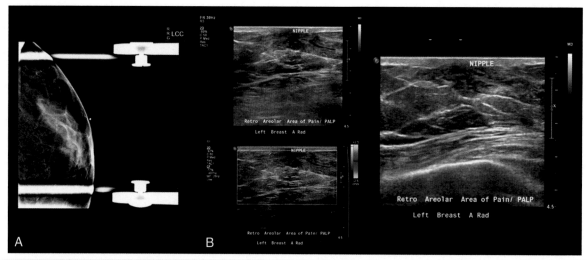

Fig. 5.28 Male breast: gynecomastia. (A) Spot compression view of area of palpable thickening and pain demonstrates typical "flame-shaped" appearance of the glandular tissue as it extends laterally back from the nipple. Mammography is diagnostic of this condition. When a classic mammographic appearance occurs such as in this case, ultrasound does not need to be performed. (B) Ultrasound static images in the same male patient with complaint of a lump demonstrates hypoechoic tissue directly behind the nipple with ducts that extends laterally similar in appearance to the mammogram.

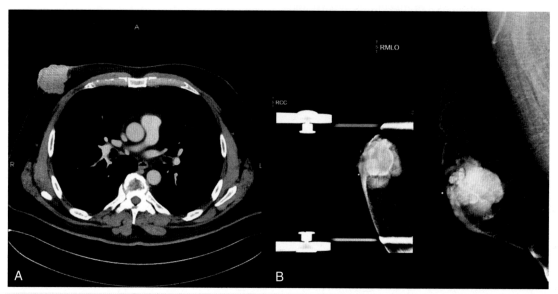

Fig. 5.29 Male breast: male breast cancer. (A) Computed tomography scan of a male patient was performed for shortness of breath. An asymmetric enhancing soft tissue mass was identified in the right retroareolar region with overlying skin thickening. Findings are suspicious and a mammogram was recommended. (B) Unilateral mammogram and spot compression views over the palpable mass in the right breast demonstrates a hyperdense partially obscured mass suspicious for malignancy. An ultrasound biopsy confirmed a diagnosis of invasive ductal carcinoma.

a benign mass while irregular, antiparallel orientation, and indistinct margins describe a suspicious mass.

TISSUE COMPOSITION

Breast parenchyma echotexture is described in the second edition of echotexture in the second edition of the ultrasound BI-RADS lexicon. The three ultrasound descriptors for tissue composition patterns are homogeneous background echo texture: fat, homogeneous background echotexture-fibroglandular, and heterogeneous background echotexture. Heterogeneous background shows an admixture of hypoechoic and more echogenic areas. Of particular importance, heterogeneous background composition may exhibit

scattered areas of shadowing, potentially impacting the ability to interpret the ultrasound examination (Fig. 5.30).

MASSES

A distinct advantage of real-time scanning is the capability of differentiating a mass from the surrounding normal tissue. A mass is a space-occupying lesion identified in two different planes. Ultrasound has the resolution to improve mass characterization (solid or cystic) and margin analysis previously described on mammography. For example, a margin may appear as circumscribed on mammography but show indistinct or microlobulated margins with ultrasound interrogation. Margins that are not circumscribed

Table 5.5 Ultrasound Features of Solid Breast Masses: Malignant Versus Benign

Malignant
- Irregular shape
- Not-parallel orientation (taller than wide)
- Not-circumscribed margin (indistinct, angulated, microlobulated, and spiculated)
- Very hypoechoic
- Acoustic shadowing
- Microcalcifications
- Duct extension
- Branch pattern
- Hard elasticity assessment

Benign
- No malignant characteristics
- Oval shape
- Parallel orientation (wider than tall)
- Circumscribed margin
- Intense homogeneous hyperechogenicity
- Four or fewer gentle lobulations
- Thin echogenic pseudocapsule/ellipsoid shape

Modified from Stavros AT, Thickman D, Rapp CL, et al: Solid breast nodules: use of sonography to distinguish between benign and malignant lesions, *Radiology* 196:123–134, 1995.

are worrisome and correlate to a higher positive predictive value (PPV) for malignancy than circumscribed masses (Fig. 5.31).

It is essential to be familiar with specific sonographic characteristics that may carry a higher suspicion for malignancy than others. Stavros et al. published data in 1995 with an update to guide interpretation and management of solid breast masses (Box 5.1). Some findings may indicate

suspicion based on the surface, shape, and internal characteristics of a mass. Management is made based on the most suspicious characteristic since most masses have more than one of these imaging features. With the proper use of the BI-RADS lexicon descriptors, breast masses are correctly categorized as benign, probably benign, or suspicious (Table 5.6).

Shape

Masses can be oval, round, or irregular in shape (Fig. 5.32). An oval mass is elliptical and may contain two or three gentle lobulations but must also be wider than tall to keep this classification. A common occurrence is an oval gently lobulated fibroadenoma (Box 5.2). Round masses have a dimension that is the same in the anterior-posterior and transverse direction. Rounded masses are unusual and should be viewed with suspicion. Round masses require further interrogation since they are considered antiparallel in orientation. A mass classified as irregular in shape has characteristics that are neither round nor oval and should prompt a biopsy.

Orientation

Orientation is unique to ultrasound and characterizes the longest axis of the lesion (Fig. 5.33). Most benign masses grow along the direction of the tissue plane and are parallel to the skin surface. Masses that are larger in anterior-posterior (AP) dimension than in the horizontal plane are growing in an antiparallel orientation, suggesting an infiltrative process and rapid growth. Antiparallel orientation has been described as taller-than-wide and is suspicious for malignancy. This finding should prompt further interrogation of the mass evaluating shape and margin to exclude cancer. Obliquely oriented masses should be classified based on their long axis and relationship to the skin (see Fig. 5.3).

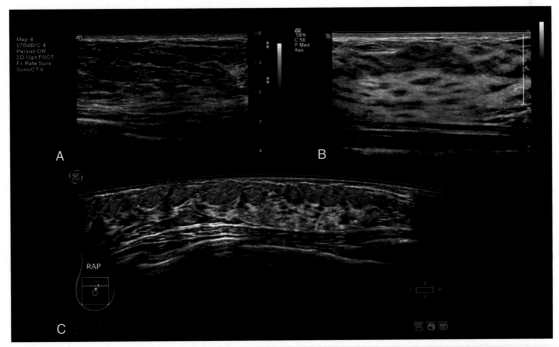

Fig. 5.30 Image interpretation: ultrasound tissue composition. (A) Homogenous background echotexture-fat, (B) homogenous background echotexture-fibroglandular, and (C) long field-of-view (FOV) heterogenous background echotexture. Heterogenous background demonstrates an admixture of hypoechoic and echogenic areas.

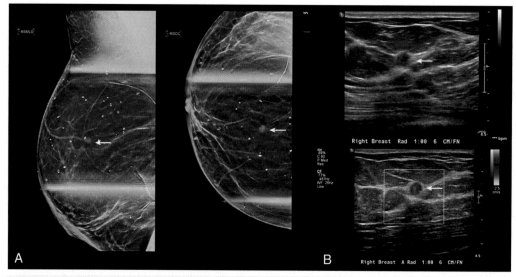

Fig. 5.31 Mass. (A) Spot views of a mass in the right upper inner breast demonstrates a circumscribed round mass *(arrow)*. (B) Further interrogation with ultrasound demonstrates that the mass is solid *(internal vascularity)* with a microlobulated border *(arrow)*. Not having circumscribed margins increases level of suspicion for malignancy. Pathology diagnosis was an intermediate grade invasive ductal carcinoma.

Box 5.1   American College of Radiology Recommendations for Breast Ultrasound Labeling

- Right or left breast
- Mass position in terms of clock face or quadrant
- Number of centimeters from the nipple
- Scan plane (radial/antiradial and transverse/long)
- Initials of person performing the scan
- Orthogonal images of mass without and with measuring calipers

Margin

Mass margins are classed as circumscribed or not circumscribed. Unlike mammography, mass margin must be visualized in its entirety on ultrasound to be classified as circumscribed. Such margins are well defined and have an abrupt transition from the surrounding tissue. Masses with this margin characteristic are oval or round (Fig. 5.34).

Mass margins categorized as not circumscribed have margins that are indistinct, angular, microlobulated, and spiculated (Fig. 5.35). A mass can have more than one margin characteristic demonstrated, consistent with histopathological heterogeneity in one breast cancer. Indistinct margins have no clear boundary with the surrounding tissue and may have an associated echogenic rim representative of tumor infiltration or inflammatory change (Fig. 5.36B and Box 5.3). Masses with a scalloped edge depicting short undulations are classified as microlobulated (Fig. 5.37). Angular mass margins form acute angles, and spiculated margins have radiating lines extending from the mass. All not circumscribed margins are suspicious, although spiculated and angular margins have the highest positive predictive value for malignancy (see Fig. 5.36). Management of all lesions should rely on the most suspicious feature (Box 5.4).

Table 5.6   Breast Imaging Reporting and Data System (BI-RADS) Assessment Categories and Management Recommendations

Assessment	Management	Likelihood of Cancer
Category 0: Incomplete; need additional imaging evaluation	Recall for additional imaging	N/A
Category 1: Negative	Routine screening	Essentially 0% likelihood of malignancy
Category 2: Benign	Routine screening	Essentially 0% likelihood of malignancy
Category 3: Probably benign	Short-interval (6-month) follow-up or continued surveillance	>0% but ≤2% likelihood of malignancy
Category 4: Suspicious	Tissue diagnosis	>2% but <95% likelihood of malignancy
Category 4 A: Low suspicion for malignancy	Tissue diagnosis	>2% but ≤10% likelihood of malignancy
Category 4B: Moderate suspicion for malignancy	Tissue diagnosis	>10% to ≤50% likelihood of malignancy
Category 4 C: High suspicion for malignancy	Tissue diagnosis	>50% to <95% likelihood of malignancy
Category 5: Highly suggestive of malignancy	Tissue diagnosis	≥95% likelihood of malignancy
Category 6: Known biopsy; proven malignancy	Surgical excision when clinically appropriate	N/A

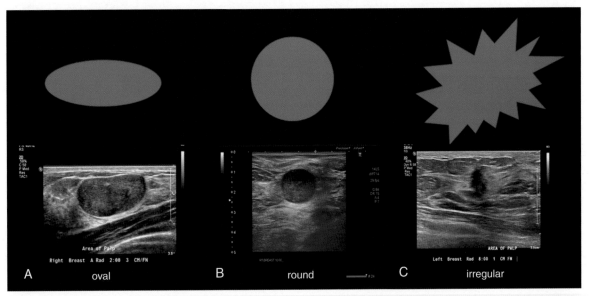

Fig. 5.32 Mass shape: (A) oval, (B) round, (C) irregular. A round mass has an anterior to posterior (AP) dimension that equals its transverse dimension and is categorized as antiparallel. If a round mass is not a simple or complicated cyst, it should be treated with suspicion.

Box 5.2 Differential Diagnosis of Round or Oval Solid Breast Masses

- Fibroadenoma
- Phyllodes tumor
- Invasive ductal cancer, not otherwise specified
- Medullary cancer
- Mucinous (colloid) carcinoma
- Papillary carcinoma
- Metastasis (not breast primary)
- Papilloma

Echo Pattern

Echo pattern is unique to ultrasound and is defined relative to the subcutaneous fat. Four echo patterns describe a mass: hyper-, hypo-, iso-, and anechoic (Figs. 5.34, 5.38–5.40). Masses illustrating both cystic (anechoic) and solid components are classified as complex cystic and solid (Fig. 5.41).

In comparison, heterogenous masses are solid masses with varying echo patterns (Fig. 5.42). The echo pattern alone has little specificity as malignancies can show features consistent with all the above patterns.

Posterior Features

Posterior acoustic feature is interpreted as a mass description and refers to the attenuation of the ultrasound beam. There are four types of attenuation features described in the BI-RADS lexicon: no posterior features, posterior acoustic enhancement, shadowing, or a combined pattern. The transmission is evaluated just behind the mass and compared with tissue at a similar depth. When there is no identifiable evidence of shadowing or enhancement deep to the lesion, the mass is classified as having no posterior features (Fig. 5.43). Posterior acoustic enhancement appears as a bright (echogenic) line deep to the lesion, appearing as if a flashlight is shining through the lesion (Fig. 5.44). In contrast, shadowing is attenuation that appears as a dark

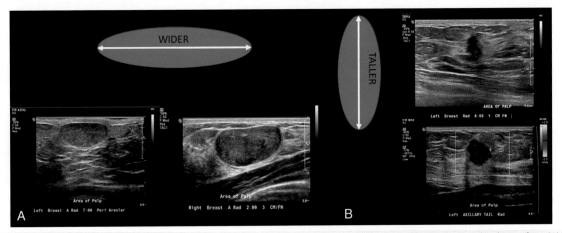

Fig. 5.33 Mass orientation: parallel and antiparallel. Orientation is based on the relationship of the long axis of a mass to the skin surface. (A) Two horizontal or parallel oriented hypoechoic circumscribed masses are representative of benign fibroadenomas. (B) Two antiparallel "taller than wide" masses with angular and indistinct margins are consistent with malignancy. Pathology diagnosis of invasive ductal carcinoma (IDC) in both cases.

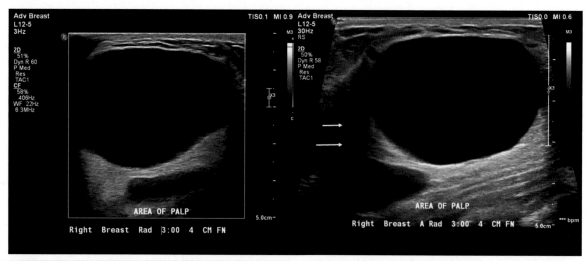

Fig. 5.34 Margin analysis: circumscribed. Benign simple cysts are anechoic with imperceptible walls. They can be round or oval with a circumscribed margin and enhanced posterior acoustic features. Color or power Doppler will not demonstrate internal vascularity (*left image*). Internal vascularity in an apparently anechoic mass should be considered as suspicious and biopsy should be recommended. Notice the refraction edge shadowing that is present at the edge of curved surfaces (*arrows*).

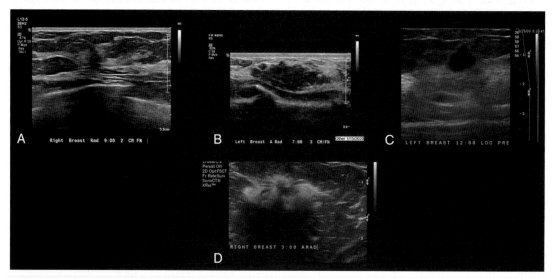

Fig. 5.35 Margin analysis: not circumscribed. (A) Indistinct margin: Mass margin demonstrates no clear boundary between the lesion and the surrounding tissue. (B) Microlobulated: Mass margin has multiple short undulating lobulations. (C) Angular: Mass margin forms an acute angle. (D) Spiculated: Mass margins have lines radiating from the mass and may or may not have architectural distortion associated with it. More than one descriptor may apply to a mass, any of which should prompt a suspicious assessment.

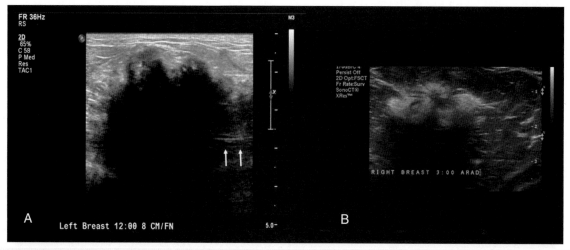

Fig. 5.36 Margin analysis: not circumscribed—spiculated. (A) A 52-year-old woman with new palpable lump. Ultrasound demonstrates an irregular spiculated hypoechoic mass with posterior acoustic shadowing. Spiculations consist of multiple linear hyperechoic and hypoechoic lines radiating from the edge of the lesion (*arrows*). A finding that is highly suspicious for malignancy and should prompt tissue sampling. Patient diagnosed with diabetic mastopathy. (B) Ultrasound in a different patient demonstrates an indistinct spiculated hypoechoic mass with a surrounding echogenic rim consistent with tumor invasion and desmoplastic reaction. True measurements of this lesion should include the echogenic rim.

- Invasive ductal cancer
- Invasive lobular carcinoma
- Primary or secondary non-Hodgkin lymphoma
- Fat necrosis
- Pseudoangiomatous stromal hyperplasia
- Abscess

- Invasive ductal carcinoma
- Invasive lobular carcinoma
- Tubular cancer
- Postsurgical scar
- Radial scar
- Fat necrosis (atypical)

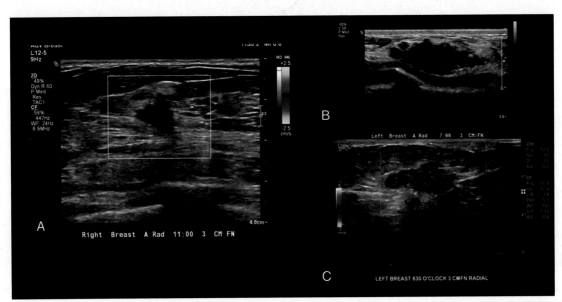

Fig. 5.37 Margin analysis: not circumscribed—microlobulated, short cycle undulations, scalloped margin. Pathology diagnosis, DCIS (A–B). Invasive ductal cancer (C). Microlobulated margin can also be identified in benign findings such as clustered microcysts and fibroadenomatoid change.

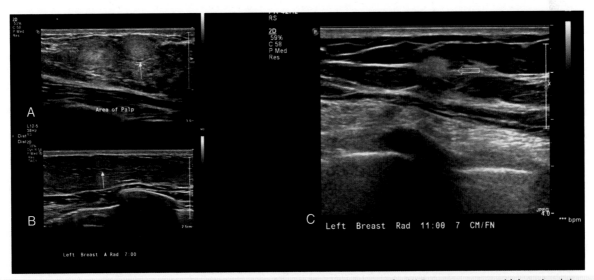

Fig. 5.38 Echo pattern: hyperechoic. The echo pattern is increased relative to the subcutaneous fat. (A) Pregnant woman with lactational changes and galactocele (*arrow*). The fat content in the breast milk makes the palpable masses hyperechoic with respect of the subcutaneous fat at ultrasound. (B) A small lipoma (*arrow*) almost isoechoic to the adjacent tissue. Lipomas are hyperechoic in the breast. (C) A hyperechoic invasive ductal carcinoma, grade 2 (*open arrow*).

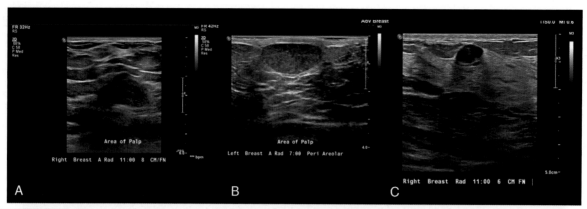

Fig. 5.39 Echo pattern: hypoechoic. The echotexture is lower than the subcutaneous fat and contains low level echoes throughout the mass. A, B, and C have a pathologic diagnosis of a fibroadenoma. Each one demonstrates a varying degree of posterior acoustic features.

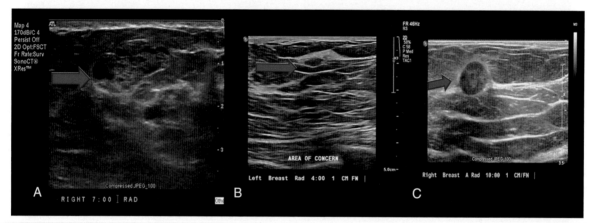

Fig. 5.40 Echo pattern: isoechoic. Echotexture is similar to the subcutaneous fat. (A) Complex fibroadenoma (*arrow*); (B) Stromal fibrosis (*arrow*), a finding that would be inconspicuous if the adjacent island of fibrous tissue were not present. Patient was a call back from screening examination for a new mass, therefore biopsy was performed. If this was found on a baseline exam, BI-RADS 3 (probably benign) would be appropriate. (C) isoechoic mass (*arrow*) is antiparallel in orientation with a spiculated margin; therefore, biopsy was performed. Pathology showed fat necrosis.

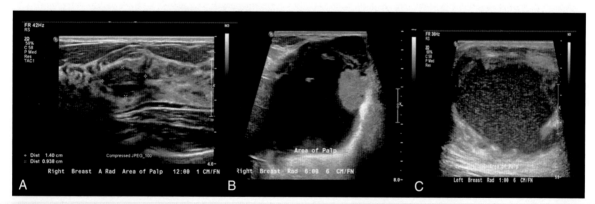

Fig. 5.41 Echo pattern: complex cystic and solid mass contains both anechoic regions (cystic) and echogenic (solid) components. Given the complexity, these lesions should be considered suspicious and tissue sampling recommended. Pathology diagnosis is (A) mucin-producing adenocarcinoma, (B) papillary neoplasm, and (C) mastitis and abscess formation.

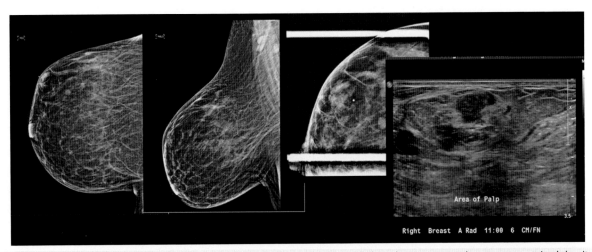

Fig. 5.42 Echo pattern: heterogenous. A 43-year-old woman with new palpable lump. Unilateral mammogram demonstrates a mixed density mass, mostly containing fat in the area demarcated by the radiopaque BB markers. Targeted ultrasound was performed and demonstrates an oval circumscribed heterogenous mass demonstrating similar size and characteristics to the mammographic finding. Compatible with a hamartoma and a benign finding. Fat is iso- and hyperechoic, and the areas of fibrosis are more hypoechoic within this fibroadenolipoma. BI-RADS 2 (benign assessment).

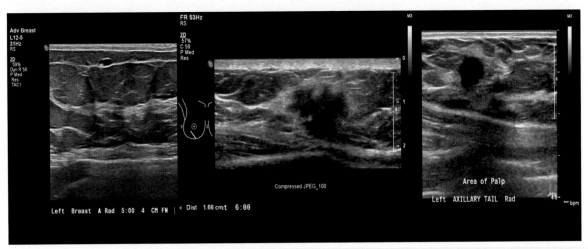

Fig. 5.43 Posterior features: no posterior acoustic features. There is no shadowing or enhancement deep to these lesions.

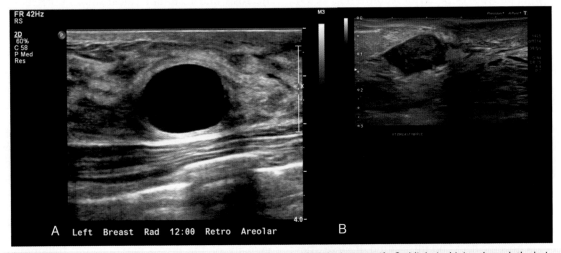

Fig. 5.44 Posterior features: enhancement. There is an echogenic band just behind the lesion as if a flashlight is shining through the lesion. A finding that is seen in this (A) simple cyst and (B) fibroadenoma.

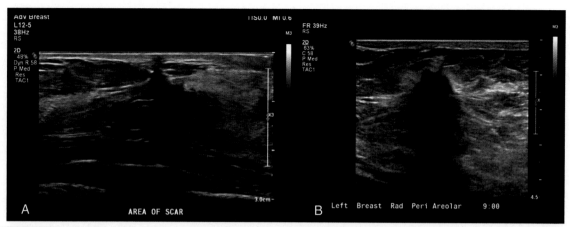

Fig. 5.45 Posterior features: acoustic shadowing. There is marked attenuation of the acoustic beam seen as a dark column compared with adjacent tissue at similar depth. This can be appreciated in benign conditions such as a surgical scar in case A and a malignancy as in case B.

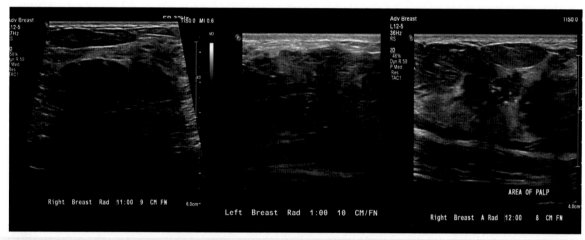

Fig. 5.46 Posterior features: combined pattern. Area posterior to mass shows a combination of no attenuation, partial shadowing, or enhanced through transmission. (A) Trapezoidal view of a fibroadenoma. (B) Handheld ultrasound of hypoechoic mass with associated calcifications biopsy proven to represent a phyllodes tumor. (C) Pathology diagnosis of invasive ductal cancer with associated calcifications.

column behind the mass and is associated with the cellular density and fibrosis of a lesion. Shadowing is worrisome but has only a moderate degree of suspicion since cancers can demonstrate all types of posterior features (Fig. 5.45). For example, triple-negative breast cancers can demonstrate enhanced through transmission. Lastly, some masses demonstrate a combined pattern of attenuation with areas that show no attenuation, partial shadowing, or enhanced through transmission (Fig. 5.46).

CALCIFICATIONS

Mammography is the modality of choice used to visualize breast calcifications. The identification of calcifications on ultrasound depends on the size of the calcifications and the heterogeneity of the background echotexture. Calcifications appear as hyperechoic foci on ultrasound and can be seen inside a mass (whether benign or malignant), outside of a mass grouped in the fibroglandular tissue, or intraductal in location (Figs. 5.47–5.48). Calcifications appear as hyperechoic foci or echogenic flecks on ultrasound. If large, they may cast a shadow. Only when microcalcifications are

grouped or numerous will they cause some attenuation. Intraductal calcifications are commonly seen in high-grade ductal carcinoma in situ (DCIS) and are the result of tumor necrosis and resultant calcification. Correlation with the mammogram is helpful.

ASSOCIATED FEATURES

Because there is no single ultrasound finding that can predict cancer with 100% accuracy, combined findings and associated imaging features are used to achieve a high PPV. The effect a mass has on the surrounding tissue is an important predictive indicator for invasive disease. Some associated findings include architectural distortion, duct changes, skin edema, skin thickening and retraction, and the presence and distribution of vascularity (Fig. 5.49). Skin edema with associated skin thickening is identified in benign and malignant diseases. For example, congestive heart failure and mastitis commonly display findings consistent with edema, such as the prominence of the skin and hyperechogenicity of the breast parenchyma. Inflammatory breast cancer demonstrates a similar appearance. Vascularity has

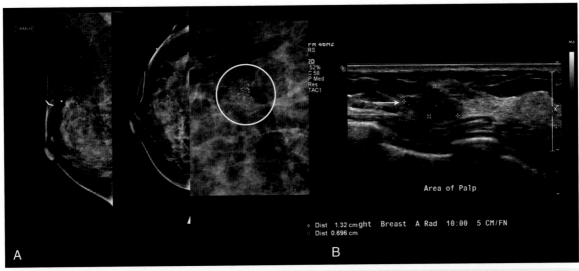

Fig. 5.47 Calcifications within a mass. (A) Mammographic views show grouped coarse heterogeneous calcifications *(circle)* associated with a palpable mass indicated by radiopaque BB marker. (B) Calcifications are seen as echogenic foci within hypoechoic mass at ultrasound *(arrow)*.

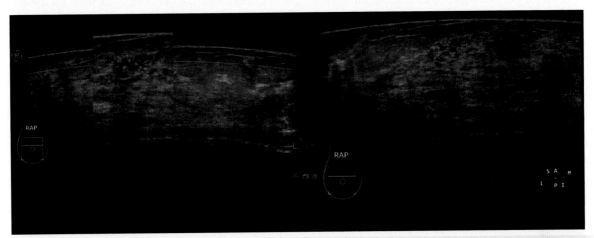

Fig. 5.48 Calcifications intraductal: calcifications appear as hyperechoic foci with little to no attenuation only when in aggregates. This patient had extensive calcifications involving the upper outer breast. Automated breast ultrasound was performed to evaluate an area of invasion. Both long field of view transverse images demonstrates duct extension filled with microcalcifications involving a similar distribution to the mammogram (not shown). No invasion was identified.

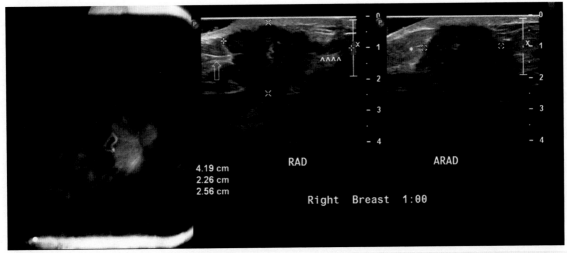

Fig. 5.49 Associated features: architectural distortion, skin thickening and retraction, edema, and duct changes. Architectural distortion seen as straightening of the Cooper ligaments *(open arrow)* and associated edema (*) from peritumoral desmoplastic reaction. Milk duct changes can also manifest as irregularities in duct caliber and presence of intraductal extension of tumor (^). Calcifications are also associated with the spiculated mass. *(left-most image)* Pathology high-grade invasive ductal carcinoma (IDC).

three assessment levels: absent, internal vascularity and marginal vessels that form around the rim of a lesion (rim vascularity) (see Fig. 5.27).

SPECIAL CASES

Special cases described in the BI-RADS lexicon have a pathognomonic appearance. Such cases are cysts (Box 5.5), which include simple cyst and clustered microcysts (Fig. 5.50). Clustered microcysts consist of grouped simple benign cysts, each measuring 2 to 3 mm with no discrete solid component or thick septations (Fig. 5.51). Management of this lesion depends on whether this is an isolated finding or identified in the screening setting. If the clustered cysts are identified on a diagnostic examination, then an assessment of BI-RADS 3 can be given to this probably benign finding. For a single cluster of microcysts identified in the screening setting, an assessment code of BI-RADS 2 benign is appropriate.

Other special cases such as complicated cysts, dermal masses in or on the skin, foreign bodies including implants, postsurgical fluid collections, fat necrosis, and lymph nodes have distinct appearances. Vascular abnormalities of the breast include arterial venous malformations

Box 5.5	Simple Cyst Criteria

- Oval or round shape with circumscribed margins
- Anechoic
- Imperceptible wall
- Enhanced transmission of sound

and thrombosed superficial veins called Mondor disease (Box 5.6).

Cysts: Simple versus Complicated versus Complex Cystic and Solid Mass

In the latest edition of the ultrasound lexicon, there is a clear distinction between complicated cysts and more complex appearing cystic masses. Complicated cysts contain mobile internal homogenous low-level echoes, presumably representing debris without evidence of a discrete solid component. Moreover, complicated cysts have all the features of a simple cyst, including imperceptible walls and enhanced through transmission (see Fig. 5.51). The use of tissue harmonics can help differentiate complicated cysts from simple

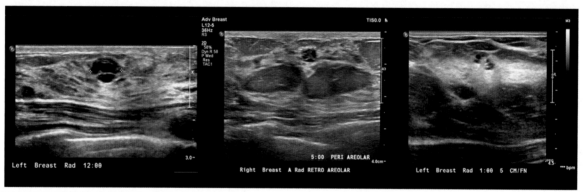

Fig. 5.50 Special cases: benign findings clustered microcysts. Each individual microcyst is benign.

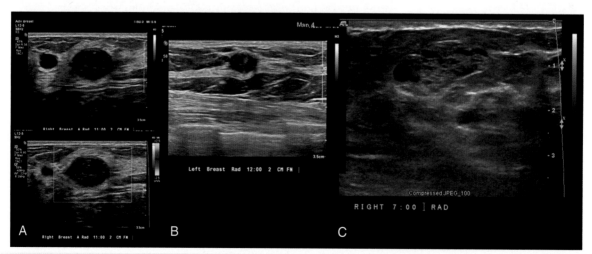

Fig. 5.51 Special cases: cyst versus complicated cyst versus complex cystic and solid versus solid mass. It is important to distinguish cystic changes from a complex cystic and solid mass. (A) Simple cyst is next to a complicated cyst with internal debris. Color Doppler was performed showing no internal vascularity. (B) Complex cystic and solid mass with thick septa and possible nondependent mural nodule. Pathology diagnosed apocrine metaplasia and fibrocystic changes. (C) Heterogenous solid mass with cystic changes. Pathology diagnosed a fibroadenoma with cystic changes.

Box 5.6   Special Cases: Pathognomonic Appearance

- Simple cyst, clustered microcysts, complicated cysts
- Dermal masses, sebaceous cysts
- Foreign body including implants
- Benign postsurgical scar
- Lymph node
- Fat necrosis
- Sebaceous cysts
- Vascular abnormalities such as arteriovenous malformations (AVMs), Mondor disease

---

Box 5.7   Differential Diagnosis of Round Masses

- Benign:
  - Cyst (includes complicated cysts)
  - Fibroadenoma
  - Lactating adenoma or galactocele in lactating women
  - Papilloma
- Benign/borderline:
  - Phyllodes tumor
- Malignant:
  - Invasive ductal cancer (uncommon form of most common cancer)
  - Medullary cancer
  - Mucinous (colloid) cancer
  - Papillary carcinoma
  - Adenoid cystic carcinoma
  - Breast metastasis

---

cysts by reducing artifactual echoes. Complex cystic and solid masses contain an intracystic or mural mass and may include thick septations and a thick wall. Benign findings such as intraductal papilloma, hematoma, and an abscess can appear as complex cystic and solid masses. Malignancy must be excluded and correlation with clinical history is helpful.

Benign versus Probably Benign Masses

An oval mass that contains three or fewer gentle lobulations is considered a BI-RADS assessment category 3 probably benign mass. These characteristics are classic for fibroadenomas, and in Stavros' 1995 study had a 99% negative predictive value. Solid-appearing masses with more than three lobulations are considered microlobulated and have a significantly lower negative predictive value and would not be appropriate to assess as probably benign.

A BI-RADS 3 probably benign assessment code recommends follow-up imaging instead of biopsy. Recommended follow up consists of two examinations at 6-month intervals followed by another examination at 12-month interval. If there is no interval change from baseline examination after 2 years of follow-up the mass can then be assessed as benign (BI-RADS category 2).

One unique type of oval mass is an intramammary lymph node appearing as a circumscribed mass with a thin echogenic pseudo capsule or rim. Intramammary lymph nodes are benign and given a BI-RADS 2 assessment. Another typically benign mass is a simple anechoic cyst. When there are uniform low-level echoes within a cyst, this is termed a complicated cyst, which should be assessed as probably benign BI-RADS 3. If there are multiple bilateral (at least three total with one in each breast) complicated cysts seen only on ultrasound, a BI-RADS 2 benign assessment code is appropriate.

Round Mass

Round is considered antiparallel in orientation and is regarded as suspicious. Anechoic cysts are one of the most common round masses in the breast; however, it must meet strict criteria to obtain a benign BI-RADS 2 assessment. If there is any internal echogenicity, then the cyst is not considered a simple and benign finding. Round hypoechoic masses are the most likely to be incorrectly characterized as probably benign BI-RADS 3 lesions (Box 5.7). There are circumscribed solid cancers, such as triple-negative breast cancers that appear anechoic to hypoechoic with no other malignant features except for round shape (Fig. 5.52 and Box 5.8). Internal vascularity is the element distinguishing this type of cancer from a simple cyst. Other round malignancies include medullary and mucinous (colloid) carcinoma. Intracystic papillary cancers also appear round. In addition, metastatic involvement of lymph nodes lose the classic oval shape and become rounder and irregular with more tumor deposition.

Additional Features of Malignancy

The risk of a false negative interpretation is greater for smaller lesions than larger masses. Masses that are less than 5 mm may be hard to characterize. The use of harmonics and compound imaging may help with internal echo pattern and margin analysis. The addition of color and power Doppler findings may help as well. There are ultrasound findings that are more suggestive of malignancy, such as angular and spiculated margins and acoustic shadowing, but further clinical context must also be considered (prior surgery). The evaluation of the surrounding tissue and its relationship with the mass can indicate a more aggressive process. The obliteration of tissue planes imitates an infiltrating or inflammatory process and appears as an echogenic rim around the lesion. Cooper ligament thickening with straightening and ductal changes are also concerning for local spread of disease (see Fig. 5.49).

BI-RADS Final Assessment for Ultrasound

BI-RADS assessment for ultrasound follows the same principles as mammography (Table 5.7). Since its first ultrasound publication in 2003, radiologists have become familiar with the descriptive terminology and algorithms defining benign

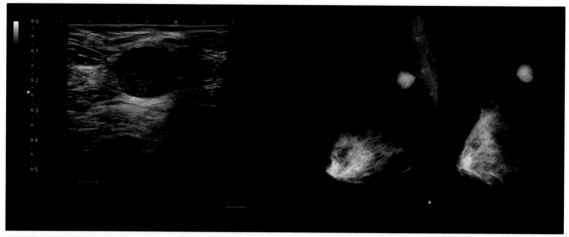

Fig. 5.52 Special cases: round cancer. A 48-year-old woman with a new palpable lump in the right breast. Mammogram demonstrates a round circumscribed mass that appears hypoechoic with enhanced posterior features on ultrasound. Pathology demonstrated an invasive ductal carcinoma estrogen/progesterone (ER/PR) receptor and human epidermal growth factor receptor (HER2) positive.

Box 5.8   Round Breast Cancer

■ The most common round breast malignancy is invasive ductal cancer. It is an uncommon form of a very common tumor.

from suspicious lesions. The lack of any malignant characteristic findings mentioned above can further categorize a mass as BI-RADS 2. If there is one suspicious feature, the other benign characteristics should be ignored. BI-RADS 3 lesions on ultrasound should have a less than 2% chance of malignancy while anything greater should prompt a biopsy.

The BI-RADS lexicon defines specific sonographic findings as appropriate for a BI-RADS 3 category, including a circumscribed, oval, solid, parallel-oriented mass (typical fibroadenoma) and a complicated cyst. If there is an interval decrease in size at follow-up for a probably benign finding, there should be a reclassification of the lesion to a benign, BI-RADS 2 category. Complete resolution of a BI-RADS 3 mass at follow-up should be given a BI-RADS 1 (negative) assessment. On the contrary, masses that increase in size at follow-up imaging (20% or more in diameter) should be considered suspicious (BI-RADS category 4) and prompt a biopsy. Considerations are made for an increase in size 1 to 2 mm, as this is thought to be related to the scan pressure and patient positioning.

Following BI-RADS for mammography, category 4 ultrasound findings can be subdivided into 4 A, 4B, and 4 C and inform the level of suspicion to the referring physicians. Category 5 is highly suggestive of malignancy and has many sonographic features described above. BI-RADS 6 is reserved for lesions already diagnosed as malignant before surgical intervention.

In summary, ultrasound is widely applied in everyday practice; its use can further characterize and diagnose breast-related disease. Proper use includes technique, and a firm understanding of sonographic normal breast anatomy can improve diagnostic capability. With a clear understanding of the two aforementioned and use of the BI-RADS lexicon descriptors, breast ultrasound can enhance the differentiation of benign and malignant disease.

Table 5.7   ACR Lexicon BI-RADS Ultrasound Mass Descriptors

Shape	Oval
	Round
	Irregular
Margin	Circumscribed
	Indistinct
	Angular
	Microlobulated
	Spiculated
Echo pattern	Anechoic
	Hyperechoic
	Complex cystic and solid
	Hypoechoic
	Isoechoic
	Heterogeneous
Orientation	Parallel
	Not parallel
Posterior features	No posterior features
	Enhancement
	Shadowing
	Combined pattern

KEY ELEMENTS

Technique
• Tissue harmonic imaging will clear up artifactual echoes and enhance real echoes.
• Compound breast imaging improves lateral resolution and margin characterization.
• Echogenicity of a mass is described relative to the subcutaneous fat.
• It is also important to scan masses in orthogonal planes and at multiple angles, preferably in real time, to assess the entire margin of a mass.
• When investigating color flow, it is important to use only modest compression of the probe and to select a sensitive frequency.

Interpretation

- Screening breast ultrasound results in an increase in cancer detection rates at the cost of high false-positive rates.
- Ultrasound can differentiate between cysts and solid breast masses, as well as characterize masses as benign or suspicious based on their sonographic features.
  ○ Assessment of a mass on ultrasound relies on shape, orientation, and margin analysis.
  ○ The entire margin must be circumscribed on ultrasound to classify a mass as circumscribed. If any portion of the margin is not circumscribed, the margin of the mass should be reported as not circumscribed.
- Complex cystic and solid mass contains both anechoic region (cystic) and echogenic (solid) components and should be considered suspicious.
- A solitary complicated cyst can be characterized as Breast Imaging and Reporting Data System (BI-RADS) category 3 (probably benign), but several or multiple benign-appearing complicated cysts or complicated cysts in combination with simple cysts should receive a BI-RADS category 2 (benign) assessment.
- An oval, circumscribed, and parallel mass with no suspicious sonographic features can safely be assessed as BI-RADS category 3 (probably benign), unless it is new on imaging that has shown the area previously.
- There is considerable overlap between the sonographic features of a postsurgical scar, fat necrosis, and malignancy.
- The most common round cancer is invasive ductal cancer, although it is an uncommon form of the most common cancer.
- Abnormal lymph nodes demonstrate cortical irregularity, cortical thickening (circumferential or eccentric), or hila replacement.

Suggested Reading

American College of Radiology, & D'Orsi CJ. *ACR BI-RADS Atlas: Breast Imaging Reporting and Data System; Mammography, Ultrasound, Magnetic Resonance Imaging, Follow-up and Outcome Monitoring, Data Dictionary.* ACR, American College of Radiology; 2013.

American College of Radiology. (2016). ACR Appropriateness Criteria Palpable Breast Masses. Reston: American College of Radiology.

American College of Radiology. (2016). ACR practice parameter for the performance of a breast ultrasound examination. Reston: American College of Radiology.

Anvari, A., Forsberg, F., & Samir, A. E. (2015). A Primer on the Physical Principles of Tissue Harmonic Imaging. RadioGraphics, 35(7), 1955–1964. https://doi.org/10.1148/rg.2015140338

Baad M, Lu ZF, Reiser I, Paushter D. Clinical significance of US artifacts. *RadioGraphics.* 2017;37(5):1408–1423. https://doi.org/10.1148/rg.2017160175.

Berg WA, Blume JD, Cormack JB, et al. Combined Screening With Ultrasound and Mammography vs Mammography Alone in Women at Elevated Risk of Breast Cancer, & Investigators, for the A. 6666. *JAMA.* 2008;299(18):2151–2163. https://doi.org/10.1001/jama.299.18.2151.

Berg WA, Zhang Z, Lehrer D, et al. Detection of Breast Cancer With Addition of Annual Screening Ultrasound or a Single Screening MRI to Mammography in Women With Elevated Breast Cancer Risk, & Investigators, for the A. 6666. *JAMA.* 2012;307(13):1394–1404. https://doi.org/10.1001/jama.2012.388.

Feldman MK, Katyal S, Blackwood MS. US Artifacts. *RadioGraphics.* 2009;29(4):1179–1189. https://doi.org/10.1148/rg.294085199.

Fowler AM, Mankoff DA, Joe BN. Imaging neoadjuvant therapy response in breast cancer. *Radiology.* 2017;285(2):358–375. https://doi.org/10.1148/radiol.2017170180.

Mainiero MB, Moy L, Baron P, et al. ACR appropriateness criteria® breast cancer screening. *J Am Coll Radiology, 14(11, Suppl).* 2017:S383–S390. https://doi.org/10.1016/j.jacr.2017.08.044.

6 Basics of Digital Breast Tomosynthesis

SARAH M. FRIEDEWALD AND SONYA BHOLE

| OVERVIEW | This chapter covers the basics of digital breast tomosynthesis (DBT), including acquisition, display, and interpretation techniques. Additionally, dose-related concerns and synthesized imaging will be explained. |

Digital breast tomosynthesis (DBT) was developed to improve on the limitations of traditional digital mammography (DM), namely the limited sensitivity in women with dense breast tissue as well as the relatively high number of patients called back from screening for additional imaging.

Many prospective and retrospective studies have demonstrated that in the screening setting, imaging with DBT results in increased cancer detection, with a simultaneous decrease in the number of false-positive examinations. Because of these advances, adoption of DBT has been rapid and is now becoming the standard of care in the United States. As of May 2020, 70% of mammography facilities have at least one DBT unit, and 40% of all accredited machines in the United States have DBT capability. Additionally, the benefits of DBT are not limited to screening. DBT facilitates interpretation in the diagnostic setting by improving lesion characterization and aiding in the localization of findings for further evaluation with ultrasound and possible biopsy.

Acquisition of Images

When DBT was first approved by the U.S. Food and Drug Association (FDA) and released for clinical use in 2014, both DM and DBT images were acquired. This was a combined examination under the same compression rather than replacement of DM with DBT. Maintaining the standard of care DM images was important to enable comparison with prior examinations and allow for assessment of symmetry between breasts. The DBT images therefore were adding information for the radiologist to review and required longer interpretation times. As new manufacturers developed equipment capable of DBT imaging, different methods were employed to maximize information while minimizing dose and interpretation times. Common to each system available today are the administration of many low-dose x-ray images through the breast, which are then reconstructed into thin "slices." However, each manufacturer of DBT machines has their own method of acquiring these low-dose images. Additionally, not all manufacturers suggest imaging the breast with the combination examination, but rather suggest imaging with DBT in only one view. Other efforts to minimize the dose involve generating a synthetic mammography (SM) to replace the need to acquire a separate DM image.

METHODS OF ACQUIRING DBT IMAGES

Similar to a standard DM acquisition, with DBT, the breast remains stationary in compression and is repositioned for each view. However unlike DM where the gantry is stationary during the exposure, DBT images are acquired while the gantry moves in an arc across the breast to obtain multiple very low-dose images at different angles. The number of projection images obtained per view are fixed (manufacturer determined) and are independent of breast thickness. The "reconstructed slices" are generated from the projection images and are the images that the radiologist interprets. The thickness of these images can be manipulated by the reader in some systems or is determined by the manufacturer. The number of reconstructed slices is dependent on the thickness of the breast (i.e., if the breast compresses to 5 cm and the reconstructed slices are 1-mm thick, then there will be 50 images to interpret for that view).

Two main methods of obtaining the projection images are the "step and shoot" method and the "continuous" method (Box 6.1). As the names imply, with the step and shoot method, the gantry comes to a full stop between each low-dose exposure. With the continuous method, the gantry sweeps across the breast in one motion and acquires multiple images during the exposure. The continuous method has a faster acquisition (and therefore less patient motion), but gantry movement during exposure results in some focal spot blur. The main advantage of the step and shoot method is decreased focal spot blur, resulting in improved signal to noise. However, because the gantry is stopping for each exposure, there is increased time of acquisition and the potential for patient motion.

Dose of DBT Compared With DM

Although the dose of the combination examination (DM + DBT) is below the FDA limit of 3 mGy for the phantom image, efforts to decrease the exposure to the patients have been

---

Box 6.1 Method of Digital Breast Tomosynthesis (DBT) Image Acquisition

- Step and shoot: decreased focal spot blur but longer exposure
- Continuous: faster acquisition, therefore less susceptible to patient motion, but has some focal spot blur

underway. One method to decrease the dose is to expose the patient to one view with DBT only and the other view to DM only. Therefore the overall dose is comparable to DM. Studies have shown that overall, this method is not inferior to standard DM imaging. Another method to decrease the dose is to generate an image that is similar in appearance to DM without the need to acquire a separate DM image. This generated image is called a *synthetic mammogram*. Fig. 6.1 shows the American College of Radiology (ACR) Phantom dose in mGy for analog film, DM, DBT plus DM, and DBT with SM only.

IMAGING WITH DBT IN ONE VIEW ONLY

Several studies have shown noninferiority of acquiring DBT in one view and DM in the other view as a dose-reduction method. Because it has been shown that cancers were rated more visible on DBT compared with DM, imaging the breast in the mediolateral oblique (MLO) view with DBT increases the opportunity for cancer detection. However, despite the improved conspicuity of findings, imaging with DBT in both views provides the greatest opportunity for lesion detection. In fact, cancers have been shown to be more conspicuous on the DBT craniocaudal (CC) view compared with the DBT MLO view, which could lead to missed cancers if DBT is only performed on the MLO view. Therefore imaging with DBT for both views is optimal.

SYNTHETIC IMAGING

The FDA has approved software advancements that generate two-dimensional (2D) SM from the DBT data set. Because several studies have demonstrated that synthetic images are nearly as good as a standard DM, a number of facilities have stopped acquiring the DM image, effectively reducing the dose of the DM + DBT to approximate that of original DM levels.

Because DBT is the source of the SM image, there is often enhanced visualization of DBT-only findings such as architectural distortion and masses. Additionally, calcifications on SM are brighter than on DM and contribute to improved interpretation speed. Importantly, because the SM images are effectively a summation of the DBT reconstructed slices, the benefit of the thin slices are not gained and overlapping tissue may still obscure findings. SM should serve as a preview of the findings on DBT and must not be a replacement for reviewing the DBT slices.

There have been several improvements over time with the quality of synthetic images. The earliest versions had problems with reconstruction that generated features of the breast that were pixelated, such as the nipple. Additionally, resolution of the morphology of calcifications was poor. Furthermore, earlier versions of SM were challenged with an artifact generated from the processing algorithm that artificially enhanced structural elements in the breast that falsely appeared to represent calcifications, termed *pseudocalcifications*. However, the most recent high-resolution synthetic images appear almost indistinguishable from a standard DM and result in very few pseudocalcifications. Research has demonstrated that the performance of synthetic images when used in conjunction with DBT approximates that of the combination examination. Additionally, better visualization of skin lines and improved conspicuity and characterization lesion margins are an added benefit of the higher resolution SM. Decreased dropout ("halo" artifact) adjacent to large calcifications or other high attenuation objects such as surgical clips is minimized. Finally, reduced background noise and image blur contribute to the image quality and approximation to DM. However, the very large file sizes of these higher-resolution SM images require significant storage and bandwidth to transfer data efficiently. Fig. 6.2 shows a DM and corresponding standard resolution and high-resolution SM for a patient.

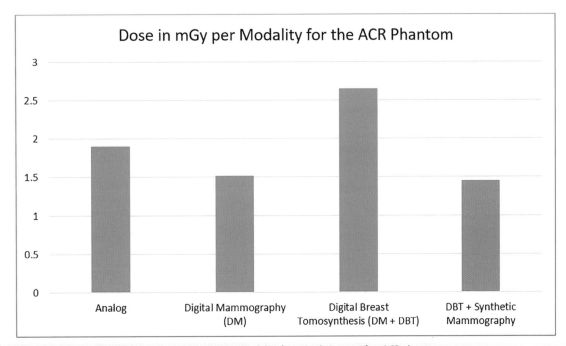

Fig. 6.1 Chart demonstrating the differences in dose (mGy) per modality for a single image of an ACR phantom.

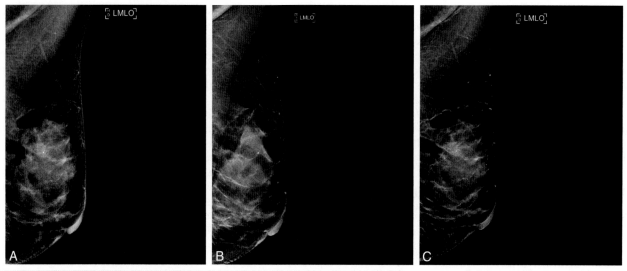

Fig. 6.2 Comparison of 2D digital mammogram with different synthetic mammograms in the MLO view. (A) Digital mammogram. (B) Standard-resolution synthetic mammogram. (C) High-resolution synthetic mammogram.

Images Available for Interpretation

Depending on the manufacturer and the preference of the breast imaging facility, multiple sets of images can be available for interpretation (Box 6.2). The combination of DM and DBT can be available for the entire examination or just for selected views. A standard 2D mammogram can be acquired under the same compression as DBT or as a separate compression and exposure (dependent on the manufacture). DM may be eliminated if synthetic imaging is available. However, DBT should not be viewed alone; either a DM or SM must accompany the DBT reconstructed slices. Finally, the projection images (raw data) may or may not

be available depending on the picture archiving and communication systems (PACS) display workstation. Fig. 6.3 shows examples of these images available for review. The DBT update to Breast Imaging Reporting and Data System (BI-RADS) fifth edition recommends that the dictated report should include the types of images that were obtained providing clarity regarding which images were obtained for interpretation.

DBT Terminology

Although the term *3D* is commonly used to describe DBT, this term is not technically accurate. Unlike in computed tomography or magnetic resonance imaging, one cannot use cross-reference lines with DBT from one view to another to determine the location of a finding. Images are not acquired isotropically but are taken at multiple different angles across the breast. Reconstruction into a plane perpendicular to DBT plane of acquisition would produce very poor fidelity images. Just as with standard 2D mammography, each DBT view (e.g., CC, MLO) is acquired after repositioning the breast. Additionally, because the breast is not a fixed shape structure, there can be significant movement of the breast tissue between images. This can cause significant movement of findings between views. Therefore, according to the DBT supplement to BI-RADS fifth edition, abbreviated terms for DBT that are acceptable are *tomo* or *tomosynthesis* and that *3D* should be reserved for discussing DBT in an informal setting such as with a patient or in colloquial speech.

DBT Display

Often included in the display window showing the DBT reconstruction slices is a slice indicator or "scroll bar" instructing the radiologist as to the specific location of the DBT slice within the stack of images. For example, the slice

---

Box 6.2   Images Available to Review

- Digital mammography (DM)
  - Standard acquisition of DM
  - Dose is in addition to digital breast tomosynthesis (DBT) data set
  - Can be acquired under the same compression as DBT or under a separate exposure (dependent on manufacturer)
- Projection images
  - Set number of low-dose images (number dependent on manufacturer) that are generated from the DBT exposure
  - Not routinely used for interpretation
  - Can be helpful to detect motion
  - May not be displayed on all picture archiving and communication systems (PACS) workstations
- Reconstruction images
  - Generated from the projection images
  - Used for interpretation
  - Often defaulted to 1-mm slices (but newer systems can have increased slice thickness)
- Synthetic mammography (SM)
  - Generated from the DBT data set
  - No additional x-ray dose (unlike DM acquisition)
  - Can be a substitute for DM images thereby reducing overall DBT dose

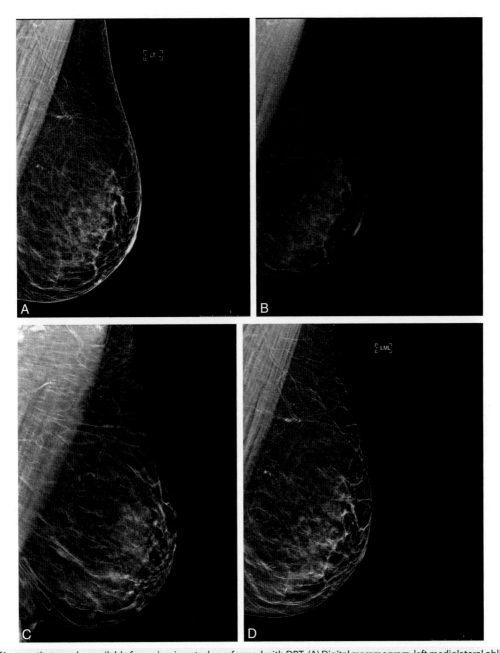

Fig. 6.3 Types of images that may be available for review in a study performed with DBT. (A) Digital mammogram, left mediolateral oblique (LMLO) view standard 2D mammogram. (B) Projection images (raw DBT data, may not be viewable on all PACS stations). (C) Reconstruction images: thin slice images reconstructed from the DBT data set. (D) Synthetic image generated from the reconstructed slices to simulate a DM.

that is being viewed will be either to the medial or lateral aspect of the central slice on the MLO view or the superior or inferior aspect of the central slice on the CC view. The scroll bar is fixed in length and demonstrates the thickest portion of the breast. The slice thickness will be indicated and sometimes can be manipulated by the radiologist. Additionally, the DBT slice number will be also displayed on the PACS workstation and can be configured to show slice 1 beginning at the side of the detector or the compression paddle. If one is describing a finding that is in focus on a particular DBT slice, it is important to include the slice number when describing the finding in the dictated report. If the PACS system does not have a visual slice indicator and relies on image numbers, it is important to adopt a consistent

standard regarding location of slice 1 (detector side versus compression paddle side) to avoid confusion. For example slice 20 of 50 on a CC projection is closer to the head if slice 1 is set for the compression paddle side, whereas slice 20 of 50 is closer to the foot if slice 1 is on the detector side. Fig. 6.4 shows different examples of slice indicators for mediolateral (ML) and lateromedial (LM) views.

Advantages of DBT

Many studies (prospective and retrospective) have demonstrated superiority of the combined DBT + DM examination versus DM alone. This is largely due to superimposition

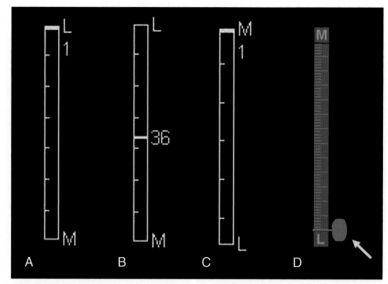

Fig. 6.4 Different examples of a slice indicator or "scroll bar." (A) ML view with the slice indicator on slice 1 set on the detector side of the DBT stack. (B) ML view with the slice indicator at slice 36. (C) LM view with the slice indicator on slice 1 on the detector side. (D) ML view on a different viewer that has the settings arranged so that the detector is on the bottom of the scroll bar. The indicator (*arrow*) at bottom of scroll bar shows slice 1 on detector side.

of breast tissue contributing to the limited sensitivity and specificity of DM. Because superimposed breast tissue is effectively removed with DBT, increased conspicuity and improved characterization of findings enable the radiologist to find more cancers and properly characterize benign findings.

REASONS FOR INCREASE IN CANCER DETECTION

Increased conspicuity of findings and improved margin characterization are hallmarks of DBT (Box 6.3). Architectural distortion is by far the most common finding that is DBT evident but DM occult (74%), followed by masses (24%). One study showed that half of DBT-only findings (DM occult) that were recommended for biopsy were malignant.

Because invasive ductal carcinoma is the most commonly encountered histologic type of breast cancer and often presents as architectural distortion, DBT has a significant advantage over DM due to the increased conspicuity of this finding. Additionally, some studies have demonstrated that

---

Box 6.3   Common Reasons for Improved Performance With Digital Breast Tomosynthesis (DBT)

- Increased cancer detection
- Architectural distortion more visible
- Increased conspicuity of a mass
- Margins of masses better appreciated
- Improved localization of findings
- Decreased recall
- Superimposed tissue
- Skin calcifications/lesions
- Nipple not in profile
- Tortuous vessels
- Lymph nodes

DBT improves detection of invasive lobular carcinoma, a notably elusive histologic subtype of breast cancer, compared with DM. Fig. 6.5 shows an example of a small cancer seen on DBT but occult on DM.

REASONS FOR DECREASE IN RECALL

Compared with other modalities that increase cancer detection, imaging with DBT has the unique advantage of simultaneously decreasing false-positive recalls from screening. This is largely because improved characterization of findings occurs at the time of screening rather than requiring additional imaging to obtain the same information. Common reasons for decreases in recall are as follows.

Vessel Turns

Occasionally serpiginous vessels can be overlapping and appear as masses on DM. Most of the time vascular structures are easily identified on DM. However, turns in the vessel can create the appearance of a mass, which accounts for a small percentage of unnecessary recalls. With DBT, one can trace the pathway of the vessel along its course and confirm that the "mass" on DM actually represents a vessel turn, obviating the need for recalls illustrated in Fig. 6.6.

Lymph Nodes

Characteristic appearances of lymph nodes include a fatty hilum with a thin (<3 mm) uniform cortex. Intramammary lymph nodes can be occasionally mistaken for a mass needing further evaluation on DM. The reniform shape and low-density center often can be more conspicuous on DBT compared with DM. Additionally, superimposed tissue can obscure margins on DM, which makes it more challenging for the radiologist to confirm the benign nature of the lymph node. DBT images can more frequently provide clear visualization of lymph node margins, reducing the need for recall. Fig. 6.7 shows an asymmetry on DM confirmed to be an intramammary lymph node on DBT and ultrasound.

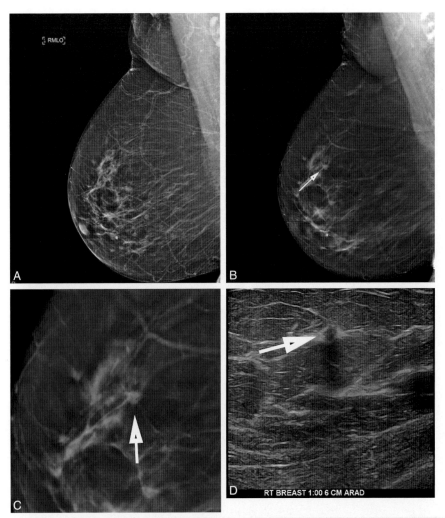

Fig. 6.5 A patient whose cancer is visible only on DBT. (A) MLO view DM image appears normal. Cancer is occult on standard 2D image. (B) DBT reveals a mass with spiculated margins in the upper right breast (*arrow*). (C) Electronically magnified DBT image of the mass (*arrow*). (D) Ultrasound image shows hypoechoic irregular mass (*arrow*) corresponding to the mammographic finding. Pathology demonstrated grade 1 invasive ductal carcinoma.

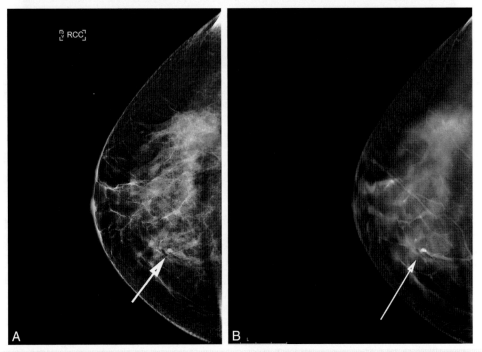

Fig. 6.6 Vessel turn simulating a mass on DM. (A) CC view DM image shows a small mass in the inner breast (*arrow*). (B) DBT image demonstrates the mass is a vessel turn (*arrow*) and does not need to be recalled.

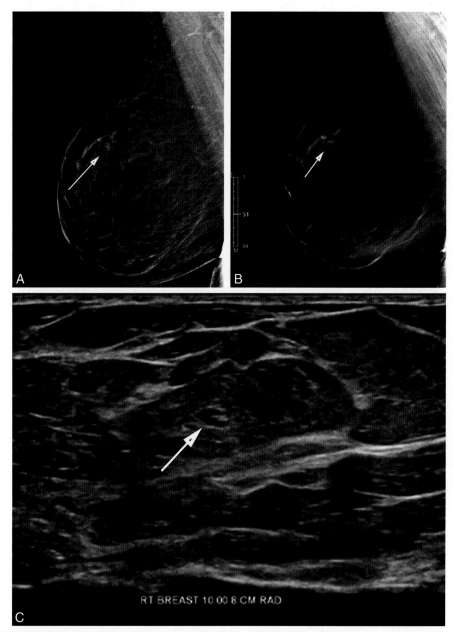

Fig. 6.7 Lymph node demonstrated on DBT. (A) MLO view DM image shows an asymmetry (*arrow*) in the upper right breast that cannot be clearly identified as a lymph node. (B) DBT image shows a fatty hilum characteristic of an intramammary lymph node (*arrow*). (C) Targeted ultrasound shows a normal intramammary lymph node (*arrow*) corresponding to the asymmetry identified on the mammogram.

Superimposed Tissue

Differentiating between true findings within the breast that need further evaluation versus overlapping normal tissue structures can be challenging with DM. However, one of the greatest strengths of DBT is the ability to correctly attribute an asymmetry to normal breast tissue elements such as Cooper ligaments, or vascular structures. Accurately identifying normal superimposed tissue provides ample opportunity for recall reduction as benign asymmetries on DM contribute to a significant number of false-positive recalls.

Decrease in Technical Recalls

Poorly positioned nipples and deodorant artifact are common reasons for technical recalls with DM. However, with DBT, the location of the nipple can be confirmed when it is in focus. Similarly, deodorant or powder artifact often appear as indeterminate, loosely grouped calcifications requiring recall. DBT allows for confirmation that the deodorant artifact is superficial to the skin and not within the breast as illustrated in Fig. 6.8.

Grouped Skin Calcifications

Grouped skin calcifications occasionally can be mistaken for breast calcifications that are suspicious for malignancy. Most of the time, skin calcifications are characteristically benign demonstrating a lucent center. However, occasionally grouped skin calcifications have a heterogeneous morphology making it challenging to diagnose, requiring further imaging to prove their skin location. With DBT the calcification

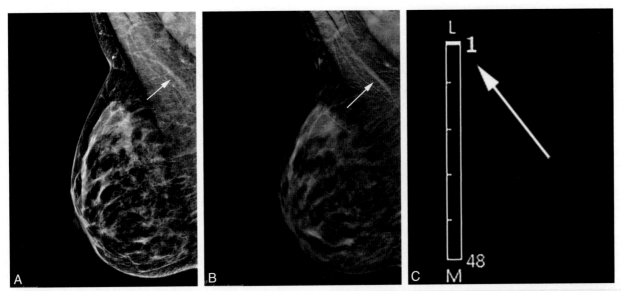

Fig. 6.8 Deodorant artifact. (A) MLO view DM image shows fine bright specs in the axilla that may be perceived as calcifications (*arrow*). (B) DBT image demonstrating that the "calcifications" (*arrow*) represent material on the skin, compatible with deodorant artifact. (C) Slice indicator demonstrating the bright specs are sharpest in the first slice. This patient does not need to be recalled.

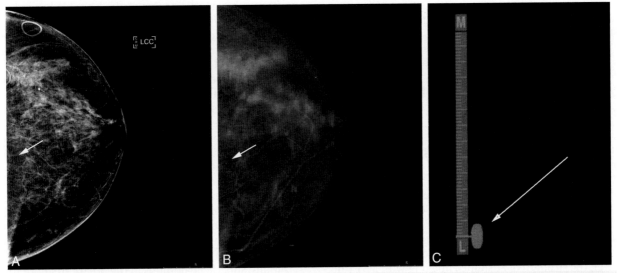

Fig. 6.9 Skin calcifications. (A) CC view DM image demonstrating indeterminate grouped calcifications in the posterior inner left breast (*arrow*). (B) DBT image demonstrating the calcifications in focus (*arrow*). (C) Corresponding slice indicator for image in B demonstrates that calcifications are in focus on the first slice adjacent to the detector confirming that they are in the skin. This patient does not need to be recalled.

location is easily determined, and if they are located within the first or last few slices of the reconstructed images, their skin location is confirmed. Fig. 6.9 shows an example of grouped calcifications localized to the skin based on DBT.

However, it is important to understand that not all skin calcifications are located in the first or last few slices of the DBT reconstructed slices. Some manufacturers reconstruct the images including and beyond the compression paddle. This is to avoid a potential inherent error in calibration of the machine and measurement of the precise thickness of the breast. If the breast thickness is under measured, it would result in exclusion of data in the reconstructed slices. However, these "extra" slices make it somewhat difficult to determine the skin location on the side of the breast

touching the compression paddle (Fig. 6.10). If the machine is calibrated perfectly, skin calcifications will be in focus at least 5 mm deeper than the last slice. Additionally, if the calcifications are located within skin that is not touching either the compression paddle or the detector, the calcifications will appear to be deeper within the tissue. Finally, skin calcifications in the anterior breast may appear deeper in the breast because the compression paddle flexes anteriorly to accommodate a thinner breast. The computer algorithm generating the reconstructed slices is parallel to the detector and will reconstruct above the breast at thinner portions. Location of calcifications within the skin can be confirmed using tangential views as described in Chapter 13: Organized Approach to Diagnostic Imaging.

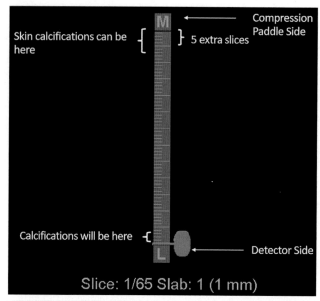

Slice: 1/65 Slab: 1 (1 mm)

Fig. 6.10 Skin calcifications can be seen on slices deeper than first or last slice in DBT reconstructed stack. Scroll bar shows five extra slices (65 slices) compared with the actual breast compressed thickness of 6 cm (which would span 60 slices, each 1-mm thick). Possible slices where skin calcifications may be seen are annotated next to the scroll bar. Suspected skin calcifications can be evaluated using the tangential view technique as described in Chapter 13: Organized Approach to Diagnostic Imaging.

Incident Versus Prevalent Screening With DBT

With the initial round of DBT screening (prevalent screen) where cancer detection is the primary advantage, studies have shown only modest decreases in recall. This is primarily due to the initial identification of both benign and malignant findings that were not previously evident with DM. Increasing detection of benign findings will contribute to increased recall, negating the benefits of improved characterization of findings at the time of screening with DBT. However, the strength of sustained imaging with DBT (incident screens) will shift the benefit more toward recall reduction. Both cancer and benign mass detection will slowly approach baseline levels (contributing to increased recall) while the ability to dismiss superimposed tissue and other benign findings will become more evident.

Special Considerations

Although DBT can be very helpful to generally localize findings in the breast, there are certain scenarios where DBT may mislead the radiologist (Box 6.4).

First, as with DM, the standard screening views with DBT are not orthogonal views. One must remember to apply triangulation principles when localizing findings using DBT. For example, lateral findings on the CC view will reside lower on the true lateral view compared with the MLO view. Conversely, medial lesions on the CC view will be identified more superiorly on the true lateral view compared with the

---

> **Box 6.4   Considerations for Localizing Findings With Digital Breast Tomosynthesis (DBT)**
>
> - Craniocaudal (CC) scroll bar slice indicator reflects the position on the lateral view, not the mediolateral oblique (MLO) view
> - The center of the breast is not always in the center of the scroll bar
> - Anterior lesions will be compressed closer to the detector because of paddle flex
> - Superficial lesions can move between views because of breast repositioning

MLO view. When a finding is identified on the CC view with DBT, the slice indicator on the scroll bar will reflect the position of the finding on the true lateral view, not the location on the oblique view, that is, the scroll bar location indicates the location of the finding on the orthogonal projection (not oblique view) of the original view. Therefore the scroll bar location on the CC view and the location of the finding in the MLO view may be inconsistent.

The second reason why the scroll bar may appear inaccurate is that the true center of the breast may not be in the center of the scroll bar. In a perfectly uniform, perfectly positioned breast, the center of the breast is located in the exact center of the scroll bar. However, due to inconsistencies with positioning and nonuniform breast thicknesses, findings that are located in the center of the breast may be in focus toward one end or the other on the scroll bar. This can be confirmed easily when the nipple is in focus on an extreme end of the scroll bar. In this scenario, the nipple can then be used as the reference for the center of the breast (rather than the center of the scroll bar).

The third reason why the scroll bar may mislead the radiologist is because the compression paddle flexes anteriorly, leading to greater compression near the nipple compared with the posterior aspect of the breast, which often includes the pectoralis muscle. Findings, therefore, will localize closer to the detector on the scroll bar in the anterior breast. This is because the true thickness of the breast is less than the fixed scrollbar length where it displays the measurement of the thickest portion of the breast.

Finally, superficial findings in the breast are more susceptible to movement and will occasionally appear in different quadrants when the breast is repositioned between views.

KEY POINTS

- Multiple low-dose images are taken of the breast to generate the digital breast tomosynthesis (DBT) reconstructed slices. The number of images taken are not dependent on the breast thickness.
- Digital mammography (DM) + DBT combined exposure is less than the FDA limit and is considered safe. However, synthetic imaging is available to further reduce the dose.
- Higher resolution synthetic imaging has improved appearance compared with older versions but has a cost of larger file sizes and slower reconstruction times.
- DBT improves cancer detection while simultaneously decreasing false-positive recalls.
- The initial benefit of DBT will be weighted toward improved cancer detection (prevalent screen). As

patients are imaged subsequently each year with DBT (incident screen), the benefits will shift toward decreased recall.
- Skin calcifications touching the detector or compression paddle will be located in the first or last few slices of the reconstructed images. However, not all skin calcifications are seen within the first or last few slices.
- The craniocaudal (CC) scroll bar slice indicator reflects the position of the finding on the orthogonal (lateral) view not the mediolateral oblique (MLO) view.

Suggested Readings

Friedewald SM, Rafferty EA, Rose SL, et al. Breast cancer screening using tomosynthesis in combination with digital mammography. *JAMA*. 2014 Jun 25;311(24):2499–2507.

Friedewald SM, Young VA, Gupta D. Lesion localization using the scroll bar on tomosynthesis: why doesn't it always work? *Clin Imaging*. 2018 Jan–Feb;47:57–64.

Korhonen KE, Conant EF, Cohen EA, Synnestvedt M, McDonald ES, Weinstein SP. Breast cancer conspicuity on simultaneously acquired digital mammographic images versus digital breast tomosynthesis images. *Radiology*. 2019 07;292(1):69–76.

Korhonen KE, Weinstein SP, McDonald ES, Conant EF. Strategies to increase cancer detection: review of true-positive and false-negative results at digital breast tomosynthesis screening. *Radiographics*. 2016;36:1954–1965.

Lee CH, Destounis SV, Friedewald SM, Newell, MS. Digital Breast Tomosynthesis (DBT) Guidance (A supplement to ACR BI-RADS® Mammography 2013) July 2019.

Ray KM, Turner E, Sickles EA, Joe BN. Suspicious findings at digital breast tomosynthesis occult to conventional digital mammography: imaging features and pathology findings. *Breast J*. 2015;21(5):538–542.

Tirada N, Li G, Dreizin D, et al. Digital Breast Tomosynthesis: Physics, Artifacts, and Quality Control Considerations. Radiographics: a review publication of the Radiological Society of North America, Inc. 39(2):413–426.

7 Mammographic and Ultrasound-Guided Breast Biopsy Procedures

KANAE KAWAI MIYAKE, ANDREW N. KOZLOV, CHRISTINE S. LO, AND DEBRA M. IKEDA

OVERVIEW *This chapter covers percutaneous mammographic- and ultrasound-guided breast needle biopsies, preoperative needle/wire and wireless localization, specimen radiography, and pathology correlation. Magnetic resonance imaging (MRI)-guided breast procedures are covered in Chapter 8: Breast MRI Indications, Interpretation, Interventions.*

Image-Guided Breast Biopsy

Image-guided percutaneous biopsy of breast lesions is an important part of breast imaging services and the current standard of care approach for obtaining tissue diagnosis. Advantages of percutaneous biopsy are that it provides a tissue diagnosis with minimal patient trauma and guides patient management and follow-up, including definitive surgery when appropriate. Surgical excisional biopsy for breast lesion diagnosis is extremely uncommon and is reserved for special scenarios when image-guided percutaneous biopsy is not feasible or inconclusive. The American College of Radiology (ACR) *Practice Parameters and Accreditation* for breast interventional procedures guidance documents are a useful reference and available on their website https://www.acr.org/.[1–3]

PREBIOPSY PATIENT WORKUP

To plan safe, accurate image-guided biopsy of breast lesions, first ensure that there has been a complete imaging workup. Do not attempt to biopsy a breast lesion if you have not confirmed it is real or if you do not know its location in the breast. For mammography, the lesion is ideally seen in craniocaudal (CC) and mediolateral (ML) or lateromedial (LM) orthogonal views. If finding is not seen on orthogonal CC and 90-degree lateral views, additional imaging (tomosynthesis, oblique views, mammograms with skin markers, ultrasound [US]) is done to ensure the lesion is real and to determine its location in the breast. Details of diagnostic workup are covered in Chapter 13: Organized Approach to Diagnostic Imaging.

Safe breast biopsies require that the patient is able to cooperate and hold still during the procedure, has no allergies to medications used during the procedure, is able to follow postbiopsy instructions that limit bleeding/infection, and will be compliant with postbiopsy follow-up (Box 7.1).

Breast Lesion Labeling

Breast lesions for which biopsy is recommended should be clearly indicated in the diagnostic report. According to Breast Imaging Reporting and Data System (BI-RADS) (D'Orsi CJ et al., 2013), a description of mammographic lesion location includes side (right or left breast), quadrant, and depth of lesion. Depth is divided into anterior, middle,

and posterior thirds. Including clockface location and distance from the nipple provides a more complete description of the lesion location. For US lesions, clockface location and distance from the nipple should be used. If more than one lesion is seen in the same US image frame, BI-RADS suggests adding a measurement of the distance from skin surface to center of lesion or its anterior aspect to help differentiate one lesion from another. Individual practices may also choose a standard numbering system or image annotation system when there are multiple lesions in the same breast.

INFORMED CONSENT AND PROCEDURAL RISKS

Informed consent is an important part of any procedure (Box 7.2). For percutaneous needle biopsy, the patient is informed of the risks, benefits, and alternatives to percutaneous biopsy (e.g., surgical biopsy) and the alternative's risks and benefits. Percutaneous breast biopsy is a safe, minimally invasive procedure. Potential risks include bleeding, infection, and need for further intervention such as repeat biopsy or surgical excision. Additional risks include unsuccessful biopsy (e.g., due to technical limitations or poor target visualization) and postbiopsy marker displacement or nondeployment. While it is common to have a small hematoma after biopsy, complications such as a significant hematoma or significant bleeding requiring surgical intervention

---

Box 7.1   Requirements for Image-Guided Breast Biopsy

Lesion is real

Lesion can be localized within the breast by mammography, tomosynthesis, ultrasound, or magnetic resonance imaging (MRI)

Lesion can be accessed safely and accurately

Patient can cooperate and hold still during the procedure

Patient is not allergic to medications used in the biopsy procedure

Blood thinning medications have been avoided if possible (biopsy may still be done with patient on anticoagulants if not reasonable to stop anticoagulation)

Patient can follow postbiopsy instructions to diminish bleeding and other complications

Patient will comply with postbiopsy imaging or surgical follow-up

---

Box 7.2	**Breast Procedural Risks**

Hematoma (common but rarely significant)
Untoward bleeding (very rarely needing surgical intervention)
Vasovagal reaction (safety concern if the procedure is done with the patient upright)
Inability to complete the needle biopsy for technical reasons
Not obtaining the target or undersampling of target even if the biopsy is performed
Postbiopsy marker clip migrated from biopsy site or marker does not deploy
Rare complications:
- Infection (with rare mastitis)
- Pneumothorax
- Pseudoaneurysm formation
- Implant rupture
- Milk fistula (if the patient is pregnant or nursing)

Possible need for surgical excision after needle biopsy for following reasons:
- Benign discordant lesion
- High-risk lesion
- Malignancy

---

are rare. Also rare are complications of infection/mastitis, pneumothorax, and pseudoaneurysm formation. Other unusual complications include implant rupture in patients with implants and milk fistula in patients who are lactating. If a rare complication is a possibility, then patient should be specifically consented for the rare event as appropriate.

For needle localization procedures on the day of surgery, the surgeon typically obtains informed consent for the surgical procedure and discusses the need for localization while the radiologist typically obtains informed consent for the localization procedure itself.

It is not uncommon that even after a thorough workup, US, magnetic resonance imaging (MRI), and mammographic findings may not be one and the same. In these cases, the patient should be informed and consented for the possibility that a second biopsy might be needed. As an example, a second biopsy would be needed if the marker placed in a lesion biopsied by one modality does not correlate with expected findings on the second modality. Specifically, a stereotactic biopsy would be needed if a mass biopsied under US does not correlate with a mammographic mass on the postbiopsy mammogram.

In addition, patients should be asked about allergies to medications used during the procedure. If postbiopsy markers or wireless fiducials are to be placed, the patient should be asked about allergies to metals and about allergies to bovine or porcine products (if the marker contains these products).

COMPLICATIONS—SPECIFIC SCENARIOS

Vasovagal reaction: For mammographic-guided presurgical needle wire/wireless localization performed on the day of surgery, vasovagal reactions are not infrequent because the patient is fasting and dehydrated. In the case of a vasovagal reaction, the patient's breast should be promptly released from mammographic compression (and any needles removed) and the patient safely placed in a supine position.

Ideally, patients who are sitting upright for the procedure may have their procedure chair reclined into a supine position without moving the patient. The patient should never be left alone during a procedure.

Bleeding: Bleeding is usually well-managed after breast biopsy via manual compression and does not pose a significant risk. The radiologist works with the patient's referring provider to determine whether any anticoagulation medication such as Coumadin (warfarin), heparin, or Plavix (clopidogrel) may be safely curtailed in order to reduce the risk of bleeding. If anticoagulation cannot be safely discontinued or bridged, biopsy may still be performed with expectation that there may be more bleeding and a need to hold pressure longer after the procedure (Melotti and Berg, 2000). In these cases, the radiologist may choose a smaller-gauge biopsy device and may apply a pressure dressing after the procedure to minimize hematoma risk. Some practices may instruct patients to stop taking all pain medications except for acetaminophen for 1 week before the biopsy because aspirin, nonsteroidal antiinflammatory drugs (NSAIDs), and other medications can inactivate platelets. Other practices do not have this restriction.

Pneumothorax: Pneumothorax is a rare complication of breast procedures. Pneumothorax can be prevented by ensuring needles are positioned parallel to chest wall. Steps to prevent pneumothorax during US-guided biopsy procedures are presented in Box 7.3. The risk of pneumothorax increases if the patient is unable to hold still or is coughing, if the angle needed to biopsy the lesion is very steep, if the lesion is on the chest wall, and if the lesion lies between ribs. When there is a possibility of pneumothorax during the biopsy, the radiologist obtains informed consent from the patient specifically for the possibility that the needle could puncture the lung and result in the need for an emergency room visit and possible stay in the hospital, which is very unusual.

Box 7.3	**Steps to Prevent Pneumothorax During Ultrasound-Guided Procedures**

Never aim the needle at the chest wall!
Roll/position patient so chest wall is parallel to needle trajectory (Fig. 7.6A–D)
Plan needle trajectory parallel to chest wall
Take into account needle trajectory/"throw" distance and tissue beyond the mass
Always visualize the entire needle shaft and needle tip by ultrasound before sampling
If you do not see the entire needle shaft and the tip, the needle is foreshortened; rescan until you see them
If unable to approach lesion parallel to chest wall, consider advancing needle with trough open and through mass with or without a coaxial needle (Fig. 7.2A but advance the needle with trough open)
Consider advancing coaxial system through mass and uncovering open needle trough (Fig. 7.3B)
Inject lidocaine below the mass (Fig. 7.6E)
Place needle into mass and lift mass away from chest wall (Fig. 7.6F)
If the biopsy is unsafe, do preoperative localization and remove the finding at surgery

Skin Sterilization, Local Anesthesia, and Skin Nicks

Most facilities routinely administer local anesthesia before percutaneous needle biopsy or preoperative localization with a 25- or 21-gauge skin injection needle. A common local anesthetic for breast biopsies is 1% lidocaine with or without epinephrine. Before giving local anesthesia, the radiologist sterilizes the breast skin with a cleansing agent, for example chlorhexidine, alcohol, or iodine-based cleansing agent. The maximum dose of 1% lidocaine with epinephrine is 7 mg/kg (3.5 mg/lb) body weight, not to exceed 500 mg. This translates to 50 mL in a 70-kg patient. The maximum dose of 1% lidocaine without epinephrine is 4.5 mg/kg (2 mg/lb), not to exceed 300 mg. This translates to 30 mL in a 70-kg patient.

To facilitate insertion of the larger needles used for core needle biopsy, a small skin nick usually is made with a scalpel. A skin nick usually is not needed for insertion of localizing wire/wireless needles for preoperative localizations.

Fine-Needle Aspiration and Core Biopsy Techniques

Percutaneous breast biopsy may be performed by fine-needle aspiration or using automated (spring-loaded) core or vacuum-assisted core biopsy techniques. The three main types of needles and scenarios in which they are commonly used are summarized in Table 7.1.

FINE NEEDLE ASPIRATION

Fine-needle aspiration (FNA) needles, usually 25- to 20-gauge, are used for cyst aspirations and for solid breast masses and axillary lymph nodes. The aspirated material requires interpretation by expert cytopathologists. FNA is usually done with US or palpation guidance with one or more needle passes using an in-and-out motion of the needle at each pass. FNA is less commonly done in the United States compared with Europe and Asia. An advantage of FNA is the availability of a preliminary, immediate interpretation of malignancy. A disadvantage of FNA is that it cannot distinguish invasive disease from ductal carcinoma in situ (DCIS). There is also potential for a nondiagnostic biopsy due to insufficient material.

AUTOMATED CORE BIOPSY

Automated core needles in 18- to 14-gauge diameters (Fig. 7.1A–B) commonly are used to biopsy masses using US or palpation guidance. In some facilities, especially outside the United States, automated core needles are used with stereotactic guidance to biopsy masses or calcifications. An automated core biopsy needle obtains a single specimen with each pass of the needle, and the needle is removed from the breast after each biopsy and then reinserted for the next sample. Because separate, repetitive insertions are required for each sample, a coaxial device (trocar and sheath) may be used to gain repeated access to the lesion, especially with US. Multiple core specimens are obtained by reinserting and refiring the needle. Each specimen is between 15 and 22 mm long depending on the needle and width, and the width depends on the needle gauge. The weight of the individual specimens is about 17 mg with 14-gauge automated cores, 37 mg with 14-gauge vacuum, 95 mg with 11-gauge vacuum, and 120 mg with 9-gauge vacuum biopsy devices. Pathologists who are comfortable interpreting surgically excised breast biopsy tissue can interpret this type of histologic material.

VACUUM-ASSISTED CORE BIOPSY

Directional 7- to 14-gauge diameter vacuum-assisted (vacuum) needles (see Fig. 7.1C) are used for stereotactic/tomosynthesis-guided, US-guided, and MRI-guided biopsies. Depending on the manufacturer, vacuum biopsy can be performed with a single insertion and multiple specimens obtained in a rotational fashion or may require repeated insertions obtaining one sample at a time. Specimens are obtained by placing the needle trough at or in the target by imaging guidance. The external part of the needle remains stationary outside of the breast while the cutting part of the needle extracts the samples inside the breast and then vacuums them out to an external collecting chamber. The radiologist points the vacuuming aperture at the target or rotates the aperture within the lesion. Vacuum-assisted devices have the advantage of obtaining larger samples than automated core biopsy samples, leading to greater confidence in the diagnosis. For stereotactic or tomosynthesis guided biopsy, 6 to 12 specimens are usually obtained, whereas fewer samples are obtained with US because US allows real-time visualization to ensure the target is sampled. Some facilities use vacuum-assisted needles to completely remove/excise benign lesions such as fibroadenomas.

All single-insertion and multiinsertion needles can be used with or without coaxial guides (Fig. 7.2). The coaxial device consists of an inner sharp stylet and an outer sheath, and provides a needle path to the target that the radiologist can use repeatedly without reinsertion through the breast

Table 7.1 Needles Used for Percutaneous Breast Biopsies

Needle Type	Gauge	Biopsy Use
Fine-needle aspiration	25- to 20-gauge	Cyst aspiration. Solid mass if highly likely to be specific benign diagnosis (ex fibroadenoma). Alternative to core biopsy of axillary lymph nodes or in patients at increased risk of bleeding. Solid mass if primary question is proving additional site of malignancy.
Automated core (includes spring-loaded core devices)	18- to 14-gauge	Ultrasound-guided biopsy. Uncommon for stereotactic biopsy in the United States but used elsewhere in the world.
Vacuum-assisted	14- to 7-gauge	Stereotactic and magnetic resonance imaging (MRI) biopsy. Ultrasound-guided biopsy alternative to automated core biopsy.

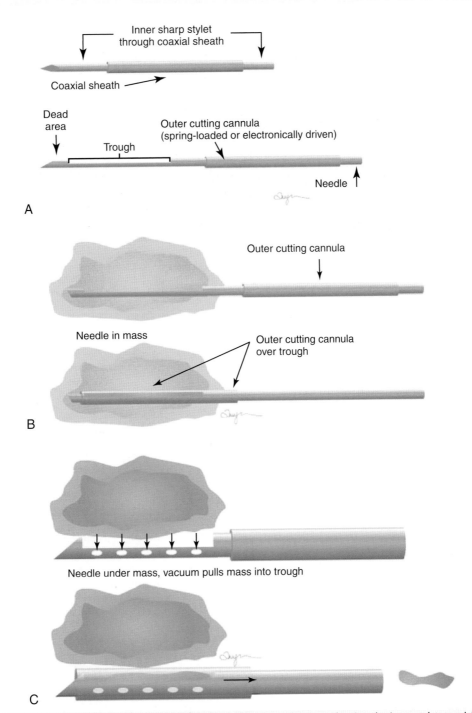

Fig. 7.1 Schematics of needle biopsy systems. (A) Schematic of core biopsy needle parts, showing the inner stylet, coaxial sheath, and needle. (B) Schematic of how to use a multifire core biopsy needle for breast biopsies. The outer cutting cannula shoots over the trough and cuts the mass. The entire needle is removed each time. (C) Schematic of a vacuum-assisted probe for needle core biopsy. The outer cutting cannula shoots over the trough and cuts the mass. The vacuum transports the specimen to the needle end for removal. There may be one or multiple insertions, depending on the vendor.

tissue. The radiologist places the coaxial device through the breast tissue so that the stylet tip/sheath edge is at or in the lesion. Then the radiologist removes the stylet, leaving a sheath "tunnel" through the breast tissue directly to the lesion. The radiologist can repeatedly place the biopsy needle through the sheath into the lesion and take samples without having to disturb the surrounding breast tissue. Coaxial biopsies are done with the sheath near the mass so the needle can fire through the mass (Fig. 7.3A) or the sheath placed through the mass so that the open trough

of the needle may be uncovered for sampling while inside the mass (Fig. 7.3B). This technique is especially helpful for lesions at the chest wall.

CYST ASPIRATION

Mammographic masses often prompt requests for breast US-guided aspiration to see if the mass is a cyst. To do a cyst aspiration, the radiologist advances a fine needle into the cyst and aspirates the fluid under real-time US guidance

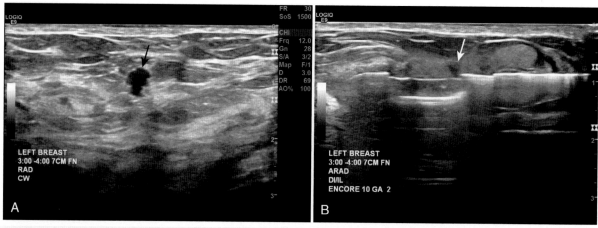

Fig. 7.2 A 51-year-old woman with a 5-mm mass for vacuum-assisted ultrasound biopsy. (A) Ultrasound shows 5 mm irregular hypoechoic mass (*arrow*) in the 4 o'clock position of the breast. (B) Single ultrasound image shows the mass (*arrow*) in the biopsy trough. Vacuum-assisted needle has been placed adjacent to the mass and draws the mass into the vacuum-needle biopsy trough. Then the outer cutting cannula is fired, obtaining the sample into the trough as the vacuum continues to draw tissue into the trough (not shown). Pathology showed usual ductal hyperplasia columnar change and apocrine metaplasia.

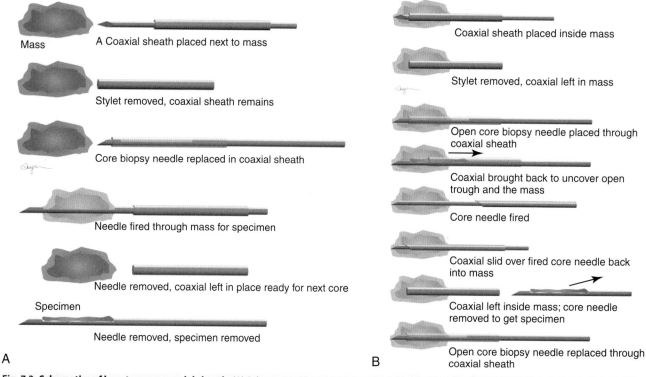

Fig. 7.3 Schematics of how to use a coaxial sheath. (A) Schematic of how to use a coaxial sheath next to a mass for ultrasound-guided core biopsies. The radiologist places a coaxial containing a sharp, inner stylet through the breast tissue next to a mass. The radiologist removes the stylet, places a core biopsy needle through the coaxial sheath, fires the needle through the mass, and withdraws the needle. The coaxial sheath is left adjacent to the mass, providing a tunnel through the breast tissue. The radiologist removes the specimen from the needle and can replace the needle through the coaxial sheath for the next core. (B) Schematic of how to use a coaxial sheath inside a mass for ultrasound-guided core biopsies. The radiologist places a coaxial containing a sharp, inner stylet into a mass. The radiologist removes the stylet, places an open core biopsy needle through the coaxial sheath, withdraws the coaxial to expose the biopsy trough inside the mass, and fires the needle to take the sample. Before withdrawing the biopsy needle, the radiologist threads the coaxial sheath over the fired needle and leaves the sheath inside the mass. The core biopsy needle can now be replaced into the sheath to take the next sample.

until the cyst disappears (Fig. 7.4). Cyst aspiration also can be done by mammography guidance using a fenestrated compression plate and mammography.

If the cyst fluid is clear, yellow, blue or green, it is considered normal and is discarded. Cytologic evaluation of

cyst fluid is recommended if the fluid is bloody or if there was an intracystic mass seen on the US. If fluid is sent for cytologic evaluation, a biopsy marker should be placed for future localization purposes if needed. If there is an intracystic mass, core biopsy or FNA biopsy of the mass

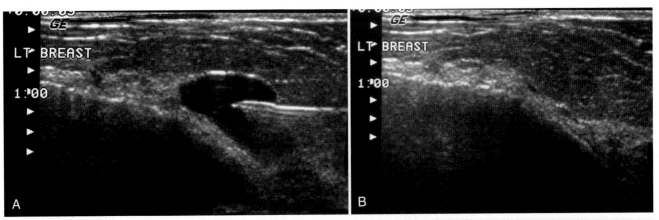

Fig. 7.4 Cyst aspiration. (A) Ultrasound shows a needle in a cyst near an implant. (B) The follow-up ultrasound shows that the cyst is gone.

should be performed under US guidance instead of cyst aspiration.

A *pneumocystogram* is a mammogram obtained after a radiologist injects air into a cyst cavity following cyst aspiration. The pneumocystogram of an air-filled cyst cavity on the mammogram proves that any mass prompting biopsy on the mammogram corresponds to the aspirated cyst (Fig. 7.5). A normal pneumocystogram should show an air-filled, thin-walled, round, or oval cavity without intracystic solid masses or mural nodules. This procedure is rarely performed if breast US is available.

It is important to obtain postaspiration mammograms after US-guided cyst aspirations to determine whether the mammographic mass (presumed cyst) disappears. If the mass persists on the postaspiration mammogram, the aspirated cyst is not the mammographic correlate and the mammographic mass needs further investigation and potentially a stereotactic biopsy.

PALPATION-GUIDED PERCUTANEOUS NEEDLE BIOPSY

FNA or core biopsy can be performed on palpable masses. There is no visualization of the lesion or needle during the biopsy, which is guided by palpation alone. The physician places a needle into the lesion under palpation guidance. The lesion must be discreetly palpable and well away from the chest wall for the biopsy to be done with accuracy and safety. This procedure is usually reserved for cysts and solid masses that are almost definitely malignant or benign by imaging and palpation criteria. Because there is no imaging guidance, palpation-guided biopsy may be performed by the breast surgeon, pathologist, or other physician.

ULTRASOUND-GUIDED PERCUTANEOUS NEEDLE BIOPSY

US-guided biopsy uses readily available equipment, is well-tolerated by patients, and is cost-effective. In the diagnostic setting, US is often used for palpable lumps and to evaluate mammographic masses and asymmetries. Correlating a mass seen at US to the mammographic mass can be tricky since the mass may move quite a bit from the upright

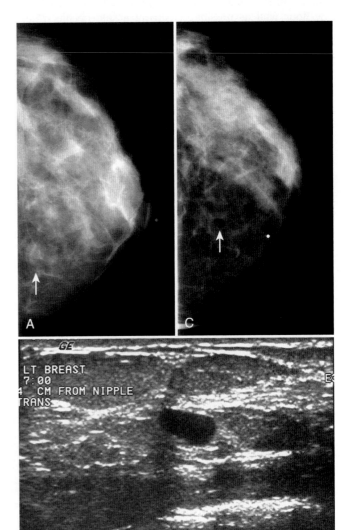

Fig. 7.5 Pneumocystogram. (A) A craniocaudal (CC) mammogram shows an oval breast mass in the inner portion of the breast. (B) Ultrasound shows a complicated cyst versus a solid oval mass. After cyst aspiration under ultrasound guidance, air was placed in the cyst cavity. (C) CC pneumocystogram mammogram shows air (*arrow*) replacing fluid in the mass, which confirms that the finding on the mammogram represents a cyst that was aspirated.

mammogram to the supine US image. This is because the breast falls dependently onto the chest wall when the patient lies down in supine position for the US examination. Thus one can understand why the mass looks far away from the chest wall on the upright compressed mammogram but lies next to the pectoralis muscle on the US (Fig. 7.6).

Pneumothorax is an important, preventable complication of US-guided biopsy. Unlike upright or prone mammography-guided procedures, supine US-guided biopsies may not have needle trajectories parallel to the chest wall. Further complicating matters, some core biopsy needles "throw" the needle tip 2.5 cm further into the tissue from its initial position. Thus, planning a safe US needle biopsy trajectory must take into account the needle tip, the needle "throw" trajectory, and the tissue beyond the tip (see Box 7.3).

To perform a safe procedure, the radiologist rolls the patient on the table so that the chest wall is as parallel to the floor wall as possible, ensuring a safe needle trajectory through the mass that does not angle steeply toward the lungs. Patient positioning can take some time, but

it is worth the few minutes to position the patient so that the biopsy is safe. One way to keep the needle away from the chest wall is to inject anesthetic or saline underneath the targeted mass to lift it away from the pectoralis muscle. Alternatively, the radiologist may insert the biopsy needle tip into the mass to lift it into a safer trajectory before firing the needle (Fig. 7.7). Yet another technique is to insert a needle that does not require a throw and opens inside the mass to sample it. If the mass cannot be biopsied safely, the mass should be localized and excised.

For US-guided FNA, the radiologist introduces a needle in the plane of the transducer axis to show the entire shaft of the needle, its tip, and the lesion. Once the needle is within the lesion, the radiologist aspirates the mass with a vigorous to-and-fro movement to obtain material for cytologic evaluation and then withdraws the needle (Fig. 7.8). Ideally, the material should be analyzed immediately so that additional passes may be obtained as needed to ensure adequate cellular material for diagnosis. After aspiration, direct pressure is applied to the biopsy site to obtain hemostasis. Depending

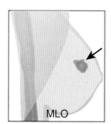
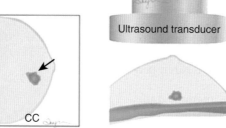
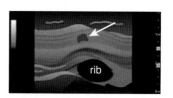

MLO   CC

A   Patient is upright on mammogram, mass compressed away from chest wall

Supine patient, the mass drops down toward the chest wall

Ultrasound shows mass near chest wall

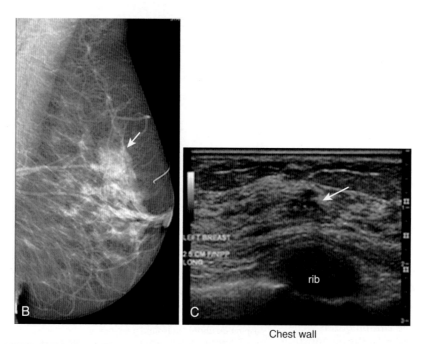

Chest wall

Fig. 7.6 Masses appearing to be far away from the chest wall on mammography may be found near the chest wall on ultrasound. (A) Schematic mammograms show a mass in the upper inner quadrant that appears to be far from the chest wall. However, mammograms are obtained with compression with patient in upright position; when the patient lies supine, the mass falls dependently against the chest wall. On ultrasound, the mass may be closer to the chest wall than expected from the mammogram. (B–C) A representative example case. Left mediolateral oblique (MLO) mammogram (B) shows a mass (*arrow*) appearing to be far away from the chest wall, but the corresponding ultrasound (C) shows the mass (*arrow*) near the chest wall.

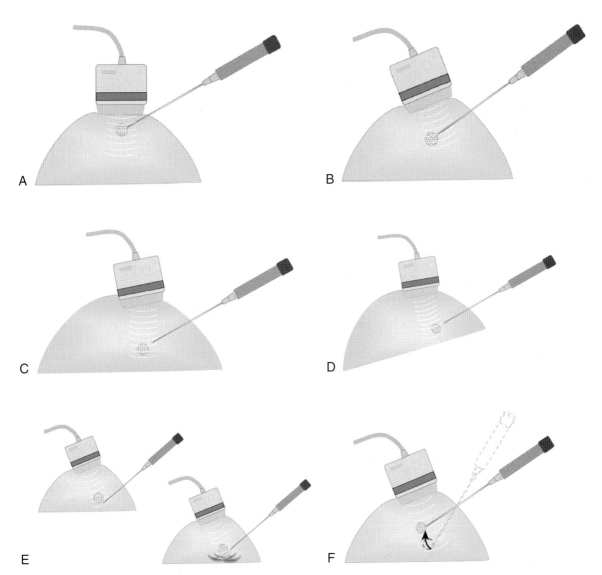

Fig. 7.7 Schematics of how to keep the needle tip away from the chest wall on ultrasound-guided core biopsy. (A) With superficial lesions, the needle tip and throw are usually far away from the chest wall. (B) With deeper lesions, the needle angle is steeper, and the radiologist judges whether the needle "throw" will penetrate the lung. (C) When the patient is flat and the lesion is even deeper, the needle trajectory can point toward the chest wall (risking pneumothorax). (D) To change the needle trajectory, the patient can be angled so that the chest wall parallels the needle track/throw. (E) Injecting anesthetic underneath the lesion can lift it away from the chest wall for biopsy. (F) Inserting the needle tip into the lesion and redirecting the throw of the needle avoids placing the needle tip into the chest wall. (Courtesy Dr. Sunita Pal, Stanford Radiology, Stanford, CA.)

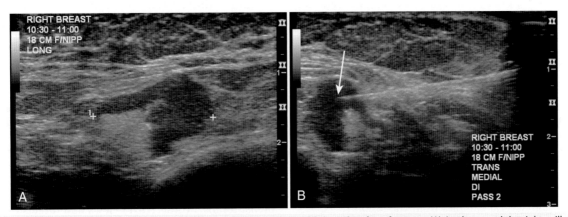

Fig. 7.8 Fine-needle aspiration of axillary lymphadenopathy in a patient with invasive ductal cancer. (A) At ultrasound the right axillary lymph node (marked by calipers) has an irregular, thickened cortex and a compressed fatty hilum. (B) Ultrasound shows the fine-needle tip (*arrow*) in the lymph node cortex. Cytology showed metastatic disease from invasive ductal cancer.

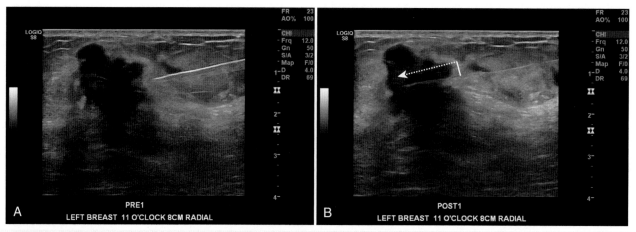

Fig. 7.9 Illustration of automated core biopsy needle "throw." A 53-year-old woman with invasive ductal cancer. (A) Ultrasound in the prefire position shows automated core biopsy needle with the tip adjacent to the mass. (B) Postfire ultrasound shows the needle through the mass. Note that the needle tip has traversed through the mass (*dashed arrow indicates distance of "throw" from prefire position*). This biopsy device automatically opens the trough, cuts the sample and recloses the trough; thus the trough is not seen.

on the clinical scenario, a marker may also be placed into the lesion after FNA biopsy.

To perform an automated core biopsy under US guidance, the radiologist localizes the lesion by US and chooses the course of needle insertion that offers the most accuracy and safety. While anesthetizing the core biopsy track under direct US guidance, the radiologist uses the anesthesia needle to get an idea of how dense the breast tissue feels and to see the needle trajectory. The radiologist calculates the core needle throw to determine where to place the core needle tip "prefire" so the core trough will be in the middle of the lesion "postfire" (Fig. 7.9). The radiologist also takes care that the postfire needle trajectory does not damage vital structures or produce a pneumothorax.

Then, under direct US visualization, the radiologist introduces the automated core biopsy needle into the breast. If the lesion is large enough, the radiologist introduces the needle tip into the edge of the lesion to hold it in place. The radiologist may then push the needle through the mass with the trough open for sampling. Otherwise, the radiologist may choose to fire the needle through the mass with or without a coaxial system (Fig. 7.10). In all cases, the radiologist fires the biopsy core needle under direct visualization and removes the needle each time to harvest the cores. Optimally, three to six tissue specimens are obtained from different parts of the mass. After sampling, the radiologist places a marker into the mass, removes the needle, and applies manual pressure for hemostasis. After hemostasis is established, the technologist bandages the wound and takes orthogonal mammograms to show the marker and any residual mass (if mammographically visible).

A vacuum biopsy is similar to an automated core biopsy, but the vacuum needle is usually placed under or inside the lesion. The probe "vacuums" tissue into the trough, cuts a sample, and carries it to a container outside the breast so that multiple samples can be obtained with one insertion. The radiologist concentrates on aiming the trough at the mass to obtain several samples from the lesion (Figs. 7.2 and 7.11). Afterward, the radiologist places a marker in the lesion. This can be done either through the probe or by using a marker that is inserted via its own separate needle. The vacuum technique carries a special caveat regarding the skin. If the probe is too close to the skin, the skin can be vacuumed into the trough and sampled, causing skin injury requiring a suture or, in extreme cases, a skin graft.

STEREOTACTIC AND TOMOSYNTHESIS-GUIDED PERCUTANEOUS NEEDLE BIOPSY

Stereotactic and tomosynthesis-guided biopsy is performed for suspicious calcifications or for a mass, asymmetry, or architectural distortion seen on mammography or tomosynthesis. Targets for stereotactic biopsy usually are not visualized by US. Stereotactic and tomosynthesis targeting methods use a mammographic compression device with a small aperture and an x-ray tube that has the ability to take either a tomosynthesis view or two stereotactic views plus 15 degrees and minus 15 degrees off perpendicular. Details for optimal technical standards, biopsy and stereotactic accreditation are detailed in the *ACR Practice Parameter for the Performance of Stereotactic-Guided Breast Interventional Procedures* (https://www.acr.org/-/media/ACR/Files/Practice-Parameters/Stereo-Breast.pdf) and the ACR Stereotactic Breast Biopsy Accreditation Program (https://www.acraccreditation.org/modalities/stereotactic-breast-biopsy).

For stereotactic or tomosynthesis biopsy, the patient is placed in a prone, upright, or decubitus position with the breast compressed by a fenestrated compression paddle (Fig. 7.12). The radiologist reviews prebiopsy mammograms to determine the lesion's location on orthogonal views. The breast is then firmly compressed with the compression paddle aperture placed on the skin surface closest to the breast lesion.

After taking a straight-on (0-degree) scout view that visualizes the lesion, the technologist takes two stereo views or a tomosynthesis-view of the lesion (Fig. 7.13). The radiologist locates the lesion on the stereotactic or digital breast tomosynthesis (DBT) views and targets the finding. A computer calculates the X-, Y-, and Z-coordinates from the images and directs a computer connected to a needle on

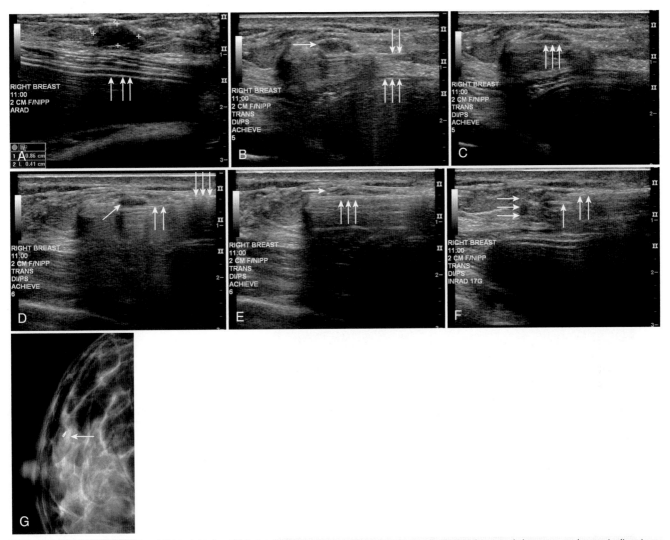

Fig. 7.10 Use of a coaxial system for ultrasound biopsy to core a mass adjacent to an implant. (A) Ultrasound shows an oval mass (*calipers*) on top of a breast implant (*triple arrows*), for which core biopsy was recommended. (B) Ultrasound-guided core biopsy shows the trough of the needle (*double arrows*) traversing an oval mass (*single arrow*) on top of an implant (*triple arrows*). (C) Postfire ultrasound shows the needle traversing the mass. At this point, a coaxial (*triple arrows*) was placed over the needle, securing the needle's original position within the mass. (D) The needle was replaced in the coaxial sheath and the coaxial (*triple arrows*) was withdrawn to expose the trough (*double arrows*) and allow the mass (*single arrow*) to fall within it. (E) Postfire ultrasound with the coaxial sheath extended over the needle shows both the needle and coaxial (*triple arrows*) traversing the mass (*single arrow*). (F) Ultrasound showing a needle threaded through the coaxial sheath (*double arrows*) placing a marker (*single arrow*) in the mass (*triple arrows*). (G) Cropped implant-displaced digital lateral mammogram shows dense tissue and the marker (*arrow*). Histology showed fibroadenoma.

the stereotactic or tomosynthesis unit to these coordinates. After cleaning the skin, the radiologist anesthetizes the skin and the deeper breast tissue at the coordinates and may take repeated views to check the target was not shifted by the local anesthetic. The depth to administer anesthetic should account for the entire length of the sampling aperture and needle tip and not stop at the Z-coordinate (center of the sampling aperture).

After verifying target coordinates, the radiologist passes a needle into the breast to the computer-calculated depth. For stereotactic biopsy, the technologist takes two prefire stereotactic images (see Fig. 7.13) or one tomosynthesis image which should show the tip of the biopsy needle at the edge of the target lesion (Fig. 7.14). The radiologist then fires the needle deeper into the breast and reviews postfire images to ensure that the needle sampling trough is within the breast lesion and samples the target.

Not all targeting in stereotactic or tomosynthesis-core biopsies go smoothly. After firing, the needle may be in the wrong position, for example to the left or the right, above or below, or too deep or too shallow to the target. Fig. 7.15 shows how to direct the needle or adjust needle position to obtain a sample from the target if the needle trough is within or to the side of the lesion. For example, if the target is to the side of the needle and a vacuum device is being used, then the vacuum-sampling trough may be directed toward the target to successfully biopsy the lesion.

The radiologist collects multiple specimens from the lesion. If using an automated core biopsy needle, biopsies are taken from different parts of the lesion and the needle is reinserted each time. If a vacuum needle is used with the needle trough in the center of the lesion, the collection trough of the vacuum needle is rotated 360 degrees to acquire tissue from different parts of the lesion. If the needle trough is at

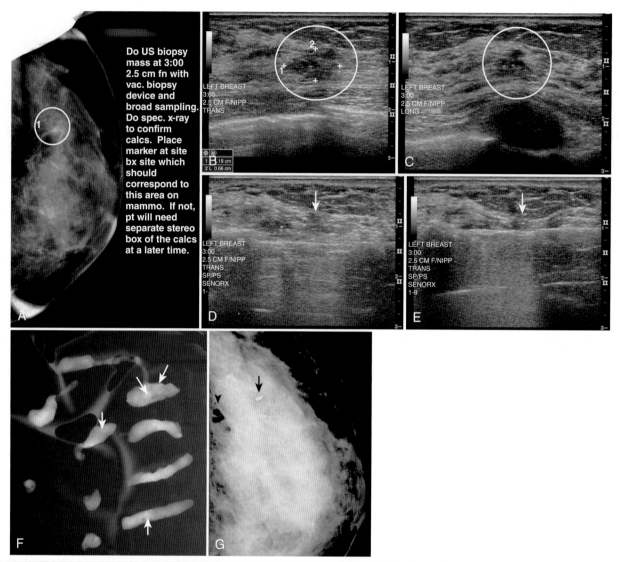

Fig. 7.11 Ultrasound-guided core biopsy of calcifications with core specimen radiography. (A) Craniocaudal mammogram shows calcifications (*circle*) in the outer left breast. Note the radiologist has annotated the mammogram with instructions on how to manage this patient. (B–C) Ultrasound later showed a mass and calcifications in this location. Transverse (B) and longitudinal (C) ultrasound images show a 1.1-cm hypoechoic mass containing calcifications (*circles*). (D) The ultrasound shows the vacuum-assisted core needle trough below the mass and calcifications (*arrow*). (E) Nine samples were obtained by vacuum-assisted core biopsy, and the ultrasound image shows less of the mass and calcifications (*arrow*) above the trough. (F) Specimen radiograph of core biopsy samples show the calcifications (arrows) first seen on the mammogram. (G) Postbiopsy mammogram shows the marker (*arrow*) in the outer breast, absence of the calcifications, and air (*arrowhead*) near the chest wall from the biopsy. Biopsy showed DCIS.

the side of the lesion, the trough is aimed at the finding and the lesion is sampled directionally. After sampling, the core samples are radiographed while the needle or probe is still at the target site in case more biopsy samples are needed (see Fig. 7.13). If the core specimen radiographs show the calcifications or mass, the tissue specimens are placed in formalin and labeled to be sent to the pathology laboratory. The radiologist then deploys a marker into the biopsy cavity through the biopsy probe and pulls the probe back slightly, and the technologist takes an additional image to confirm marker placement. The probe is then fully removed, the patient is released from compression, and hemostasis is achieved with direct manual pressure over the biopsy site.

Subsequently, immediate postbiopsy upright CC and lateral projection mammograms are obtained to document marker placement and its position relative to the targeted findings (see Fig. 7.13). Residual targeted calcifications or residual portions of the mass may also be seen, although it is possible that biopsy site changes may obscure visualization. Usually, the marker is located in or near the biopsy site. If the marker is some distance away from the site, the radiologist should report the marker's location with respect to the original target; for example: "After biopsy, the marker is displaced 3 cm lateral to the original location of the calcifications." If the original biopsy site must be removed and the postbiopsy maker is far away from the site, the radiologist may use both landmarks from the prebiopsy mammogram and the displaced marker to guide localization of the original biopsy site. Because postbiopsy hematomas may form at locations away from the original target site, a hematoma alone should not be relied on as the sole target for localization. If feasible to wait until the biopsy site has healed, a repeat diagnostic mammogram may reveal a residual target lesion to localize for surgery.

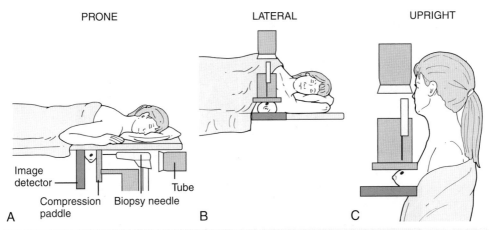

PRONE   LATERAL   UPRIGHT

Image detector

Compression paddle   Biopsy needle   Tube

A   B   C

Fig. 7.12 Schematics of stereotactic biopsy unit and positioning. (A) Prone position. The patient lies prone on the table with unilateral breast hanging dependently though a hole, compressed against the detector underneath the table with a compression paddle containing an open aperture, through which radiologists perform stereotactic-guided biopsy. This is the dedicated prone stereotactic biopsy table. (B–C), Add-on stereotactic device to upright conventional mammographic units. In this scenario, the stereotactic views are obtained from a conventional mammography unit that has the biopsy needle added on with the patient in the lateral decubitus position with the breast compressed from the side (B) or with the patient sitting in the upright position in a chair with compression in the craniocaudal direction (C) or lateral direction (not shown).

Jackman and Marzoni (2003) discuss various techniques used to successfully perform stereotactic biopsy lesions in technically challenging situations. For example, if the technologist is struggling to visualize calcifications within the biopsy field of view, skin surface fiducial markers can be used as a guide. The technologist places skin markers on the planned entry side of the breast, closest to the expected location of the calcifications, and takes a scout mammogram in a standard mammography unit in the projection in which the biopsy will take place. By looking at the scout mammogram obtained with skin markers, the technologist decides which of the skin markers is closest to the target calcifications and can adjust location of the biopsy grid to center on the calcifications (Fig. 7.16).

A method to overcome a thin breast uses a second open grid taped onto the detector. Using this technique, a technologist tapes an open grid onto the detector so that the back paddle allows the posterior breast tissue to puff out of the grid aperture during compression (see Fig. 7.16). The technologist sterilizes the anterior and posterior breast skin in case the needle traverses through the entire breast depth. The breast is placed into compression, and the target is localized in the usual manner. However, care is taken to ensure that the needle does not traverse the entire breast or hit the detector. Usually, manual advancement of the probe is wise, as well as watching the needle enter the breast from the side to prevent these events.

Another option available on some manufacturer units is a "lateral-arm" for sampling in a thin breast. In this case a "lateral-arm" attachment allows insertion of the biopsy needle parallel to the detector, also termed a "lateral-needle" approach (in contrast to the usual needle approach perpendicular to the detector).

CORE SPECIMEN RADIOGRAPHY

Core biopsy specimen radiography is mandatory to ensure the calcifications, mass, or other target lesions are adequately sampled or removed (see Figs. 7.11 and 7.13). If the target has not been adequately sampled, the radiologist usually obtains additional material and reimages the new specimens. Core specimen radiographs are not usually done after US-guided biopsy unless the biopsy target contains radiographically detectable calcifications. Occasionally, the radiologist may be uncertain if the specimen radiograph shows the target, especially if the target was a mass or asymmetry. Then, the radiologist compares the specimen radiograph to the diagnostic mammogram and immediate postbiopsy mammograms, determining whether the lesion was sampled or removed and where the postbiopsy marker is located. As needed, additional diagnostic mammography may be performed after biopsy site changes have resolved to evaluate for a residual targeted lesion.

If calcifications are the biopsy target, then calcifications should be seen on core specimen radiographs for the imaging and histologic findings to be concordant. Most, but not all, calcifications seen on a specimen radiograph are seen on histologic slides. If the radiologist was targeting calcifications and there are no calcifications on the specimen radiograph, specimen pathology results will not be representative of the calcifications prompting biopsy (which are probably still inside the breast). However, the pathology report may still describe calcifications even if they are absent on the core specimen radiograph because pathologists can see tiny calcifications on breast specimen slides that cannot be seen by core specimen radiography. These calcifications are usually smaller than 100 μm and are likely incidental. Thus patients undergoing biopsy for calcifications who have no calcifications on specimen radiographs need rebiopsy, if the pathology report describes microscopic calcifications which are too small to be seen at mammography. Careful radiologic-pathologic correlation is critical to ensure proper patient management and follow-up. To avoid this pitfall, experienced breast pathologists will generally not report these microscopic incidental calcifications as correlating to radiographically visible calcifications.

Calcifications seen on the specimen radiograph may not be seen at pathology for several reasons, detailed below and in Box 7.4.

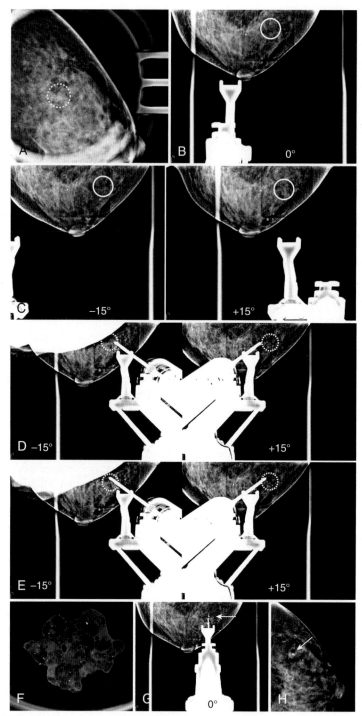

Fig. 7.13 A Images from stereotactic core biopsy in a 50-year old woman with suspicious calcifications. (A) Spot Compression magnification craniocaudal (CC) mammogram shows pleomorphic calcifications (*dashed circles*). (B–C), Straight-on (B) and ±15 degrees stereotactic views (C) show the target (*dashed circles*) in the middle of the compression plate aperture. (D) Prefire stereotactic views show the needle pointing at the calcifications (*dashed circles*). (E) Postfire stereotactic views show the needle traversing the calcifications (*dashed circles*). (F) Specimen radiography shows the calcifications in the sample. (G) Postmarker placement view shows the marker (*arrow*) at the biopsy site. (H) Photographically enlarged postbiopsy CC mammogram shows air and biopsy marker (*arrow*) at the biopsy site. Pathology showed invasive ductal cancer.

First, the calcifications may be composed of calcium oxalate and are seen on the slides only with polarized light (Tornos et al., 1990). Unlike calcium phosphate calcifications, which are easily seen on hematoxylin and eosin (H&E) staining and standard light, calcium oxalate is not visualized with H&E staining and requires a special polarized light to show the calcifications.

Second, the calcifications still may be in the paraffin blocks. During specimen processing, thin breast tissue samples are embedded in paraffin blocks, which are then sliced and placed on slides for staining. Each block is several millimeters thick, but each slide contains only micromillimeters of paraffin and tissue. Thus the calcifications may still be in the block and may never have been placed on a slide for

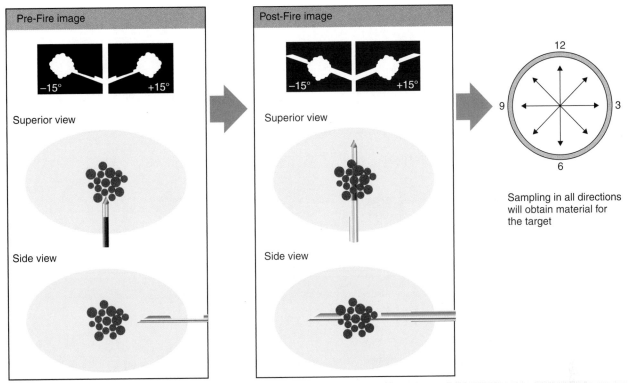

Fig. 7.14 Schematic of perfect positioning on stereotactic biopsy. Two prefire stereotactic images 15 degrees off perpendicular show the tip of the biopsy needle at the edge of the lesion aiming toward its center. Two postfire stereotactic images show that the trough of the needle is centered within the breast lesion. Because the needle is perfectly placed centrally in the target, samples may be obtained 360 degrees around the needle trough.

Box 7.4   Reasons Why Targeted Calcifications Are Not Seen on Pathology Slides

Calcifications are composed of calcium oxalate (need polarized light)
Calcifications still in paraffin blocks (radiograph the paraffin blocks)
Calcifications removed from tissue by microtome during sectioning
Calcifications were in milk-of-calcium cysts and washed out of the breast specimen
Calcifications are still in the breast (repeat mammogram)

---

review. A radiograph of the blocks may show the calcifications, and resectioning of that particular block will show the calcifications (Fig. 7.17).

Third, the calcifications may be removed from the specimen if the microtome cutting device that slices the tissue/paraffin block for slides pushes large calcifications out of the specimen at the time of sectioning. Another reason the calcifications may not be in the specimen is if the calcifications were in milk of calcium within tiny benign cysts and were washed out of the breast specimen when the tiny cysts were ruptured by sectioning.

If the targeted calcifications are seen on the specimen radiograph but no calcifications are found in the pathology slides or in the paraffin blocks, a repeat mammogram can determine whether the calcifications are still in the breast and were not removed at surgery. One also needs to correlate the calcifications' appearance seen on the mammogram with the calcifications seen in the specimen radiograph because, very rarely, the specimen contains incidental calcifications and not the ones that were targeted.

PLACEMENT OF BIOPSY SITE MARKERS

This section will discuss the placement of biopsy site markers. Wireless fiducials for preoperative localization will be discussed in the later section "Preoperative Needle Localization with Hookwire or Wireless Methods" in this chapter. The methods of wireless fiducial placement are the same as for placement of postbiopsy markers.

Radiologists place metallic or nonmetallic markers, or wireless fiducials, into targeted lesions or the biopsy site immediately after image-guided biopsies to mark the biopsy site/lesion in case there is need for surgical excision. Biopsy site markers are placed in the residual mass, calcifications, enhancement or in the biopsy site even if the finding is removed. If there are two or more biopsy targets in the same breast, a unique marker shape is used for each target to differentiate the biopsy sites (Fig. 7.18). Some practices use specific marker shapes for specific imaging guidance techniques (stereotactic, MRI, US). The marker then indicates what imaging guidance was used to biopsy specific targets (examples: M-shaped markers used only for stereotaxis or tomosynthesis, circle shapes used only for MRI, omega shapes used only for US). Lastly, specifying the marker shape placed in a specific biopsy location for a specific lesion in the report leaves no questions regarding the meaning of specific biopsy marker shapes on the postbiopsy mammograms (e.g., "A ribbon-shaped marker was placed in the US-biopsied mass 3:00 position 4.5 cm from the nipple, left breast").

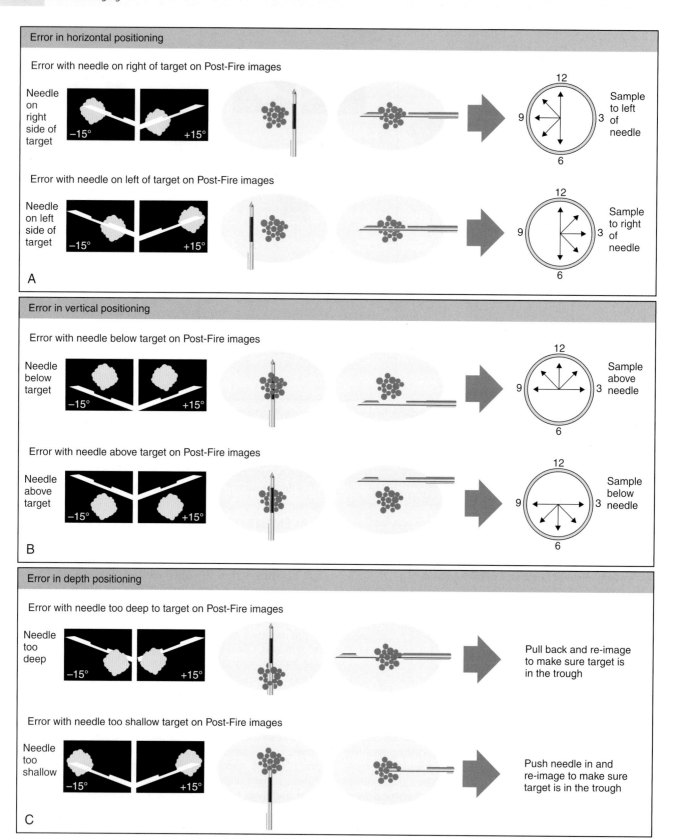

Fig. 7.15 Schematics of errors in needle positioning on stereotactic biopsy. (A) Two types of errors in horizontal positioning, one with needle to the right of target, one to the left of target. (B) Two types of errors in vertical positioning, one with needle below target, one with needle above target. (C) Two types of errors in depth positioning, one with needle too deep to target, one with needle to shallow to target. In each situation, the correction in biopsy needle sampling or placement is different to biopsy the target.

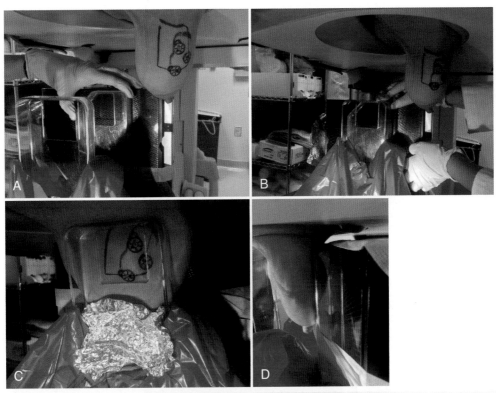

Fig. 7.16 Use of a reversed compression back paddle to increase the breast thickness in thin breasts. (A) The technologist tapes a back paddle with an aperture directly on the stereotactic image detector so that the aperture matches the stereotactic biopsy aperture. Picture illustrates the technologist placing the back paddle on the detector so that the open apertures will align. The breast hangs dependently to the side with three skin markers showing the location of calcifications and a black skin ink markings showing where the compression paddle aperture should be placed. (B) After sterilizing the breast skin, both front and back, the technologist will place the breast in the compression paddle so that the open apertures will align as shown. (C) Breast in compression, repositioned after resterilization with radiopaque skin BB markers showing location of faint calcifications. Aluminum foil was added to help with exposure. (D) Seen from the side, the compressed breast tissue extends both forwards and backward from the apertures thereby increasing the breast thickness. Adapted from Jackman RJ and Marzoni FA Jr. Stereotactic histologic biopsy with patients prone: technical feasibility in 98% of mammographically detected lesions. *AJR Am J Roentgenol.* 2003;180:785–794.

The radiologist determines whether the marker is deployed in the correct place after any imaging-guided biopsy. For example, after stereotactic or DBT marker placement, the radiologist reviews stereotactic images to be sure the marker is at or near the biopsy site before removing the probe and may deploy a second marker if the first marker is not seen. For US-guided biopsies, US-visible markers are used to be sure the marker has deployed accurately. After MRI-guided biopsy, it is hard to be sure if the marker has deployed accurately, but usually a signal void from the metallic marker will show the biopsy marker location with respect to the biopsied area. Some facilities will obtain an immediate post-biopsy, noncontrast T1-weighted MRI to identify the marker location with respect to the intended target and biopsy site. A post-MRI procedure mammogram will show the immediate postbiopsy location of the marker relative to biopsy site changes.

There are various markers composed of stainless steel, titanium, or other metals either alone or embedded in plugs of Gelfoam, bovine or porcine collagen, suture-type material, or other materials. If markers containing bovine or porcine collagen are used, the patient should be asked about allergies to either beef or pork before deploying the markers. Nonmetallic markers are also available.

A marker deployed at time of biopsy may not successfully localize the biopsy site for several reasons as summarized in Box 7.5. Nondeployment is uncommon but can occur in

stereotactic/tomosynthesis-guided biopsies using vacuum-assisted probes when the marker is placed through the probe itself. For vacuum-assisted needles, the marker can get stuck on a retained tissue fragment in the vacuum needle, so it is important to vacuum the needle prior to deploying the marker and to check that the marker has deployed before removing the probe. If the introducer sheath is still in place, a second marker can be placed if the initial marker deployment was unsuccessful. For markers that are inserted using their own needle, the main problem is marker deployment too deep or too shallow in the Z-axis.

Usually US echogenic markers can be seen during US deployment, and if the marker does not deploy or deploys in an inaccurate location, a second marker can be placed immediately. US visible markers are increasingly important in breast imaging since facilities may use US for preoperative localization or surgeons may use US in the operating room aid breast lesion removal. Thus more and more facilities are placing US visible markers after biopsy of any type of guidance (stereotactic/tomosynthesis, US, MRI, palpation biopsy prior to neoadjuvant chemotherapy) to allow the possibility of using US for localization.

Common marker problems are initial inaccurate marker placement or later marker movement, particularly with stereotactic/tomosynthesis-guided biopsies. Both inaccurate initial placement and delayed migration usually occur along the Z-axis or axis of the needle insertion. Delayed marker

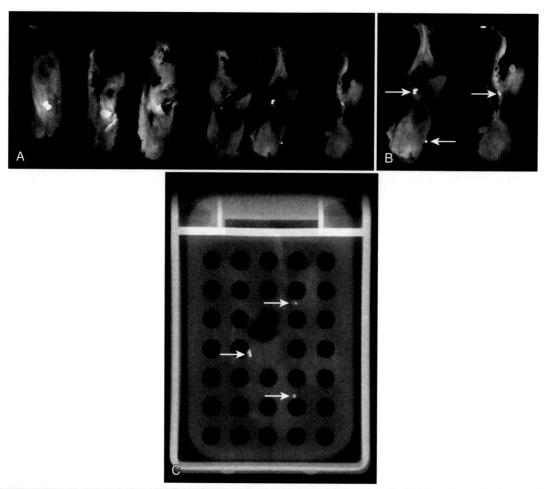

Fig. 7.17 Tissue specimen radiography in pathology department. (A) Radiograph of six tissue specimens sectioned from an excisional breast biopsy performed for calcifications. Calcifications are found in all six specimens. (B) Magnified view of two tissue specimens containing calcifications (*arrows*). (C) Pathology technologists place the tissue pieces in paraffin in a plastic tissue cassette. This paraffin block radiograph shows the calcifications (*arrows*) from the two tissue specimens shown in part B. Pathology showed fibrocystic change and calcifications. If the slides from this cassette did not show calcifications, the pathologists would have taken additional samples from this cassette. (Images Courtesy Dr. Gerald Berry, Stanford University, Palo Alto, CA.)

Box 7.5 Possible Postneedle Biopsy Marker Problems

Nondeployment (rare and recognized on stereo/tomosynthesis views while the breast is still in compression, occasionally during ultrasound-guided marker placement during real-time scanning)

Inaccurate initial deployment/clip migration (common, recognized on postbiopsy mammograms on day of biopsy)

Delayed migration from initial deployment site (rare, recognized on mammograms taken days to months after biopsy)

---

movement is uncommon and refers to marker migration from its initial placement to a different site in the breast.

Delayed marker movement and inaccurate marker placement affects preoperative localization planning. Because there is no way to predict delayed marker migration, we advise radiologists to review the postbiopsy CC and ML mammogram views immediately before mammographically guided needle/wireless fiducial localization of biopsied lesions and markers. If the marker was initially inaccurately deployed or moved away from an original biopsy site, the radiologist determines the original targeted lesion's location by using breast architecture and landmarks. The goal of localization is to target the biopsy site and any residual cancer, not just the marker. Using the mammogram, the radiologist then determines whether the marker has moved and whether the marker or the original site, or both, need to be localized for surgery.

Biopsy site markers placed by stereotaxis, tomosynthesis, US, or MRI may be imaged subsequently by MRI. Thus both MRI marker safety and degree of MRI marker signal void artifact are important to consider. Accordingly, all facilities should use MRI-conditional metallic markers and wireless fiducials when markers are placed with any modality because MRI may be performed later. Both metallic markers and wireless fiducials cause a signal void on MRI, and the size of the signal void varies according to the marker type and pulse sequence (Fig. 7.19). Some markers are MRI conditional but still cause large artifacts of up to 2 cm, thus rendering the MRI less readable than when using other markers. MRI testing of markers for artifacts by using phantoms on the facility's pulse sequences is a simple way to determine the marker artifact and the size of the signal void. Placement of wireless fiducials for pre-operative localization can also be timed

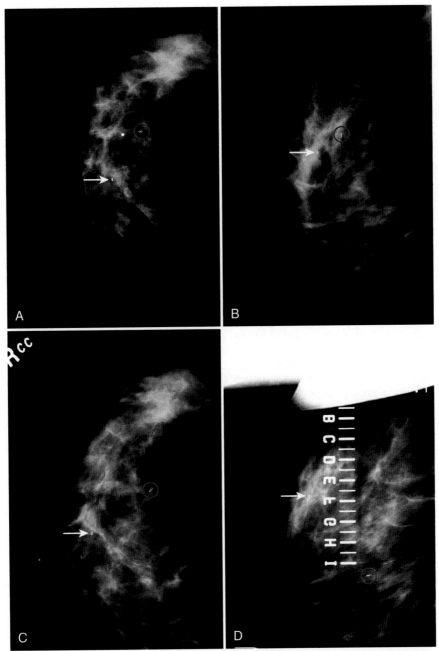

Fig. 7.18 Value of two different types of markers for two stereotactic biopsy sites and example of marker migration. Because this patient had two suspicious microcalcification groups, two different markers were placed at stereotactic biopsy. (A–B) Craniocaudal (CC) (A) and mediolateral (B) mammograms show the difference in marker configuration, which clearly identifies different biopsy sites (*circle, arrow*). If the same type of marker had been placed in both sites, it would be difficult to determine the location of each biopsy site on subsequent mammograms. Cancer was found in the upper biopsy site (*circle*), and the lower biopsy site (*arrow*) was benign. (C–D) Two months later, preoperative CC (C) and lateral (D) views show that the upper marker has migrated to the inferior portion of the breast (*circle*). Because cancer was taken from the upper biopsy site, breast architecture was used to target the original upper biopsy site for excision because the marker (*circle*) was seen in a different quadrant at time of localization. Second marker (not localization target) still visible within the breast (*arrow*). This case shows the importance of correlation of the prestereotactic biopsy scout mammogram, the immediate postmarker placement mammogram, which documents location of the marker relative to the biopsy site, and scout mammograms before preoperative needle localization.

for after breast MRI to avoid MRI artifact impacting image quality.

CARBON BREAST TISSUE MARKING AND TATTOO INK MARKING OF AXILLARY LYMPH NODES

This method to mark *breast lesions* for excisional biopsy uses activated charcoal USP (Mallinckrodt, Phillipsburg, NJ)

sterilized and suspended as a 4% weight/weight aqueous suspension. It is mixed with 0.3 mL sterile saline or water and injected in a to-and-fro motion after core biopsy along the stereotactic or US needle track to yield a dark line of carbon particles in the breast. This line of carbon particles can be used as a guide for excisional biopsy days to weeks after the percutaneous biopsy. It is used as an alternative to a postbiopsy metallic marker or wireless fiducials for intraparenchymal

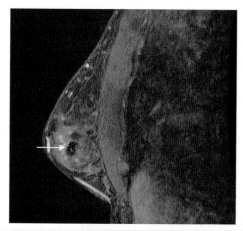

Fig. 7.19 Signal void on breast magnetic resonance imaging (MRI) due to metallic markers placed from stereotactic core biopsy. Postcontrast three-dimensional spectral-spatial excitation magnetization transfer (3DSSMT) breast MRI shows a signal void from a metal marker as a dark area (*arrow*) in a patient after stereotactic core biopsy.

breast lesions, mainly in Europe, and also reported in Korea (Ko et al., 2007).

Tattoo ink marking of *axillary lymph nodes* is an imaging-guided method to mark biopsied axillary lymph nodes showing metastasis for subsequent surgical excision during axillary sentinel lymph node biopsy (SLNB) (Patel et al., 2019) (Box 7.6). Using this method, a tattoo is placed in a BI-RADS 5 lymph-positive node at initial biopsy or after pathology demonstrates metastasis, ensuring its subsequent removal. With this method, the node to be marked is injected with 0.3 to 0.5 mL of sterile tattoo ink both in the lymph node cortex surface and in the immediate breast parenchyma adjacent to the node where the surgeon will make the incision (Fig. 7.20). This is so the surgeon may see the stained breast tissue and lymph node tattoo at the time of axillary surgery and remove it. Do not inject too much ink as this will stain the axilla and the surgeon will not be able to see the tattooed lymph node. Do not inject ink while withdrawing the needle as this may tattoo the skin. The surgeon will remove the tattooed lymph node along with any palpable, radioactive, or blue sentinel lymph nodes during axillary sentinel lymph node biopsy.

Note a potential pitfall is that patients with extensive arm, neck, and upper body tattoos may exhibit tattoo ink staining of nonsentinel lymph nodes, causing a false-positive lymph node identification.

PATIENT SAFETY AND COMFORT AFTER BIOPSY

Patient education regarding wound care is an important part of biopsy procedures (Box 7.7). After needle biopsy, hemostasis is achieved by direct pressure. Postbiopsy dressing varies by facility but a general principle is to keep biopsy site clean and dry. For large-core vacuum biopsies or in case of prolonged bleeding, a dressing that binds the breast with wraparound bandages or a pressure dressing may be used. After core biopsies, patients are also instructed to apply ice to the biopsy site periodically for several hours to reduce inflammation and pain.

Afterward, patients are given verbal and written postbiopsy wound care instructions and a phone number to call for problems. Patients are instructed on where and how to obtain their biopsy result.

Pain control is part of recovery. If not allergic to acetaminophen and in the absence of liver problems, the patient may take acetaminophen initially and then every 6 hours as needed, up to 4 g/day. Aspirin or NSAIDs are avoided right after biopsy to decrease the risk of bleeding. Most patients do well after biopsy. A courtesy phone call later in the day or

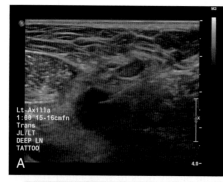
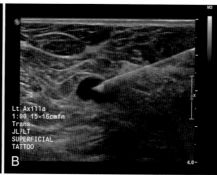
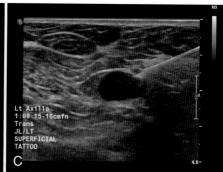

Fig. 7.20 Fine-needle aspiration of abnormal lymph node and tattoo marking. A 51-year-old woman with invasive ductal cancer and metastatic lymphadenopathy. (A) Ultrasound shows fine-needle aspiration of an abnormal left lymph node which showed metastatic breast cancer. (B) Tattoo dye placed in the superficial cortex of the lymph node. (C) Tattoo dye placed at the surface of abnormal lymph node.

Teach patient how to "hold pressure" on the biopsy site in case of oozing or bleeding

Keep the wound dry

Steri-Strips and Opsite will fall off in 4 to 7 days

Expect a quarter size blood spot on the bandage (core biopsy)

A lump may form under the bandage (hematoma, it is not a growing tumor)

Ice pack on top of paper towel over wound 10 to 20 minutes per hour as needed

Acetaminophen as needed per package instructions

Avoid aspirin or nonsteroidal antiinflammatory drugs (NSAIDs) for several days after biopsy if possible

Instruct how and where to obtain biopsy results

Phone number for patient questions

Courtesy call same day or next day

the next day is helpful to see how the patient is doing after biopsy and to answer any questions.

RADIOLOGIC-PATHOLOGIC CORRELATION AFTER BREAST BIOPSY

Imaging/pathology correlation after image-guided biopsies is critical to ensure that the histologic findings explain the imaging findings. If not, pathology results are discordant with imaging and additional tissue sampling is usually warranted in order to avoid falsely negative biopsy results and a delayed diagnosis of cancer. The decision to proceed with surgical excision or to perform another percutaneous biopsy is made based on the details of the individual case. Examples of when repeat percutaneous biopsy may be appropriate include when there are discordant FNA or core biopsy pathologies or when there are undersampled calcifications at stereotactic biopsy. Radiologic-pathologic correlation for malignant, high-risk, and benign breast lesions are covered in detail in Chapter 9: Breast Pathology and Radiologic-Pathologic Correlation.

All biopsies in which the target has been missed are considered discordant because the target has not been sampled. One can determine whether the target has not been sampled if the target is either (1) not in the specimen or (2) still in the breast on subsequent imaging. Another example of discordance is if not enough of the target has been included in the sample, for example, if too few calcifications within a calcification group have been included in the biopsy sample to be considered representative of the finding. In the latter instance, too few calcifications in the sample would make it unclear whether pathology was truly representative of the entire calcification group, and, accordingly, the pathology would be considered discordant.

Concordant imaging/pathology result examples include simple cysts (which resolve completely with benign cyst fluid in the syringe), circumscribed oval masses that are fibroadenomas, spiculated masses that are postbiopsy scars in the right clinical setting, and lymph nodes that have a typical imaging appearance. Concordant or discordant pathology correlations are harder to determine with other mass lesions, non-mass lesions, or focal or global asymmetries, which may have a more nonspecific pathology. In these cases, one must rely on the accuracy and the volume of the needle biopsy, the pathology result, and the clinical context.

Preoperative Needle Localization With Hookwire or Wireless Methods

The intent of image-guided preoperative localization is to provide surgeons a "road map" to find lesions inside the breast. This is because surgeons cannot see or feel suspicious nonpalpable masses or calcifications inside the breast to remove them. The technique of preoperative needle localization uses imaging to guide a percutaneously placed needle into the breast so that its tip is in the breast target. With hookwire techniques, the radiologist threads a metallic wire with a hook on its end through the needle such that the hookwire hooks into, or through and beyond, the suspicious nonpalpable target. Alternatively, the radiologist may place a wireless fiducial marker though the needle into the breast in or near the target. Both wire and wireless localization may be guided by two-dimensional (2D) mammography, stereotaxis, tomosynthesis, US, or MRI, all of which are discussed in this section. We note that, using any method, prelocalization planning in conjunction with the breast surgeon is critical for successful localization and excision.

2D MAMMOGRAPHIC–GUIDED NEEDLE/ HOOKWIRE OR WIRELESS LOCALIZATION

This technique uses 2D mammograms to target the lesion with the patient's breast compressed by a compression paddle that contains a hole surrounded by letters and numbers (an *alpha-numeric grid*). To perform this procedure, the radiologist reviews the original orthogonal mammograms to identify the shortest distance to the target from the skin surface. The technologist positions the patient in the mammographic unit and, with the alpha-numeric grid over the skin closest to the lesion, compresses the breast. The edges of the aperture may be marked with an ink marker at its contact with skin to detect if the patient moves. After taking a single mammogram image, the technologist leaves the patient's breast in compression while the radiologist checks the image (Fig. 7.21). The mammogram should show the lesion within the open aperture. The radiologist finds the target coordinates on the mammogram, then cleans the breast skin and administers superficial and deep anesthetic at target coordinates, then passes a needle into the target, making sure the needle is parallel to the chest wall. As a useful reference to ensure that the needle path is straight, the radiologist checks that the needle hub's shadow (cast by built-in procedural light) lies directly over the needle shaft during insertion. The technologist repeats a mammogram with the needle in place, and this mammogram should show that the needle shaft projects over the lesion. Once the radiologist confirms that the needle is through the lesion, breast compression is released being careful to not displace the needle. Then the breast is placed in orthogonal compression for another mammogram. The radiologist adjusts the needle depth so that the hook or wireless

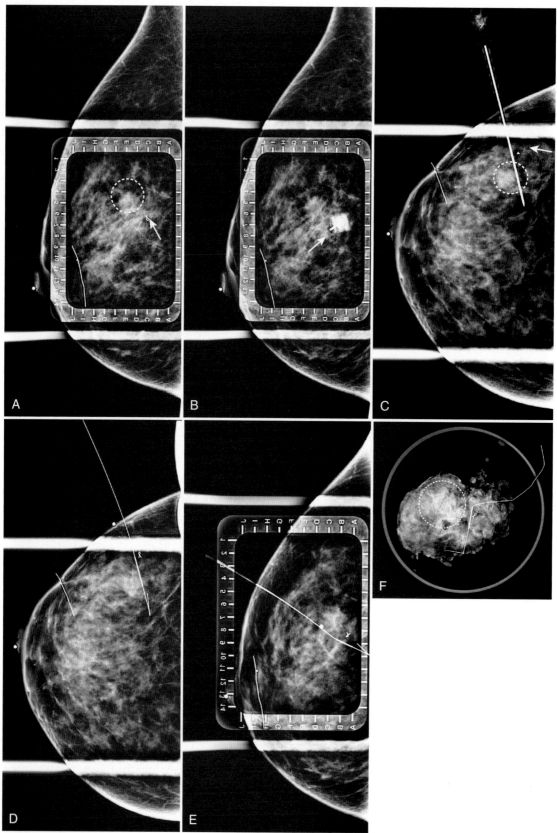

FIG. 7.21 Mammography-guided preoperative needle localization. A 36-year-old woman who underwent ultrasound-guided core biopsy showing invasive ductal cancer with a ribbon marker placed. (A) Lateromedial (LM) mammogram obtained using open compression paddle with an alpha numeric grid (E) shows a mass (*dashed circle*) and the ribbon marker (*arrow*) at location C.0, 6.5. (B) Lateromedial mammogram with needle in place shows hub of the needle (*arrow*) directly over the marker and inferior to the mass. (C) Craniocaudal (CC) mammogram with needle in place shows needle traversing the marker (*arrow*) and the mass (*dashed circle*). (D) Craniocaudal (CC) mammogram shows needle has been withdrawn and wire placed with marker and mass near the wire-stiffener and the hook beyond the marker and mass. (E) Lateromedial (LM) mammogram performed with the wire placed through the open aperture of a compression plate and light compression so that the wire would not be pushed further into the breast during the mammogram. Initial view (B) with needle hub and shaft projecting over target lesion may be used instead of (E) as the orthogonal view to avoid risk of wire migration. (F) Breast biopsy specimen radiograph shows the hook wire in its entirety as well as the marker and the mass (*dashed circle*). Pathology showed invasive ductal cancer.

fiducial will be deployed at or beyond the target (for wire localization), or at or near the target (for wireless fiducials). If a wireless fiducial is to be placed, the radiologist places the wireless fiducial through the needle and removes the needle, leaving the fiducial at or near the target.

If a hookwire is to be placed instead of a wireless fiducial, and if the surgeon desires a small injection of sterile blue dye through the needle to stain the tissue around the lesion, then the radiologist injects dye through the needle at this point. The surgeon will later look for the tissue stain in the operating room. The radiologist then places a hookwire through the needle and removes the needle, leaving the hook in or near the target and the rest of the wire sticking out of the skin. The radiologist bends the wire at the skin surface and secures external portion of wire to the skin so that the wire does not migrate into or out of the breast during patient transportation. After any wire or wireless placement by imaging guidance (mammography, US, or MRI), orthogonal mammograms are annotated to show the relationship of the target, the hookwire tip/wireless fiducial, and their location in the breast with respect to the nipple and other breast structures for the surgeon to use in the operating room (Box 7.8). For wire localizations, mammographic imaging orthogonal to the wire carries the risk of postlocalization wire displacement with mammographic compression. Thus the initial view with needle hub and shaft projecting over target lesion is generally used as the orthogonal view to avoid risk of wire migration. Alternatively, an orthogonal view using minimal compression may be obtained with the wire placed in a grid to reduce risk of advancing the wire during compression.

Box 7.8   Annotation of Postlocalization Mammograms

- **Circle/outline:** only targeted mammographic findings/area and localization devices that **should be included/seen in the specimen radiograph**
- Annotations on the postlocalization craniocaudal (CC) and mediolateral (ML) mammograms
    - Lesion laterality and numeric designation if previously used (e.g., R1 or L1)
    - Lesion location in clockface and distance from the nipple (e.g., 10 o'clock 7 cm FN)
    - **Visible**, targeted mammographic findings (not magnetic resonance imaging [MRI] or ultrasound findings), with size, and any **markers (specify shapes) that should be included/ seen** in the specimen radiograph (e.g., 0.8 cm grouped calcs with ribbon marker)
    - If no mammographic findings (no residual calcs/mass, no marker at site, MRI finding) describe target as "tissue" w/details (e.g., tissue at site of prior biopsy, tissue at site of MRI finding)
    - Pathology of prior core biopsy (e.g., atypical ductal hyperplasia [ADH], ductal carcinoma in situ [DCIS], invasive ductal carcinoma [IDC], invasive lobular carcinoma [ILC])
    - Location of localization device relative to target (e.g., wireless marker 0.6 cm anterior to 0.8 cm grouped calcifications with ribbon marker)
    - Other relevant details: other findings/adjacent markers not localized (e.g., top hat marker from prior benign biopsy not localized)
- Example annotation: "R1, 10 o'clock 7 cm from the nipple, wireless marker 0.6 cm anterior to 0.8 cm grouped calcifications with ribbon marker, DCIS. Top hat marker prior benign biopsy not localized."

The patient is sent to the operating room after wire localization (or sent home to return for subsequent excision in the case of wireless localization). A breast specimen is imaged subsequently at time of excision.

"Bracketing" wires/wireless fiducials guide surgeons removing a large area of breast tissue (Fig. 7.22). This happens when the target(s) extend over too wide an area to be localized by one device. In this situation, the radiologist places two or more wires/wireless fiducials in the breast to mark the boundaries of the volume of tissue to be removed. The brackets help the surgeon remove the lesion(s) between and around the multiple devices in toto. Breast specimens excised after brackets should include all bracketing wires/wireless fiducials, postbiopsy markers, and mass(es) or calcifications between or around them.

TOMOSYNTHESIS-GUIDED NEEDLE/HOOKWIRE OR WIRELESS LOCALIZATION

With this technique, the radiologist localizes the lesion using an upright mammographic unit capable of tomosynthesis, a compression paddle with or without an alpha-numeric grid and tomosynthesis to guide the needle into the target (Fig. 7.23). The localization technique is the same as for 2D preoperative needle localization except that the orthogonal mammogram does not have to be obtained because the depth is calculated by the tomosynthesis view. Errors in hookwire or wireless fiducial placement using tomosynthesis calculations instead of the orthogonal view are usually along the trajectory of the needle (in the Z-axis). If the depth is not calculated by tomosynthesis, the orthogonal view of the needle can be obtained with 2D imaging or tomosynthesis.

STEREOTACTIC-GUIDED NEEDLE/HOOKWIRE OR WIRELESS LOCALIZATION

With this technique, the radiologist localizes the lesion under stereotactic guidance, as described for stereotactic core biopsy. The radiologist places a needle into the breast, obtains stereotactic views to make sure the needle is in the middle of the lesion, may inject blue dye, and inserts the hookwire or wireless fiducial. The patient is removed from the stereotactic device and undergoes standard orthogonal mammograms, with the same caveat regarding compression perpendicular to a wire as discussed in prior section on mammographic-guided localizations. The usual problem with stereotactic wire/wireless placements are errors of the final position of the hookwire tip/wireless fiducial along the trajectory of the needle (in the Z-axis), just as in tomosynthesis localizations.

ULTRASOUND-GUIDED NEEDLE/HOOKWIRE OR WIRELESS LOCALIZATION

To do US localization, the patient lies supine, rolled, or angled on the table so the needle path is directed safely away from the chest wall to prevent pneumothorax (Fig. 7.24). Using sterile technique and direct US visualization, the radiologist anesthetizes the skin and deep breast tissue, keeping the entire shaft of the needle, the needle tip, and the target in the same plane. The anesthesia needle insertion is a "trial run" to judge the safety of the needle path and the difficulty of needle insertion. Then the radiologist inserts the preoperative localization needle into the lesion

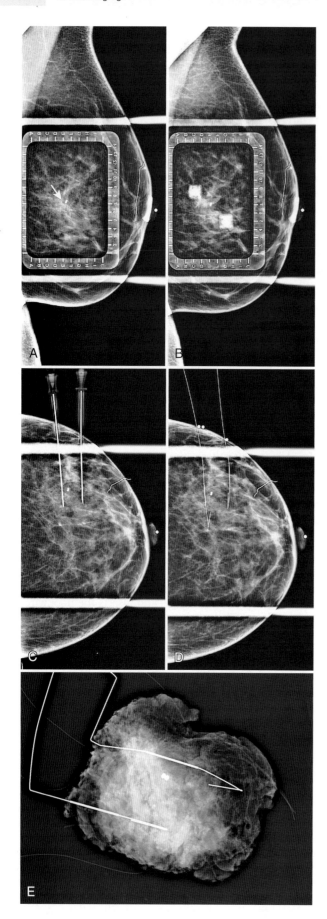

Fig. 7.22 Preoperative bracket needle localization under x-ray guidance. A 49-year-old woman who underwent stereotactic-guided core biopsy showing ductal carcinoma in situ (DCIS) with a dumbbell marker placed. (A) Mediolateral mammogram shows the alphanumeric plate with the dumbbell marker (*arrow*) at location E.5, 7.0. (B) Mediolateral mammogram shows two needles bracketing the marker and residual calcifications. (C) Craniocaudal (CC) mammogram with needles in place shows needles traversing the marker. (D) CC mammogram after the needles have been withdrawn shows the wires bracketing the marker and surrounding the residual calcifications. (E) Breast specimen shows the two intact wires and the marker and residual calcifications. Pathology showed DCIS.

under real-time US guidance, injects blue dye if needed by the surgeon, inserts a hookwire or wireless fiducial, and removes the needle. If desired, a round metallic skin marker such as a radiopaque BB marker, may be placed at the wire skin entry site, and two radiopaque skin BB markers plus an indelible ink "X" may be placed on the skin directly over the US target to mark the underlying lesion when the patient arrives in the operating room. The technologist then takes orthogonal mammograms showing the US-placed wire/wireless fiducial within the breast and any skin markers, the radiologist annotates the images for the surgeon and subsequently interprets images of the breast specimen to ensure target and devices have all been removed.

TYPES OF WIRELESS FIDUCIAL DEVICES

Wireless localization uses fiducial devices (e.g., radioactive seeds, inducible magnetic seeds, radiofrequency identification devices, infrared radar devices, and novel ring devices) that may be placed days/months prior to surgery, depending on the device and lesion type. Because the surgeon locates the wireless device in the operating room using a hand-held probe on a day separate from the localization procedure, all wireless techniques share distinct advantages over same-day wire localizations (Box 7.9). Wireless localization allows for greater scheduling flexibility because the localization procedure is decoupled from the surgical procedure in time. The surgical approach is not affected, as there is no wire to retrieve, with the potential benefit of minimizing nontarget tissue removal and improved cosmesis. Similarly, the radiologist can select an optimal skin entry site regardless of the surgical approach. There is improvement in patient comfort, as no portion of the device is external to the patient and patients are not fasting for the procedure if not going to the operating room on the same day, thus reducing incidence of vasovagal reactions. Additionally, some wireless fiducials may be placed at the time of initial core biopsy, obviating the need to subsequently localize breast lesions or lymph nodes for surgery at a later time. This is especially advantageous in biopsies done prior to neoadjuvant chemotherapy, allowing cancer or metastatic lymph node removal even if there is a complete imaging response and the targets are no longer seen. Because MRI is often used for assessing tumor response to neoadjuvant therapy, degree and type of artifact from biopsy marker and wireless fiducial should be considered at time of initial biopsy. Types of wireless fiducials and localization devices are listed in Table 7.2.

Types of wireless localization fiducial techniques include radioguided occult lesion localization (ROLL), which uses injection of a radio tracer or percutaneous needle placement of a depleted radioactive seed into the

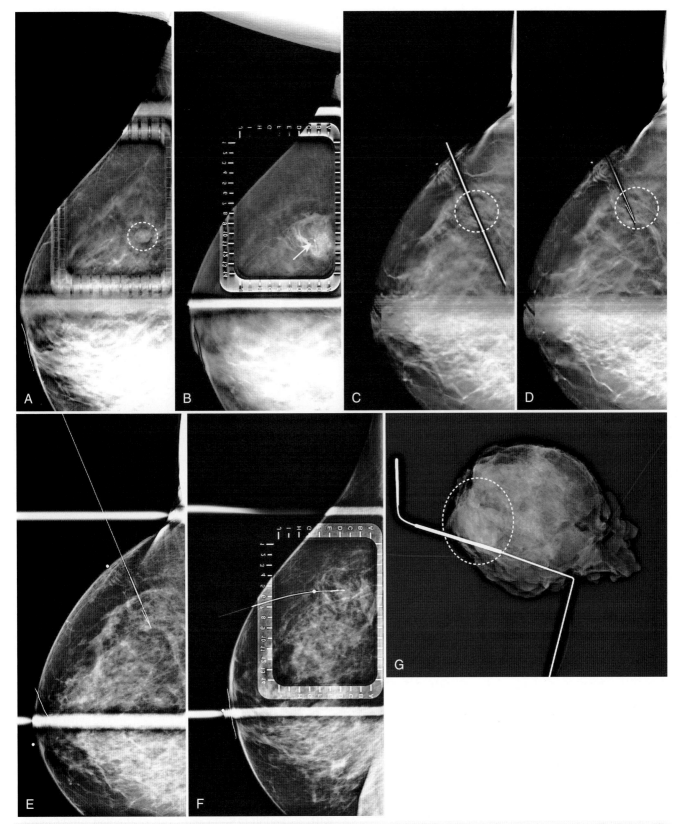

Fig. 7.23 Tomosynthesis needle localization. A 55-year-old woman with a 1.2 cm right upper outer quadrant mass on tomosynthesis not well seen on two-dimensional (2D) mammogram or ultrasound. (A) Lateromedial tomosynthesis slice image shows the mass (*dashed circle*) in the localization compression plate aperture. Location was noted at B.5, 11.0. (B) Tomosynthesis slice image after needle placement shows the needle as a dot en face in cross section (*arrow*) but the mass is obscured by adjacent lidocaine. (C) Craniocaudal (CC) tomosynthesis slice shows the mass (*dashed circle*) at the midportion of the needle. (D) The needle was withdrawn and the wire placed showing the mass (*dashed circle*) near the wire tip. (E) CC view mammogram and (F) lateromedial view mammogram with an alpha numeric grid after wire placement show the wire tip at the mass. (G) Specimen radiograph shows the mass (*dashed circle*) and intact hookwire. Pathology showed fibroadenoma with myxoid stromal change.

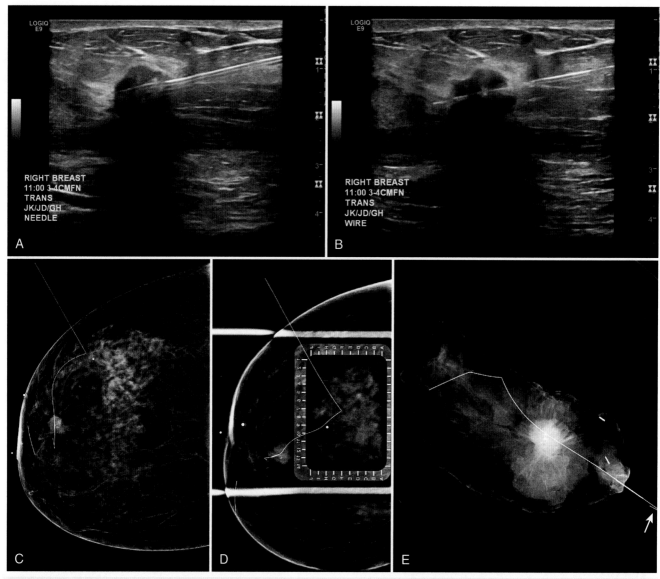

Fig. 7.24 Ultrasound-guided needle localization. A 59-year-old woman with a right upper outer quadrant mass with central calcifications shown to be invasive ductal carcinoma (IDC) by core biopsy. (A) Ultrasound image shows ultrasound needle traversing the mass. (B) Ultrasound shows the wire traversing the mass after needle removal. (C–D) After wire placement, craniocaudal mammogram (C), and lateromedial mammogram with an alpha numeric grid (D) show the wire traversing the mass. (E) Specimen radiograph shows the mass included in its entirety with surgical clips placed at the medial edge, and the hookwire is partly seen but included (*arrow*). Pathology showed IDC.

Box 7.9 Wireless Fiducial Advantages and Disadvantages

Advantages
Avoidance of dislodged/transected wires
Decoupling of radiology and surgery schedules
No operating room start time delays
Increased surgical options for cosmetic approach
Continuous intraoperative monitoring of the target
May be performed 30 days or more prior to surgery

Disadvantages
Increased cost of fiducial, detector, and console
Learning curve for radiologist and surgeon
Radioactive material (if radioactive seed)
Lack of ability to reposition fiducial once deployed

target which is later detected by surgeons in the operating room using a gamma probe (to detect radioactivity) (Fig. 7.25A–D). Nonradioactive wireless fiducials include inducible magnetic seeds detected with a hand-held magnetometer (Fig. 7.25E–G), near infrared reflective marker identified with an electromagnetic wave hand piece, a radiofrequency identification (RFID) tag that transmits a unique ID when triggered by an electromagnetic pulse from a hand held probe) (Fig. 7.25H–J), and a "wired" wireless device composed of a nitinol-ring with a flexible 25-cm wire tail preloaded on 16-gauge introducer needle (Fig. 7.25K–L).[1] Though external to the patient, the wire from the latter device can be coiled and secured to the skin with a bandage for up to 3 days prior to surgery.

Table 7.2   Wireless Methods for Preoperative Localization: Advantages and Disadvantages

Localization Technique	Advantages	Disadvantages
Surgeon-operated intraoperative ultrasound[1]	▪ Simple ▪ Real-time guidance	▪ Operator dependency accuracy ▪ Learning curve ▪ Marker/target visibility
Hematoma ultrasound-guided localization (HUG)[2]	▪ Eliminates the need for another preoperative procedure ▪ More cost-effective ▪ No radioactivity or toxic heavy metals ▪ No external component	▪ Operator dependency ▪ Need to perform the surgery within 5 weeks to avoid hematoma reabsorption
Radioactive seed localization (RSL)[3]	▪ No external component	▪ Radioactive material (may limit staff who are working) ▪ Strict nuclear regulatory rules for handling and disposal ▪ Staff and patient exposure to radioactive material
Radioguided occult lesion localization (ROLL)[4]	▪ No external component	▪ Radioactive material (may limit staff who are working) ▪ Strict nuclear regulatory rules for handling and disposal ▪ Technetium 99 m has short half-life (6 hours)
Sentinel node and occult lesion localization (SNOLL)[5]	▪ No external component	▪ Radioactive material (may limit staff who are working) ▪ Strict nuclear regulatory rules for handling and disposal
Carbon marking/tattoo[6]	▪ Visible up to 130 days and longer ▪ No radioactivity or toxic heavy metals ▪ No external component	▪ Marking must be determined visually by surgeon without help from probe or wire
Radiofrequency identification tag (RFID)[7]	▪ No radioactivity or toxic heavy metals ▪ Audible tone feedback during probe reading ▪ No external component	▪ Cannot be used in patients with pacemakers or defibrillators
Near infrared radar/reflector (Savi Scout)[8]	▪ Nonferromagnetic ▪ Little signal void on MRI ▪ Patients with implants not excluded ▪ Audible tone feedback during probe reading ▪ No radioactivity or toxic heavy metals ▪ No external component ▪ Approved for permanent placement in breast/axilla	▪ Hematoma interference ▪ Inaccessibility to lesions which are >4.5 cm with first-generation console ▪ Migration ▪ Easily cracked ceramic probe ▪ Stronger operating room console/probe than x-ray department probe ▪ Interference from operating room lights (if halogen) ▪ Cannot use in patients with nickel allergy ▪ Precaution with pacemakers/implanted chest wall device
Magnetic susceptometry (Magseed)[9]	▪ Audible tone feedback during probe reading ▪ Real-time distance measurement ▪ No interference with operating room equipment ▪ No radioactivity or toxic heavy metals ▪ No external component ▪ Approved for permanent placement in soft tissues	▪ Nonferromagnetic surgical instruments must be used ▪ Cannot use electrocautery ▪ Cannot use in patients with nickel allergy, pacemakers, implanted chest wall devices, metal implants ▪ Large signal void on MRI
"Wired" wireless localization (Perl)[10]	▪ May be placed up to 3 days prior to surgery ▪ Surgeons are familiar with wire localization ▪ No radioactivity or toxic heavy metals	▪ External wire component present, must be taped onto skin and kept sterile ▪ Patient must return for placement 3 days prior to surgery ▪ Sharp leading edge of ring may pierce skin if lesion is superficial (pathology technologist should be alerted of sharp edge) ▪ Composed of nitinol, not for use in patients with nickel allergy

[1]Karadeniz Cakmak G, et al. Surgeon performed continuous intraoperative ultrasound guidance decreases re-excisions and mastectomy rates in breast cancer. *Breast.* 2017;33:23–28; [2]Arentz C, et al. Ten-year experience with hematoma-directed ultrasound-guided (HUG) breast lumpectomy. *Ann Surg Oncol.* 2010;17: 378–383; [3]Ahmed M, et al. Radioactive seed localisation (RSL) in the treatment of non-palpable breast cancers: systematic review and meta-analysis. *Breast.* 2013;22:383–388; [4]Barentsz MW, et al. Radioactive seed localization for non-palpable breast cancer. *Br J Surg.* 2013;100:582–588; [5]Thind CR, et al. Sentinel node and occult (impalpable) lesion localization in breast cancer. *Clin Radiol.* 2011;66:833–839; [6]Patel R, et al. Pretreatment Tattoo Marking of Suspicious Axillary Lymph Nodes: Reliability and Correlation with Sentinel Lymph Node. *Ann Surg Oncol.* 2019;26:2452–2458; [7]Dauphine C, et al. A prospective clinical study to evaluate the safety and performance of wireless localization of nonpalpable breast lesions using radiofrequency identification technology. *AJR Am J Roentgenol.* 2015;204:W720–W723; [8]Mango VL, et al. Beyond Wires and Seeds: Reflector-guided Breast Lesion Localization and Excision. *Radiology.* 2017;284:365–371; [9]Lamb LR, et al. Evaluation of a Nonradioactive Magnetic Marker Wireless Localization Program. *AJR Am J Roentgenol.* 2018;211:W202; [10]Kozlov AN, Ikeda DM. First experience with a novel "wireless" wire localization device. *Breast J.* 2020;26:1838–1840.

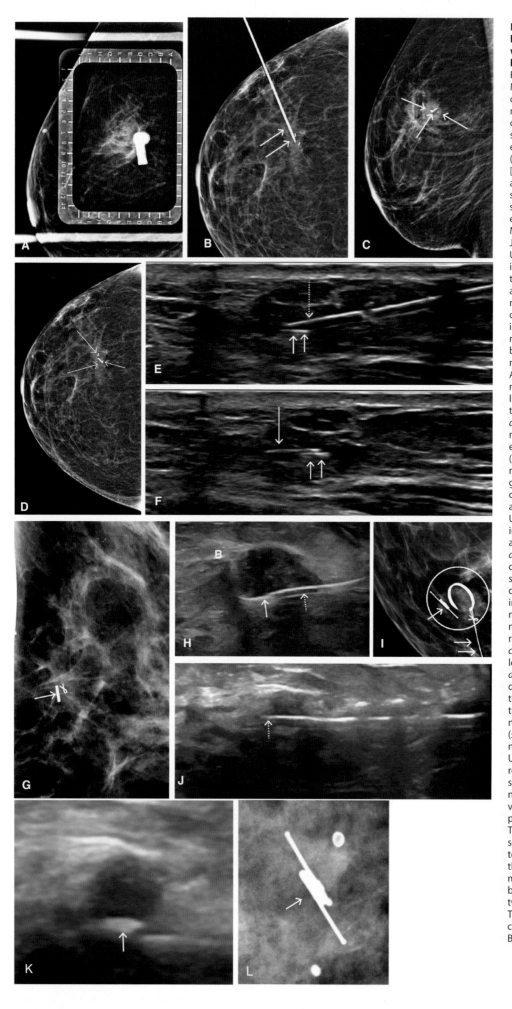

Fig. 7.25 Types of wireless fiducials and "wired wireless" preoperative localization devices. (A–D) Radioactive seed placement. Mediolateral (ML) (A) and craniocaudal (CC) (B) mammograms show a needle containing a radioactive seed (arrows) near two markers at biopsied calcifications (atypical ductal hyperplasia [ADH]). (C–D) Right ML (C) and CC (D) mammograms show the linear radioactive seed next to the biopsy markers (*arrows*). (images courtesy Marissa Gossweiler, DO, and James Covelli, MD). (E–G) Ultrasound-guided inducible magnetic seed localization. (E) Ultrasound shows a magnetic seed introducer needle tip (*dashed arrow*) in a cancerous breast mass; there is a linear bright reflector representing a postbiopsy ribbon marker adjacent to the needle tip (*double arrow*). (F) After deployment the linear magnetic seed is shown as a linear reflector (*arrow*) near the ribbon marker (*double arrow*). (G) Postlocalization mammogram shows the linear magnetic seed in the mass (*solid arrow*) near the ribbon marker. IDC. (H–I) Ultrasound-guided "wired" wireless device composed of a nitinol ring and flexible attached wire. (H) Ultrasound shows a needle introducer (*dashed arrow*) in a cancer with the ring (*solid arrow*) being deployed in the cancerous mass. Note the sharp leading end of the ring is deep to the skin to avoid piercing the skin during deployment. (I) Postlocalization mammogram shows the wired ring within the mass (*solid circle*) with its flexible wire leading to the skin (*double arrows*). The wire will be taped down to the skin. As this was the surgeon's first time using the wired wireless device, a near infrared wireless reflector (*solid arrow*) also was placed near the mass. IDC. (J–L. Ultrasound-guided near infrared reflector (J) ultrasound shows the reflector introducer needle tip (*dashed arrow*) traversing a cancerous mass and placed slightly beyond it. (K) The reflector is unsheathed so that the body of the reflector (*solid arrow*) is centered in the mass. (L) Postlocalization mammogram shows the solid body of the reflector with its two antennae (*solid arrow*). Two benign appearing calcifications are noted incidentally. Biopsy showed IDC.

SPECIMEN RADIOGRAPHY

The surgeon uses the wire/wireless fiducial location on the mammograms as a guide to find the target and excises the lesion, any markers, and hookwire/wireless fiducials. The excised tissue is called a *breast specimen*. An intraoperative breast specimen radiograph is taken to ensure that the entirety of the hookwire/fiducial localization devices and the target(s) have been removed. The radiologist reviews the specimen radiograph to see if the lesion, any markers, and the entire hookwire (with an intact hook) or wireless fiducial are included (Box 7.10). The radiologist notes whether the target is included in its entirety or if it is transected, and notes whether all markers and wires/wireless fiducials are present and calls the surgeon in the operating room with these findings. If the target(s) are not included,

the radiologist directs the surgeon to its expected location in the breast by using landmarks in the excised tissue and on the mammogram and waits for a second specimen (Fig. 7.26). If subsequent specimen radiographs still do not contain the targeted lesion(s) and/or markers/wires/fiducials, the surgeon may close the breast and obtain a mammogram to determine whether the target(s) are still in

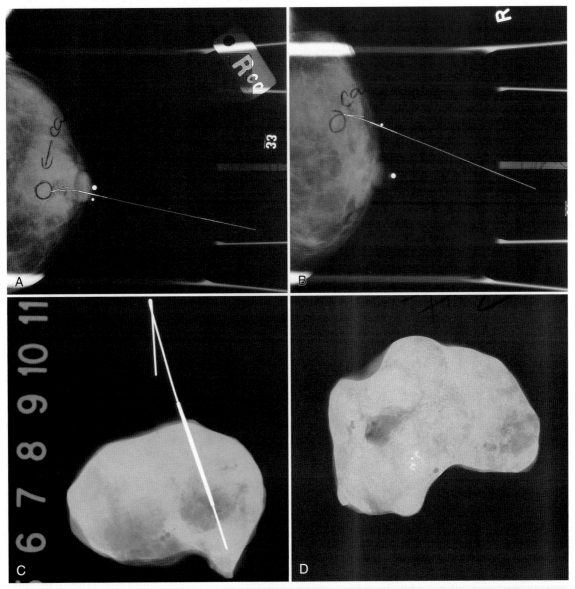

Fig. 7.26 Importance of specimen radiography. (A–B) The hookwire (analog) films from a freehand localization show the tip of the hookwire in micro-calcifications on the craniocaudal (A) and mediolateral (B) views. (C) The first specimen shows the hookwire but no calcifications. These findings were reported to the surgeon in the operating room. (D) Calcifications are seen in the second specimen. Note that freehand localization is an early localization technique no longer routinely performed and carries risk of pneumothorax when needles are advanced perpendicular to chest wall..

the breast. If specimen is interpreted after breast is closed (for example if surgeon does not request intraoperative consultation from radiology) then the radiologist should communicate any significant findings to the surgeon and a post-operative mammogram may be appropriate for documentation of target removal. The mammogram is usually done a few weeks after the surgery.

We note that specimen radiography may be obtained using a standard mammography unit or using specialized specimen radiography devices in the breast imaging suite. Alternatively, specialized specimen radiography devices may be located in the operating room with the images sent to picture archiving and communication systems (PACS) for review by the radiologist. If the findings are not seen on specimen radiographs taken in the operating room, the specimen may be transported to the breast imaging suite where additional specimen radiographs may be obtained on a mammographic unit, with or without compression, or using tomosynthesis to find the lesion (Fig. 7.27).

Tissue excised at US-guided preoperative localizations also undergoes specimen radiography, even if the finding cannot be seen on mammogram. The specimen radiograph may or may not show the US-localized finding but will show if the entire hookwire/wireless fiducial, as well as any metallic markers, was excised. If the specimen radiograph does not show the US-localized finding, the radiologist may perform specimen US to identify the mass.

KEY ELEMENTS

- Know the location of the target lesion in three dimensions.
- Do not attempt biopsy of a lesion if it is not real or if its location is unknown.
- Most nonpalpable lesions are diagnosed by image-guided percutaneous needle biopsy before surgical excision.
- Specimen radiography of mammography or ultrasound-localized surgical specimens should show the lesion, hookwire, and hookwire tip/wireless fiducials, and any associated metallic markers.
- Specimen findings are communicated to the surgeon in the operating room.
- For ultrasound-localized surgical specimens, specimen ultrasound can be done if the lesion is not seen on the specimen radiograph.

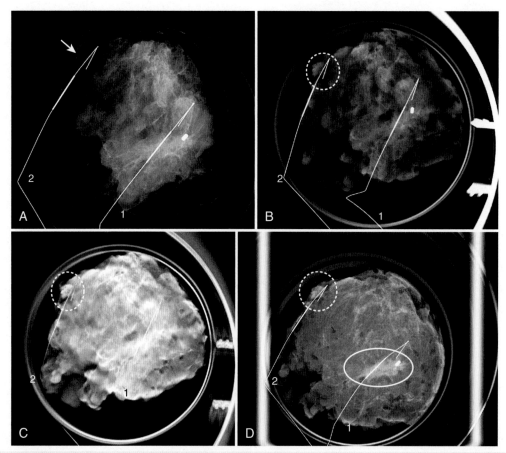

Fig. 7.27 Use of compression in specimen radiography or tomosynthesis when needed. Specimen Radiography after two x-ray-guided wire localizations for (1) stereotactic biopsy-proven atypical ductal hyperplasia (ADH) with cylinder marker and (2) an oval equal density mass in the right breast. (A) Intraoperative specimen radiograph obtained directly in the operating room without compression shows wire 1 with the marker, but wire 2 at the edge does not show the targeted mass (*arrow*), even when the image was windowed and leveled at a workstation. (B) Two-dimensional (2D) specimen radiograph on a conventional mammography unit shows the probable mass shadow (*dashed circle*) at the second wire tip. (C) Tomosynthesis through the specimen showed the mass (*dashed circle*) at the second wire tip. (D) Compression magnification specimen radiograph on the mammography unit clearly shows the mass (*dashed circle*) around the second wire tip, and postbiopsy change (*solid oval*) near first wire and the marker. Pathology showed a 3 mm focus of ductal carcinoma in situ (DCIS) at the area of ADH localized by the first wire and fibroadenoma representing the mass at the second wire.

- Reasons that calcifications may not be visualized on the histologic slides include nonremoval, calcium oxalate, location in the paraffin block, milk-of-calcium or displacement out of the specimen by the microtome.
- Risks of core biopsy include hematoma (fairly common but rarely significant), vasovagal reactions (not uncommon), and, rarely, untoward bleeding, infection, pneumothorax, pseudoaneurysm formation, implant rupture, and milk fistula (if the patient is pregnant or nursing).
- Correlation between the pathology results and imaging studies establishes concordance.
- If the specimen radiograph shows no calcifications for targeted calcifications, and yet the pathology report describes calcifications, the pathology report has described tiny, serendipitously found 100-μm calcifications that are not the mammographically visible target calcifications, and the patient needs to undergo rebiopsy.
- Marker location relative to biopsy target and accuracy for localizing target should be assessed on postbiopsy mammogram and documented in case future localization procedure is required.
- Discordant needle biopsy should prompt repeat biopsy or surgical excision depending on the individual scenario. Malignant biopsy results (invasive cancer, ductal carcinoma in situ (DCIS) should prompt surgical referral for breast cancer management. Management of high risk and other concerning pathologies is reviewed in Chapter 9: Breast Pathology and Radiologic-Pathologic Correlation.

References

1. American College of Radiology (ACR). *Practice Parameter for Performance of Stereotactic-Guided Percutaneous Breast Interventional Procedures.* https://www.acr.org/-/media/ACR/Files/Practice-Parameters/Stereo-Breast.pdf. Accessed April 25, 2020.
2. American College of Radiology (ACR). *Practice Parameter for the Performance of Ultrasound-Guided Percutaneous Breast Interventional Procedures.* https://www.acr.org/-/media/ACR/Files/Practice-Parameters/us-guidedbreast.pdf. Accessed April 25, 2020.
3. American College of Radiology (ACR). Accreditation Programs (includes mammography, ultrasound stereotactic-guided breast procedures). https://www.acraccreditation.org/. Accessed April 25, 2020.

Suggested Readings

D'Orsi CJ SE, Mendelson EB, Morris EA, et al. *ACR BI-RADS® Atlas, Breast Imaging Re porting and Data System.* Reston, VA: American College of Radiology; 2013.

Jackman RJ, Marzoni FA Jr. Stereotactic histologic biopsy with patients prone: technical feasibility in 98% of mammographically detected lesions. *AJR Am J Roentgenol.* 2003;180(3):785–794.

Kapoor MM, Patel MM, Scoggins ME. The wire and beyond: recent advances in breast imaging preoperative needle localization. *Radiographics.* 2019;39(7):1886–1906.

Ko K, Han BK, Jang KM, et al. The value of ultrasound-guided tattooing localization of nonpalpable breast lesions. *Korean J Radiol.* 2007;8(4):295–301.

Kozlov AN, Ikeda DM. First experience with a novel "wireless" wire localization device. *Breast J.* 2020;26(9):1838–1840

Melotti MK, Berg WA. Core needle breast biopsy in patients undergoing anticoagulation therapy: preliminary results. *AJR Am J Roentgenol.* 2000;174(1):245–249.

National Comprehensive Cancer Network (NCCN). *NCCN Clinical Practice Guidelines in Oncolgy; Breast Cancer Screening and Diagnosis.* Version 1.2019. https://www.nccn.org/professionals/physician_gls/pdf/breast-screening.pdf. Accessed April 25, 2020.

Patel R, MacKerricher W, Tsai J, et al. Pretreatment tattoo marking of suspicious axillary lymph nodes: reliability and correlation with sentinel lymph node. *Ann Surgical Oncol.* 2019;26(8):2452–2458.

Rebner M, Helvie MA, Pennes DR, et al. Paraffin tissue block radiography: adjunct to breast specimen radiography. *Radiology.* 1989;173(3):695–696.

Tornos C, Silva E, el-Naggar A, Pritzker KP. Calcium oxalate crystals in breast biopsies. The missing microcalcifications. *Am J Surgical Pathol.* 1990;14(10):961–968.

8 Breast MRI Indications, Interpretation, and Interventions

JING LUO AND HABIB RAHBAR

OVERVIEW *This chapter covers the fundamentals of breast MRI, including indications, technical considerations and MRI artifacts, MRI interpretation and reporting, and the basics of MRI-guided breast interventions.*

Indications

Breast magnetic resonance imaging (MRI) has higher sensitivity for detecting breast cancer compared with mammography and ultrasound. While MRI initially suffered from low specificity, more recent data suggest it is improving with recent advancement of MRI technology. Nonetheless, many benign pathologies exhibit suspicious enhancement, and implementation of breast MRI in addition to conventional breast imaging results in a greater number of biopsies. As a result, it is important that breast MRI be applied in a judicious, evidence-based manner to limit potential harms. Evidence supports the use of MRI for several clinical indications (Box 8.1). Chief among these is supplemental screening for women at high risk (≥20% lifetime) for developing breast cancer. Recent studies suggest that it may also have a role in "intermediate-risk" patients, chiefly in women with dense breasts but no other major risk factors. Breast MRI is not currently recommended as a general screening tool in the average-risk population due to its higher cost and false positive rate.

SCREENING

Breast MRI is an important adjunct screening tool for women at high risk of developing breast cancer. The American Cancer Society (ACS), American College of Radiology (ACR), and National Comprehensive Cancer Network (NCCN) currently recommend annual breast MRI in addition to annual mammogram in women with ≥20% lifetime risk. Breast cancer risk is determined by personal and family history as well as genetic predisposition (Box 8.2). Although a growing body of evidence supports screening breast MRI of intermediate-risk women, such as those with dense breasts or history of atypia on prior core biopsy, the evidence remains insufficient at this time for ACS to recommend its routine use in this setting. Although MRI has high sensitivity for detecting breast cancer, MRI is not recommended for screening in the general average-risk population due to higher costs and higher rates of benign biopsies.

Box 8.1 Indications for Breast Magnetic Resonance Imaging (MRI)

Evidence-Based Indications for Breast MRI
1. Screening for high-risk patients
2. Diagnostic imaging for women with known breast cancer
   a. Assess extent of disease for patients with newly diagnosed breast cancer
   b. Search for breast cancer in setting of metastatic axillary adenocarcinoma of unknown primary
3. Evaluation of response to neoadjuvant therapy
4. Problem solving: evaluation of suspicious nipple discharge
5. Evaluation of silicone implant integrity

Box 8.2 Guidelines for screening breast MRI

American Cancer Society 2007 Guidelines

Indications for Annual Breast MRI Screening:

- BRCA mutation carrier
- First-degree relative of BRCA mutation carrier, but untested
- Lifetime risk >20%, as defined by risk models largely dependent on family history
- Radiation to the chest between 10 and 30 years old
- Li-Fraumeni Syndrome and first-degree relative
- Cowden Syndrome and Bannayan-Riley-Ruvalcaba Syndrome and first-degree relative

Insufficient Evidence for Annual Breast MRI Screening:

- Lifetime risk <15–20%, as defined by risk models largely dependent on family history
- Lobular carcinoma in situ (LCIS) or atypical lobular hyperplasia (ALH)
- Atypical ductal hyperplasia (ADH)
- Heterogeneously or extremely dense breast on mammography
- Women with a personal history of breast cancer, including ductal carcinoma in situ (DCIS)

American College of Radiology 2018 Guidelines

Indications for Annual breast MRI Screening:

- Lifetime risk of 20% or greater
- Genetic mutation carrier and their untested first-degree relatives
- Chest radiation before 30
- Personal history of breast cancer before age 50
- History of breast cancer and dense breasts

Indication to consider annual screening breast:

- Personal history of atypia or LCIS

DIAGNOSTIC IMAGING IN WOMEN WITH KNOWN BREAST CANCER

NCCN guidelines recommend that breast MRI be considered in patients with newly diagnosed breast cancer to establish the extent of ipsilateral disease and screen the contralateral breast. Meta-analyses show that extent of disease MRI detects additional breast cancer approximately 15% of the time in the ipsilateral breast and 4% of the time in the contralateral breast.

MRI's intrinsically high tissue contrast and ability to assess dynamic enhancement patterns allow for better detection of multifocal (more than one area of malignancy within a quadrant) and multicentric (more than one area of malignancy within multiple quadrants) disease in the ipsilateral breast (Fig. 8.1). MRI assesses direct extension of disease to the overlying skin, nipple areolar complex, pectoralis muscle, and chest wall. Because MRI provides side-by-side imaging that allows for direct comparison of morphology with the contralateral side and includes all three axillae levels and the internal mammary chain, it can be helpful in assessing regional lymph node involvement. Specifically, it can identify suspicious level 1 axillary lymph nodes, for which preoperative ultrasound-guided percutaneous biopsy may be performed, as well as lymph nodes not typically visualized on mammogram and ultrasound, including level 2 axillary, level 3 axillary, and internal mammary. Finally, MRI detects clinically and mammographically occult synchronous cancer in the contralateral breast in about 4% of women with newly diagnosed breast cancer.

Rarely (<1%), breast cancer presents as metastatic axillary adenocarcinoma of unknown primary without a clinically or mammographically evident finding within the breast. In such cases, breast MRI has been shown to identify the otherwise occult breast primary malignancy in 61% of patients, which can significantly impact management approach.

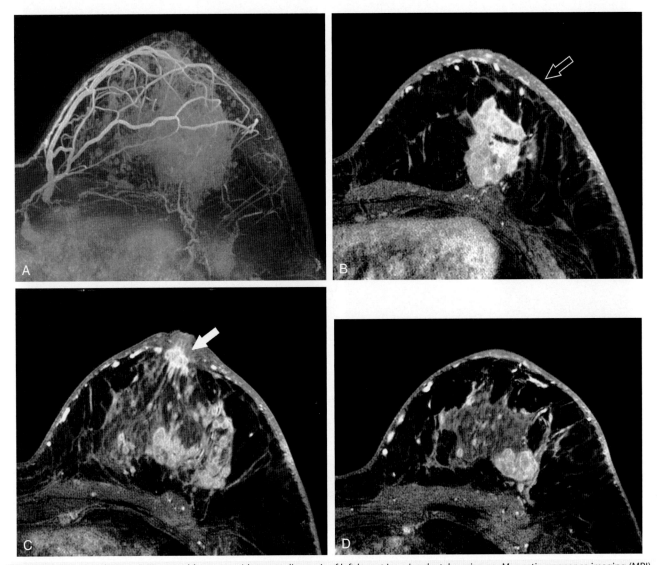

Fig. 8.1 Multicentric disease. A 52-year-old woman with recent diagnosis of left breast invasive ductal carcinoma. Magnetic resonance imaging (MRI) for extent of disease was performed. Axial maximum intensity projection images (A) and postcontrast axial T1-weighted images at three different levels (B–D) demonstrate multiple similarly appearing masses with irregular margins and heterogeneous internal enhancement, involving all four quadrants of the left breast consistent with multicentric disease. There is also associated skin thickening (*open arrow*) and nipple invasion (*solid arrow*).

EVALUATION OF RESPONSE TO NEOADJUVANT THERAPY

Breast MRI is used to assess response to neoadjuvant (presurgical) therapy for surgical and adjuvant (postsurgical) therapy planning purposes. Neoadjuvant therapy typically refers to chemotherapy, although hormonal therapy may also be used. Neoadjuvant therapy has several advantages over traditional postsurgical therapy approaches without adverse effect on overall and disease-free survival: (1) It can make breast conservation more feasible in women with locally advanced disease; (2) it can allow for in vivo assessment of the effectiveness of the selected treatment regimen;

and (3) it can allow for treatment to begin while the patient carefully considers optimal surgical and reconstruction options. MRI is an excellent imaging tool to determine neoadjuvant therapy effectiveness. Decrease in lesion size and volume and less suspicious enhancement kinetics on follow-up MRIs at various time points during chemotherapy treatment are associated with neoadjuvant treatment outcomes, such as pathologic complete response, allowing for assessment of a primary lesion's response prior to surgery (Figs. 8.2 and 8.3). For patients with poor or no response to neoadjuvant therapy, a change in treatment regimen may be indicated. Studies show that MRI is a stronger predictor of pathologic response to neoadjuvant therapy than

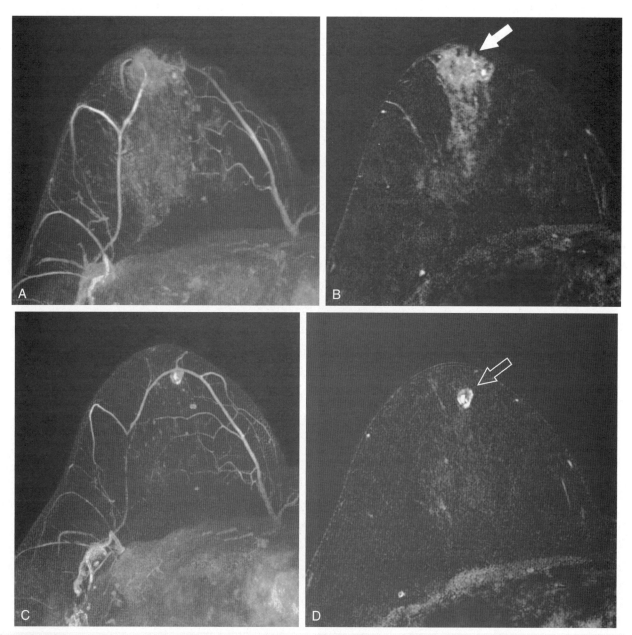

Fig. 8.2 Partial tumor response to neoadjuvant chemotherapy. A 36-year-old woman with biopsy proven grade 3 triple-negative invasive ductal carcinoma (IDC). The axial maximum-intensity projection (A) and postcontrast axial T1-weighted subtraction images (B) demonstrate an irregular mass with heterogeneous internal enhancement in the subareolar region of the right breast (*solid arrow*). There is evidence of nipple and skin invasion. The patient subsequently received neoadjuvant chemotherapy with interval decreased size of the index malignant mass (*open arrow*) on the axial maximum intensity projection (C) and postcontrast axial T1-weighted subtraction images (D), compatible with favorable response to neoadjuvant chemotherapy. Of note, in addition to the index malignant mass, there is also decreased background parenchymal enhancement likely a secondary result of neoadjuvant chemotherapy.

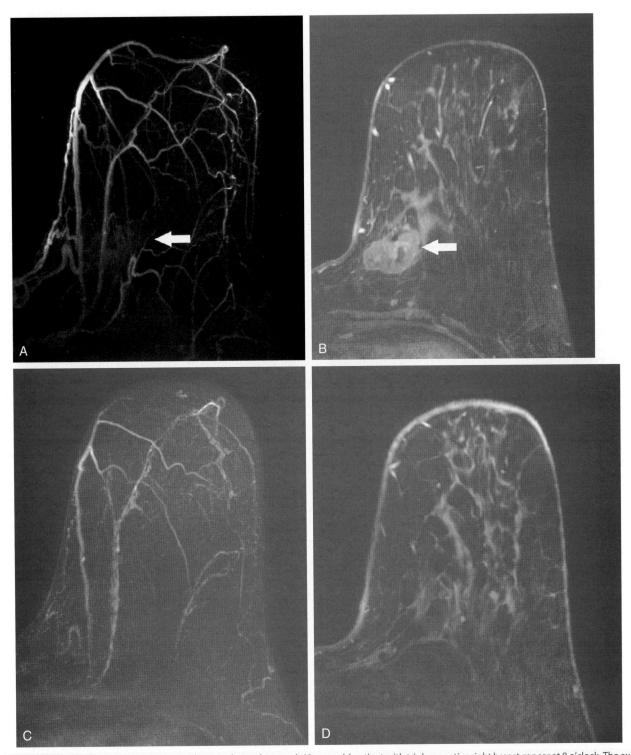

Fig. 8.3 Complete imaging response to neoadjuvant chemotherapy. A 60-year-old patient with triple-negative right breast cancer at 8 o'clock. The axial maximum-intensity projection (A) and postcontrast axial T1-weighted subtraction images (B) demonstrate an irregular mass with heterogeneous internal enhancement and irregular margins (*solid arrows*). The patient received neoadjuvant chemotherapy with interval complete resolution of the index malignant mass on the axial maximum-intensity projection (C) and postcontrast axial T1-weighted subtraction images (D), compatible with complete imaging response to neoadjuvant chemotherapy. This patient subsequently underwent bilateral mastectomies.

clinical assessment and that it is superior to mammography and ultrasound in assessing for residual disease after completion of neoadjuvant therapy. However, pathologic response to therapy at the time of surgery is still considered the gold standard. Even in cases with no residual suspicious enhancement in the breast after neoadjuvant therapy, a BI-RADS category 6 assessment should still be assigned until surgical excision is completed.

PROBLEM SOLVING: EVALUATION OF SUSPICIOUS NIPPLE DISCHARGE

The use of MRI for problem solving of equivocal mammographic or sonographic imaging findings is not supported by research, except for the clinical scenario of suspicious nipple discharge. Suspicious nipple discharge is bloody or clear in color, unilateral, spontaneous, and usually arising from a single duct. For patients over the age of 30, initial imaging workup involves mammogram and ultrasound. When both are negative, either contrast-enhanced MRI or ductography may be considered. Although ductography has historically been the examination of choice, it is invasive and requires nipple discharge to be present on the day of the procedure to allow cannulation of the appropriate duct. Ductography may only show "tip of the iceberg" as the initial obstruction prevents retrograde contrast from passing, thus missing significant upstream disease. Furthermore, ductography does not provide a means for sampling of an abnormality and can only serve as guidance for the surgeon's excision. MRI is noninvasive and has been shown in multiple studies to have higher sensitivity and specificity compared with ductography. MRI also allows for a means to biopsy the abnormality prior to surgery. This is important, since a malignant diagnosis on core biopsy prior to surgery can allow for a single operation to be performed, particularly in cases of invasive cancer where axillary lymph node sampling is required.

EVALUATION OF SILICONE IMPLANT INTEGRITY

Breast implants can be single- or double-lumen, containing saline, silicone, or a combination of both. Complications, specifically implant rupture, are common. Saline implant rupture is a clinical diagnosis and presents as rapid loss of breast volume with surrounding tissue absorbing the saline solution over several days. Silicone implant rupture is more difficult to detect on clinical examination. Mammography alone has low sensitivity for detecting silicone implant rupture, especially intracapsular implant rupture. MRI is considered the gold standard for diagnosis of intracapsular silicone implant rupture with high sensitivity and specificity. Implant evaluation is discussed in further detail in the "Augmented and Reconstructed Breast" chapter (Chapter 18).

Technical Considerations and MRI Artifacts

TECHNICAL CONSIDERATIONS

Although breast MRI acquisition protocols vary between institutions, there is a set of generally agreed-upon minimum standards and technical considerations. Examinations are performed with patients in the prone position, and breasts are positioned within a dedicated breast surface coil. The use of dedicated breast surface coils helps maximize signal, and the greater number of coil elements allows for higher spatial resolution and reduction of scan time via parallel imaging. Both breasts are imaged, which allows for assessment of symmetry, establishment of bilateral background parenchymal enhancement, and determination of bilateral benign findings. The field of view should include bilateral axillae and chest wall.

Because adequate signal-to-noise ratio (SNR) is required to achieve high imaging quality, and SNR is directly proportional to the strength of the main magnetic field B0, breast MRI is typically performed with a 1.5 T or higher strength magnet. Higher magnetic field strength also allows for better magnetic field homogeneity and more uniform fat suppression.

Although there are emerging noncontrast techniques such as diffusion-weighted imaging (DWI), clinical breast MRI currently requires administration of gadolinium-based contrast for detection of breast cancer, injected intravenously using a power injector at a dose of 0.1 mmol/kg followed by a 20 mL saline flush at a rate of 2 mL/s.

High temporal and spatial resolution is crucial for detection and characterization of lesions on breast MRI. High spatial resolution allows for assessment of small morphologic features such as spiculations and dark internal septations. The ACR Breast Magnetic Resonance Imaging Accreditation Program (BMRAP) requires all T1-weighted images to be acquired with slice thickness of 3 mm or less and a maximum in-plane pixel dimension of 1 mm^3. High temporal resolution during postcontrast sequences provides information on enhancement kinetics with invasive cancers typically demonstrating early-phase fast enhancement followed by delayed-phase washout. Because achieving high spatial resolution requires longer imaging time, spatial and temporal resolutions must be balanced when designing the imaging protocol. In general, spatial resolution is more important because it allows for improved depiction of lesion morphology, which is the most important feature for determining Breast Imaging Reporting and Data System (BI-RADS) assessment and the probability of malignancy (see interpretation algorithm below).

Fat suppression is essential in order to avoid the intrinsic high signal on T1-weighted images from obscuring enhancing abnormalities. Fat suppression can be achieved with spectral fat suppression during image acquisition or through subtraction techniques during postprocessing. Newer techniques such as the multipoint Dixon technique, which relies on chemical shift phenomena, can provide even more homogeneous fat suppression but are less commonly used due to time penalties and other artifacts (e.g., fat-water swapping).

KEY PULSE SEQUENCES

Conventional clinical breast MRI includes a precontrast fluid-sensitive sequence and a T1-weighted dynamic contrast enhanced (DCE) series consisting of precontrast, initial postcontrast, and at least one delayed postcontrast acquisitions. In most protocols, the initial postcontrast

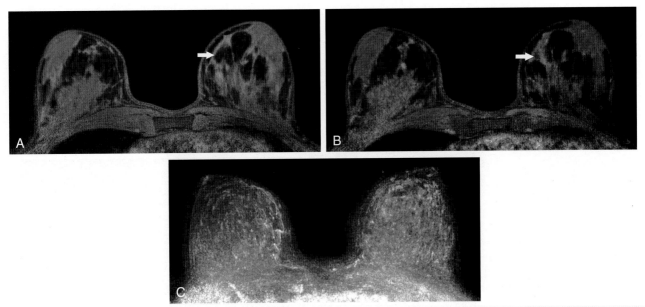

Fig. 8.4 Interscan and intrascan motion. Precontrast (A) and postcontrast (B) T1-weighted fat-saturated images demonstrate difference in fibroglandular tissue pattern when comparing images at the same slice level (*solid arrows*), indicating interscan motion. There is also mild intrascan motion in the left breast. This causes pseudoenhancement on the subtracted maximum-intensity projection image (C).

acquisition also serves as the "peak" series, which refers to the approximate time point where most breast cancers will exhibit the greatest level of enhancement. Typically, this "peak" series should have a k-space centered at approximately 90 to 120 seconds after injection. Most commonly, the T1-weighted dynamic series will employ spoiled gradient-recalled echo (GRE) to allow for efficient acquisition that balances both spatial and temporal resolution needs. Fat suppression is important and may be achieved actively for all series acquired through frequency selective pulses or passively through subtraction.

The precontrast fluid-sensitive sequence requires the use of spin-echo (T2-weighted), fast spin-echo (T2-weighted), or short tau inversion recovery (STIR) types of pulse sequences. STIR sequences provide homogeneous fat suppression by nulling T1 signal below fat but do not provide a "pure" T2 signal, since the contrast achieved is additive from T1, T2, and proton density. For this reason, and because STIR can result in poorer signal-to-noise ratio, spin-echo/fast spin-echo based approaches may be preferred for fluid signal. With this approach, fat suppression is typically performed (e.g., active fat saturation or Dixon), although some sites prefer to obtain T2-weighted images without fat suppression.

Reconstructed subtraction images are useful for distinguishing true enhancement from intrinsic T1 signal, regardless of whether active or passive fat suppression is utilized. Useful series include a "peak" axial subtraction images (obtained by subtracting the precontrast DCE sequence from the "peak" postcontrast DCE sequence) and maximum-intensity projections (MIP) reconstructed from the subtraction images. Orthogonal plane reformats in sagittal and coronal orientations are helpful for lesion localization and characterization. Minimizing intra- and interscan motion is important for avoiding significant pseudoenhancement on subtraction series.

ARTIFACTS

Motion artifact is one of the most common challenges to performing high-quality breast MRI (Fig. 8.4). The breasts are in close proximity to the heart, lungs, and great vessels, which are organs with intrinsic motion. Periodic motion, such as the heart beating, produces discrete image ghosts occurring cyclically along the phase-encode direction. Nonperiodic motion, such as esophageal peristalsis, results in diffusely increased image noise propagating along the phase-encode direction. Setting the phase-encode direction to the right/left minimizes obscuration of breast anatomy by cardiac and respiratory motion. Careful instruction to patients helps minimize patient-specific intra- and interscan motion, which in turn minimizes pseudoenhancement on subtraction series.

Wrap-around artifact is an example of aliasing and occurs when the dimensions of the anatomy being scanned exceeds the field of view (FOV). Wrap-around, as the name indicates, produces images with anatomic parts folded over and superimposed onto the region of interest. Mitigation usually consists of increasing the FOV and number of phase-encode steps, although this incurs the cost of increased imaging time.

Susceptibility artifact results from local distortion of the magnetic field, most often seen surrounding metallic objects such as biopsy clips (Fig. 8.5). Susceptibility produces signal loss through T2* effects and causes geometric image distortion, resulting in spuriously high or low signal. The artifact is helpful for localizing surgical and biopsy marker clips. Susceptibility artifact is more pronounced with higher magnetic field strength and may be mitigated by using thinner image slices, increasing gradient strength for a given FOV, and increasing bandwidth.

Magnetic field inhomogeneity occurs due to local differences in the strength of the main magnetic field within the anatomic region being imaged. Various artifacts result

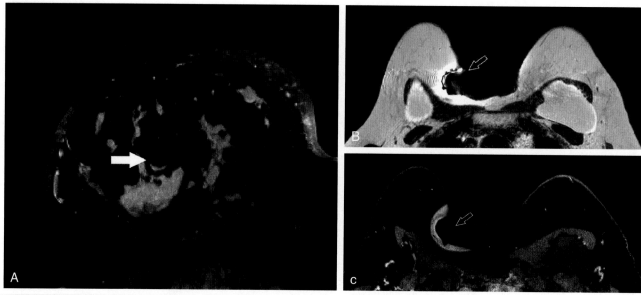

Fig. 8.5 Susceptibility artifact. Postcontrast T1-weighted fat-saturated images (A) demonstrate susceptibility artifact from the biopsy marker clip (*solid arrow*). Precontrast T1-weighted (B) and postcontrast T1-weighted fat-saturated images (C) demonstrate incomplete fat saturation and loss of signal near the right anterior chest wall due to presence of a port catheter (*open arrow*).

Table 8.1   Common Artifacts in Breast MRI

Artifact	Mitigation Techniques
Wrap around	Increase field of view (FOV) and phase-encode steps
Motion (pulsation)	Phase-encoding set to right-left direction
Pseudoenhancement	Patient coaching and positioning to avoid macromotion
Incomplete fat saturation	Shimming
Moiré fringe artifact	Reposition patient

from inhomogeneity, including shading, spatial distortion, curved slice profiles, and zebra banding (moiré fringe). One of the most important effects of poor homogeneity in breast imaging is poor spectral fat suppression, which can falsely cause lesions to appear enhancing. Inhomogeneity may be mitigated by shimming or repositioning the patient within a more uniform portion of the magnetic field.

See Table 8.1 for a summary of common artifacts on breast MRI and mitigation techniques.

Breast MRI Interpretation and Reporting

APPROACH TO MRI INTERPRETATION

A systematic approach to interpreting breast MRI improves accuracy and clinical relevance of reporting to referring providers. The ACR BI-RADS Atlas standardizes interpretation and reporting of breast MRI, which increases consistency of reporting and recommendations between radiologists and institutions. The first step in interpreting

MRI is to understand the patient's clinical and surgical history. For example, location of known cancer, histologic type of cancer, history of hormonal therapy, and current plans for treatment are all important to consider in order to provide a clinically relevant interpretation and recommendation to the referring clinician. The next step is to evaluate images systematically using the BI-RADS lexicon. This process is described in detail in the following section.

MRI BI-RADS LEXICON

Breast MRI BI-RADS terminology shares many terms with mammography and ultrasound lexicon, with some important distinctions and additions. For every MRI, the amount of fibroglandular tissue (FGT) and the amount of background parenchymal enhancement (BPE) should be assessed. Furthermore, suspicious enhancing lesions (foci, masses, and non-mass enhancement) should be characterized with lesion-specific terminology, as described in more detail below.

Amount of Fibroglandular Tissue

The amount of FGT on MRI is analogous to breast density on mammography and best assessed on precontrast T1-weighted images. According to the BI-RADS lexicon, it is divided into four categories: almost entirely fat, scattered, heterogeneous, and extreme (Fig. 8.6).

Amount of Background Parenchymal Enhancement

Normal breast parenchyma demonstrates variable physiologic enhancement depending on phase of the menstrual cycle, menopausal status, age, history of radiation, and hormone replacement or suppression therapy, which is termed BPE. BPE is best assessed on the "peak" postcontrast T1-weighted images, with k0 typically centered around 90 to 120 seconds after contrast injection. BPE typically increases over a dynamic series, and evaluating BPE on a

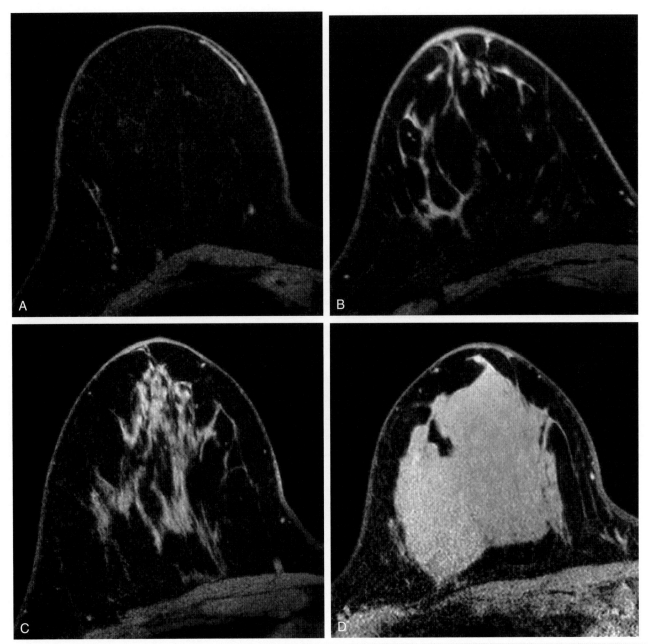

Fig. 8.6 Breast composition. Four categories of the amount of fibroglandular tissue on precontrast T1-weighted axial images: almost entirely fatty (A), scattered fibroglandular tissue (B), heterogeneous fibroglandular tissue (C), and extreme fibroglandular tissue (D).

later dynamic phase may lead to an overestimation of BPE levels. According to the BI-RADS lexicon, BPE is divided into four categories: minimal, mild, moderate, and marked, which is a subjective combined assessment of the volume of FGT demonstrating enhancement and its intensity of enhancement (Fig. 8.7).

BPE is usually symmetric between breasts. Benign asymmetric BPE is most often due to prior breast cancer treatment due to decreased FGT in the affected breast and/or radiation therapy effects or asymmetric lactational changes (Fig. 8.8). If asymmetric enhancement is present, the radiologist should carefully assess for the presence of suspicious non-mass enhancement (NME) prior to dismissing the finding as BPE.

BPE is known to have cyclic variations in premenopausal women such that on serial examinations, the amount of BPE present can vary between all four categories. BPE is also known to be lower on average in women who are postmenopausal, on endocrine therapy (e.g., Tamoxifen), or have undergone oophorectomy.

Elevated levels of BPE had been thought to adversely affect the accuracy of MRI interpretation due to the potential to "mask" an enhancing abnormality. However, recent research has demonstrated that BPE has little to no effect on MRI sensitivity. It is possible that BPE does adversely affect specificity and abnormal interpretation rate. Some authors have demonstrated BPE is lower in the early phase of a woman's menstrual cycle; however, it is also not clear

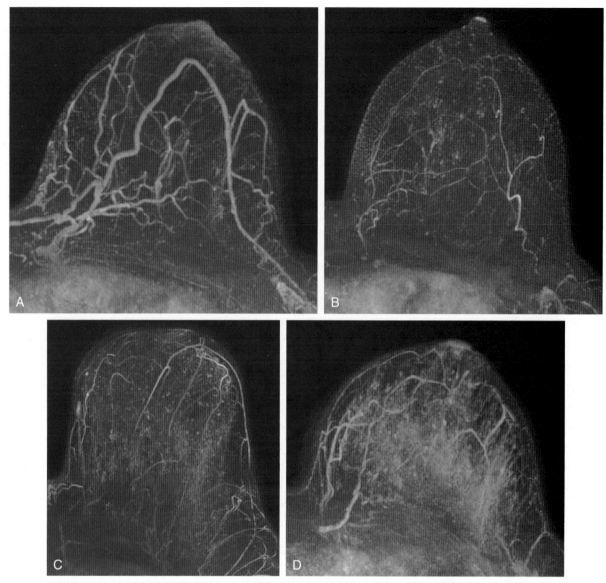

Fig. 8.7 Background parenchymal enhancement. Four categories of background parenchymal enhancement on maximum intensity projection images: minimal (A), mild (B), moderate (C), and marked (D).

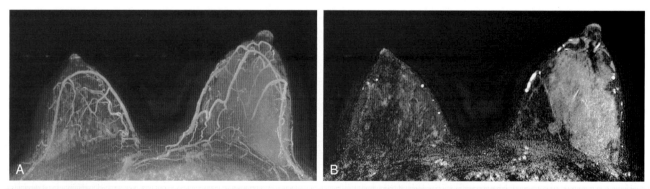

Fig. 8.8 Asymmetric lactation changes. A 34-year-old *BRCA2* mutation carrier presenting for a high-risk screening magnetic resonance imaging (MRI). According to clinical history, the patient is lactating, left breast more than right. Maximum-intensity projection (A) and postcontrast T1-weighted subtraction images (B) demonstrate mild background parenchymal enhancement (BPE) in the right breast and marked BPE in the left breast, consistent with asymmetric lactational changes.

that "timing" MRIs in any particular phase leads to a consistently lower BPE level. Thus, imaging facilities may vary in their protocols or recommendations that breast MRIs be "timed" to early menstrual cycle phases. Some argue that strict "timing" decreases access and does not provide a clear interpretation benefit.

Recent studies have shown BPE to be an independent predictor of breast cancer risk and treatment outcome; elevated BPE levels are associated with a greater risk of developing breast cancer. This is an area of active research and does not have a direct clinical application at the time of writing.

Lesion Type, Morphology, and Internal Enhancement Characteristics

A lesion on breast MRI is an enhancing finding that is unique and different from BPE. The BI-RADS lexicon describes three lesion types on breast MRI: focus, mass, and NME. Lesion can further be described based on morphology, internal enhancement characteristics, and enhancement kinetics. Among these features, morphology is the most important factor for distinguishing benign lesions from those suspicious for malignancy.

A *focus* is a unique enhancing lesion without specific morphology (margin or shape) that has no corresponding finding on precontrast T1-weighted images (Fig. 8.9). Foci are often less than 5 mm in size, although the BI-RADS lexicon does not impose a size limit on foci. A focus is most often benign and may represent a variant of background parenchyma enhancement, an intramammary lymph node, or fibrocystic changes. Imaging features that make a focus suspicious include appearance distinct from BPE, absence of fatty hilum, low signal on T2-weighted images, worrisome kinetic features (washout on delayed phase), and

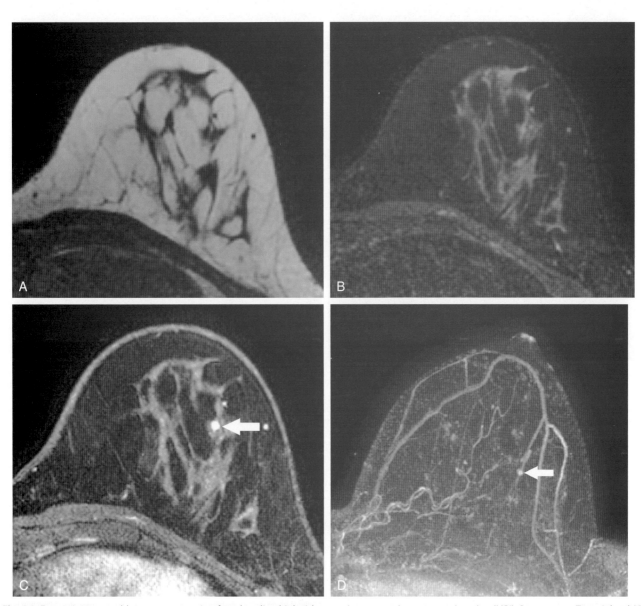

Fig. 8.9 Focus. A 37-year-old woman presenting for a baseline high-risk screening magnetic resonance imaging (MRI). Postcontrast T1-weighted (C) and maximum-intensity projection images (D) demonstrate a 4-mm enhancing focus at the 5 o'clock position (*solid arrow*). Note, there is no correlate of this finding on precontrast T1-weighted (A) and T2-weighted images (B). This finding was interpreted as BI-RADS 3 (probably benign), and a follow-up MRI in 6 months was recommended.

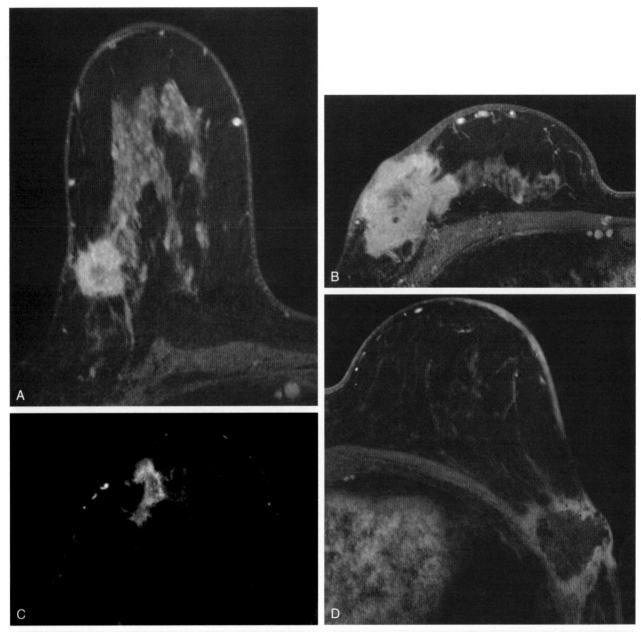

Fig. 8.10 Mass. Postcontrast axial T1-weighted images in four different women demonstrate a round mass with irregular margin and heterogeneous internal enhancement in a 48-year-old woman with invasive ductal carcinoma (IDC) (A), an irregular mass with irregular margin and heterogeneous internal enhancement with associated skin invasion in a 41-year-old woman with IDC (B), an irregular mass with spiculated margin and heterogeneous internal enhancement with associated nipple invasion and retraction in a 69-year-old woman with IDC (C), and an irregular mass with irregular margin and rim enhancement with associated skin and chest wall invasion in a 64-year-old woman with IDC status postlumpectomy with locoregional recurrence (D).

interval appearance or increased size compared with prior examinations.

A *mass* is a space-occupying lesion with convex-outward contour (Fig. 8.10). Morphologic features (shape and margin) are used to determine level of suspicious for malignancy. Because most breast cancers demonstrate fast initial enhancement, the early or peak postcontrast T1-weighted images should be used to evaluate morphology. Mass shape may be oval, round, or irregular per BI-RADS lexicon. Mass margin may be circumscribed or not circumscribed (subdivided into irregular and spiculated). In general, circumscribed masses are more suggestive of benign lesions and noncircumscribed masses are more concerning for malignancy.

Masses can demonstrate homogeneous (confluent and uniform) or heterogeneous (nonuniform) internal enhancement with heterogeneous enhancement more suggestive of malignancy. There are two special enhancement patterns: rim enhancement and nonenhancing dark internal septations. Rim enhancement of a solid mass, with enhancement more pronounced at the periphery of the mass, is particularly suspicious for malignancy except in definite cases of inflamed cyst or fat necrosis, which can be determined based on other imaging features such as high T2 signal and presence of fat, respectively (Fig. 8.11). Dark internal septations is suggestive of fibroadenoma, especially if other benign morphologic and kinetic features are present, although caution is advised as malignancy can have overlapping imaging features.

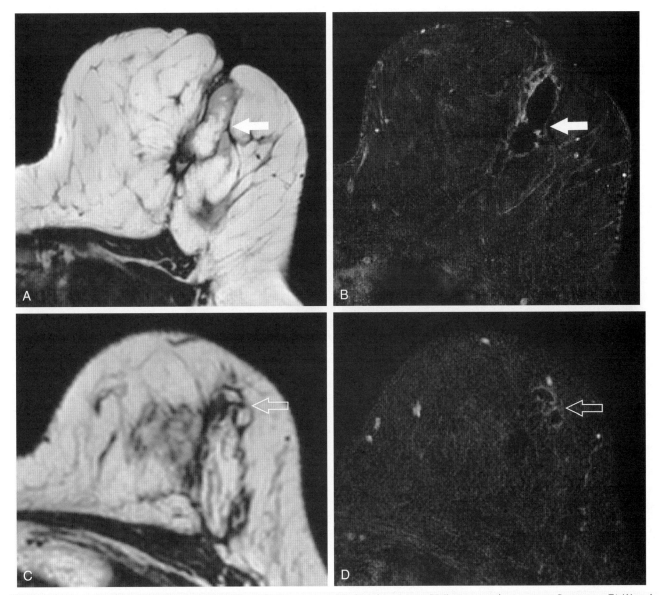

Fig. 8.11 Fat necrosis. A 40-year-old woman with history of left breast invasive ductal carcinoma (IDC) status postlumpectomy. Precontrast T1 (A) and postcontrast T1-weighted fat-saturated subtraction images (B) demonstrate a fat-containing mass with rim enhancement, consistent with fat necrosis (*solid arrows*). A 60-year-old woman with history of left breast ILC status postlumpectomy. Precontrast T1-weighted (C) and postcontrast T1-weighted fat-saturated subtraction images (D) demonstrates two adjacent fat-containing masses with rim enhancement, consistent with fat necrosis (*open arrows*).

Non-mass enhancement (NME) is a pattern of enhancement distinct from BPE but is not space-occupying and does not fit the definition of a mass or focus (Figs. 8.12 and 8.13). NME is classified according the distribution of the enhancement (Table 8.2). Linear and segmental NME are most suspicious for malignancy, while regional, multiple regions, and diffuse NME are more characteristic of a benign process, although multicentric cancer can have overlapping imaging features.

Internal enhancement characteristics of NME can be described as homogeneous, heterogeneous, clumped, or clustered ring. Among these descriptors, clumped enhancement (aggregate of enhancing foci in a cobblestone pattern) is most suggestive of malignancy. As clustered ring enhancement (thin rings of enhancement clustered around the ducts) also implies a suspicious finding, often described with ductal carcinoma in-situ.

However, as it is a newer term, there are less data assessing its predictive value.

Contrast Kinetic Features

Kinetic features should always be interpreted in the context of other imaging features such as lesion morphology. Suspicious lesions can be differentiated from normal breast parenchyma and benign findings by evaluating lesion type and morphology the majority of the time. For the remaining equivocal cases, kinetic features should be taken into consideration.

Examples of equivocal lesions include unique focus not bright on T2-weighted images, morphologically benign-appearing mass, and equivocal NME versus asymmetric BPE.

Because the rate and quantity of intravenous gadolinium contrast agent injection are constant, the rate of contrast

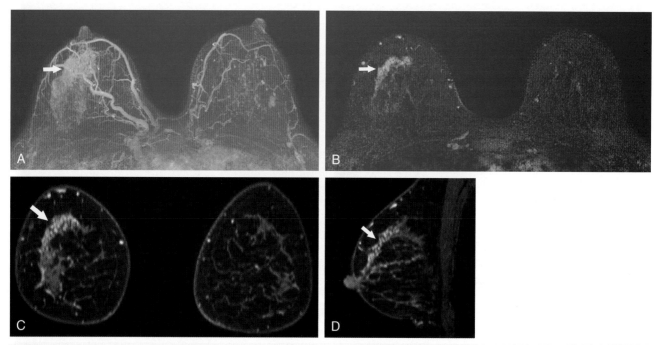

Fig. 8.12 Segmental non-mass enhancement. A 36-year-old with biopsy-proven right breast invasive ductal carcinoma (IDC). Breast magnetic resonance imaging (MRI) was performed for extent of disease. Besides the biopsy proven mass (not shown), axial maximum-intensity projection (A), postcontrast T1-weighted subtraction images in axial (B), coronal (C), and sagittal (D) planes demonstrate segmental non-mass enhancement in the upper outer quadrant with heterogeneous internal enhancement (*solid arrows*). MRI-guided biopsy of this finding revealed invasive and in situ carcinoma.

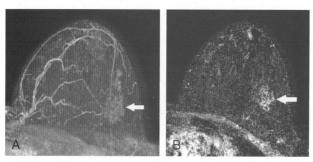

Fig. 8.13 Clustered ring non-mass enhancement. A 53-year-old woman with family history of breast and ovarian cancer presented for a high-risk screening magnetic resonance imaging (MRI). Axial maximum-intensity projection (A) and postcontrast T1-weighted subtraction images demonstrate segmentally distributed non-mass enhancement at 3 o'clock upper outer quadrant with clustered ring internal enhancement (*solid arrows*).

Table 8.2   Distribution of Non-mass Enhancement

Distribution of Enhancement	Definition
Focal	Less than a quadrant
Linear	In a line, corresponding to a single duct
Segmental	Triangular or cone-shaped with the apex at the nipple
Regional	Spans at least one quadrant; broader area than a single duct system
Multiple regions	At least two broad areas, separated by normal tissue or fat
Diffuse	Widely scattered and evenly distributed

enhancement of a lesion is dependent on perfusion and capillary permeability, which in turn is thought to reflect underlying tumor angiogenesis. In practice, breast cancers tend to enhance rapidly after contrast injection initially, followed by quick washout of contrast agent.

In order to assess kinetic features, the DCE MRI must include a precontrast series and at least two postcontrast T1-weighted series, described in more detail above. DCE features are evaluated for two phases of enhancement: initial-phase enhancement and late-phase enhancement. Currently, automated computer-aided detection (CAD) systems are used to display kinetic information in the form of graphs and color maps.

Initial-phase enhancement is classified as slow (<50%), medium (50%–100%), or fast (>100%, previously called "rapid") as defined by the percent of increase in signal intensity when comparing the first postcontrast images obtained at peak enhancement (within the first 2 minutes) to precontrast images. Delayed-phase enhancement is classified as persistent (>10% increase), plateau (within 10% increase or decrease), or washout (>10% decrease) as defined by change in signal intensity comparing delayed postcontrast images to the first postcontrast images. Most lesions demonstrate a mixture of initial-phase and delayed-phase features (Fig. 8.14). Prior studies have shown that the most valuable feature when using kinetics to problem solve an equivocal MRI finding is the "worst curve type," which refers to applying the presence of any initial and delayed phase class using the following hierarchy:

a. Initial phase: Fast > medium > slow
b. Delayed phase: Washout > plateau > persistent

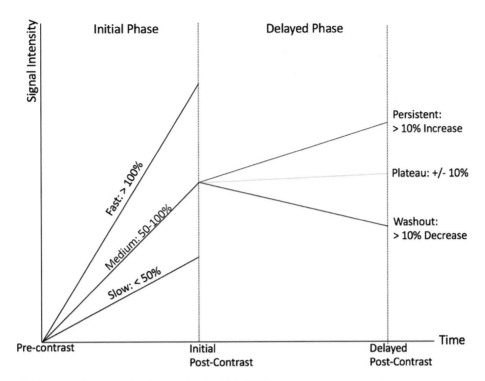

Fig. 8.14 Contrast kinetics features of breast magnetic resonance imaging (MRI).

Assigning BI-RADS Assessments on MRI

We suggest following a systematic approach for interpreting MRI of the breast. The authors' approach is as follows (Fig. 8.15). After reviewing the indication for imaging and the patient's clinical history, begin with the subtracted MIP images for an overview of BPE, symmetry, and obvious lesions. Next, use the T1-weighted DCE and subtraction images to locate suspicious findings and determine their type and morphology as well as assess the amount of FGT. Next, use the fat- and fluid-sensitive sequences to assess for entities such as cysts, lymph nodes, and fat necrosis. A BI-RADS assessment category should be assignable for most lesions using the above information. For the minority of lesions that remain equivocal, use the worst curve kinetics to inform their BI-RADS assessment. When multiple lesions are present, the BI-RADS assessment hierarchy organizes findings from the most clinically actionable to the least: 5 > 4 > 0 > 6 > 3 > 2 > 1. Finally, a BI-RADS assessment should be given for each breast. In general, unlike mammography, BI-RADS 0 and 3 are rarely given in breast MRI. In fact, most lesions should have a definitive category based on MRI alone.

Foci should be a rare finding, as most nonspecific dots of enhancement are not unique and are in fact part of BPE. A truly unique focus of enhancement can often be categorized as benign or probably benign and assigned BI-RADS category 2 or 3, particularly when they demonstrate high signal on T2-weighted images. BI-RADS category 4 should generally be reserved for foci that demonstrate low signal on T2-weighted images and suspicious kinetic features (e.g., washout on delayed phase), or if it is new or increased in size compared with a prior examination. Foci never have imaging characteristics sufficient to be characterized as BI-RADS category 5.

Masses have a wide range of suspicion for malignancy. Most suspicious or indeterminate masses should be assessed as BI-RADS category 4. A BI-RADS category 5 mass implies a very high probably (95% or greater) of malignancy and should possess multiple suspicious features including irregular shape, non-circumscribed margins, and rim or heterogeneous internal enhancement. A BI-RADS category 3 should be rarely used and implies that the mass has a less than 2% probability of malignancy. Uniform high signal on T2-weighted images is a reassuring feature for benignity when combined with other reassuring features, such as oval shape and circumscribed margins, and homogeneous internal enhancement, but should not be used in isolation to avoid biopsy. Kinetic features can be helpful to reassure that a mass is likely benign; however, they should not be used to obviate biopsy of a mass with suspicious morphologic features. A BI-RADS category 2 should be reserved for characteristically benign lesions, such as intramammary lymph nodes and fat containing lesions, described further below.

NME is most frequently assigned BI-RADS category 4. Because a spectrum of entities from benign to malignant can present as NME, biopsy is recommended in most cases. Among descriptors for NME, linear or segmental distributions and clumped internal enhancement are most suspicious for malignancy.

MALIGNANT MRI FINDINGS

Invasive Carcinoma

Among the many different histologic types of breast cancer, invasive ductal carcinoma (IDC) and invasive lobular carcinoma (ILC) are the most common. See Table 8.3 for different types of breast cancer and their characteristic features.

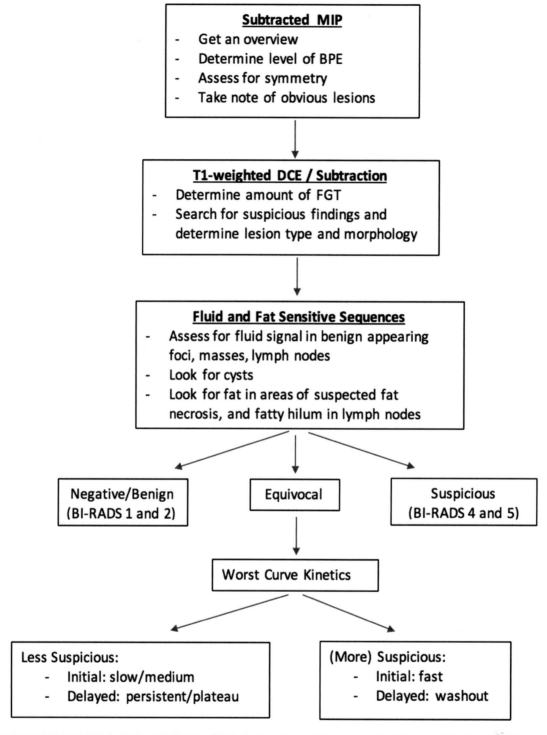

Fig. 8.15 Systematic approach for interpreting breast magnetic resonance imaging (MRI).

Ductal Carcinoma in Situ

Ductal carcinoma in situ (DCIS) is a proliferation of abnormal epithelial cells confined within the breast ducts. DCIS is a nonobligatory precursor to IDC and accounts for approximately 25% of breast cancers detected on screening mammography. MRI has higher sensitivity for detection of DCIS compared with mammography.

DCIS most commonly presents on breast MRI as segmental NME with clumped or clustered ring enhancement. Less commonly, DCIS presents as masses or enhancing foci on MRI. As opposed to its invasive counterpart, DCIS more commonly demonstrates delayed peak enhancement and washout, making the use of kinetic features potentially less reliable.

Features Associated with Malignancy

In addition to systemically evaluating each lesion on MRI, it is important to closely evaluate other anatomic structures in the FOV for associated features of malignancy (Box 8.3).

Table 8.3 Types of Invasive Breast Cancer and Its Characteristic Features

Invasive ductal carcinoma	Most common type of breast cancer (70%–90%)
	Classic appearance on magnetic resonance imaging (MRI): irregular mass with spiculated margins
	Classic kinetic features: initial fast enhancement, delayed washout
Invasive lobular carcinoma	Second most common type of breast cancer
	Infiltrative growth pattern
	Can present as mass or non-mass enhancement (NME)
	Account for a high proportion of mammographically occult breast cancers
Papillary carcinoma	Presents in older women
	Favorable prognosis
Mucinous carcinoma	Often contain areas of T2 hyperintensity (mucin)
Metaplastic carcinoma	Often contain areas of T2 hyperintensity (due to cystic degeneration)
Medullary carcinoma	Presents in younger women (60% of patients <50 years old)
	Has benign imaging features (oval or round in shape)
Malignant phyllodes*	Often are round or oval in shape with circumscribed margins (difficult to distinguish from a benign fibroadenoma)
	Rapid growth over time is an important clinical clue

*Phyllodes tumor is by definition not a breast cancer.

Important areas to assess include the nipple areolar complex, overlying skin, pectoralis muscles, axillary and internal mammary lymph node chains, chest wall (intercostal muscles and ribs), mediastinum, visualized lungs, and upper abdomen (Fig. 8.16).

For every MRI, and especially in women with known invasive cancer, it is important that the radiologist evaluate for the presence of abnormal axillary and internal mammary lymph nodes (Fig. 8.17). More details are provided in the "Lymph Node Evaluation in Breast Imaging" chapter (Chapter 17). Axillary lymph nodes provide 97% of lymphatic drainage from the breast, with the internal mammary lymph nodes accounting for the remaining 3%. Axillary lymph nodes are divided into three levels using the pectoralis minor muscle as the delineating anatomic landmark. There are no reliable size criteria for determining the

Box 8.3   Features Associated With Malignant MRI Findings

- Skin thickening, retraction, or invasion
- Nipple retraction or invasion
- Muscle invasion
- Growth through Cooper ligaments
- Architectural distortion
- Morphologically abnormal axillary and internal mammary lymph nodes

presence of absence of abnormal axillary lymph nodes. Instead, radiologists are best served to rely on asymmetry and morphologic features, such as rounding, loss of fatty hila, and cortical thickening (at least 3 mm). Internal mammary lymph nodes can be more challenging to assess given their typically smaller size. Again, symmetry and morphology, when assessable, are the most valuable features, with a general size cutoff of at least 5 mm favored by some.

BENIGN MRI FINDINGS

Cysts are common benign findings with round or oval shape and circumscribed margins (Fig. 8.18). Simple cysts have high signal on T2-weighted sequences and do not enhance. Complicated cysts with high protein content or blood products can have high T1-weighted and variable T2-weighted signal. Inflamed cysts can demonstrate thin rim enhancement without nodularity.

Duct ectasia presents as dilated and fluid-filled ducts in a branching pattern radiating from the nipple. Duct ectasia has imaging characteristics that overlap with those of cysts. It is important to evaluate for the presence of an intraductal mass, especially in the setting of a solitary dilated duct. Ductal or clustered ring enhancement raise concern for early forms of malignancy such as DCIS.

Intramammary lymph nodes are very common and usually reside in the upper outer quadrant of the breast. The presence of a fatty hilum on non-fat-suppressed T1-weighted images and high signal on T2-weighted images are the most important features for identifying a lymph node. Kinetic features are not helpful because almost all lymph nodes demonstrate initial rapid and delayed washout. Features suspicious for nodal metastasis include cortical thickening, loss of normal reniform shape, and loss of fatty hilum.

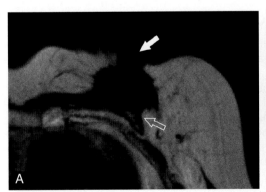 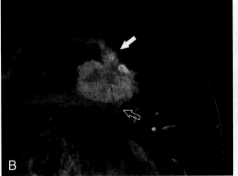 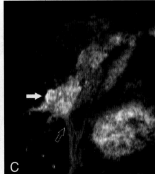

Fig. 8.16 Nipple and pectoralis muscle invasion. A 75-year-old with biopsy-proven left breast invasive ductal carcinoma (IDC). Precontrast T1-weighted (A), postcontrast T1-weighted axial (B), and sagittal (C) images demonstrate an irregular mass with irregular margin and heterogeneous enhancement. There is evidence of nipple retraction (*solid arrows*) and invasion of the pectoralis muscle (*open arrows*).

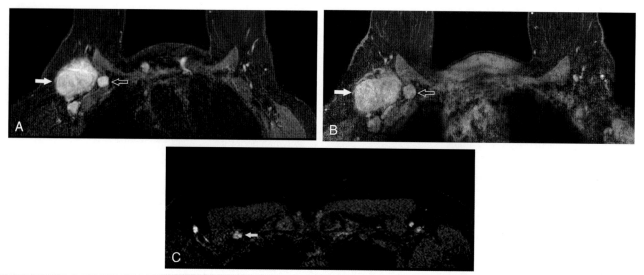

Fig. 8.17 Axillary lymphadenopathy. T2-weighted (A) and postcontrast T1-weighted axial images (A–B) in a 79-year-old with right breast triple-negative invasive ductal carcinoma (IDC) demonstrate morphologically abnormal level 1 (*solid arrow*) and level 2 (*open arrow*) axillary lymph nodes. T2-weighted axial images (C) in a 36-year-old woman with right triple-negative breast cancer demonstrate a morphologically abnormal level 3 axillary lymph node (*yellow arrow*).

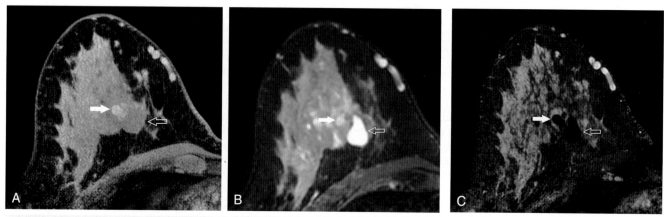

Fig. 8.18 Cysts. A 41-year-old women presented for a high-risk screening magnetic resonance imaging (MRI). Precontrast T1-weighted (A), T2-weighted (B), and postcontrast T1-weighted (C) subtraction images demonstrate multiple nonenhancing oval masses with circumscribed margin, some of which demonstrating high T1 signal and variable T2 signal (*solid and open arrows*), consistent with a combination of simple cysts and hemorrhagic/proteinaceous cysts.

Fat containing lesions, including fat necrosis, lipomas, galactoceles and hamartomas, are characteristically benign. Presence of fat can be best identified on non-fat suppressed T1-weighted images.

MRI-Guided Breast Interventions

A suspicious (BI-RADS 4 or 5) lesion identified on MRI warrants biopsy for histopathological evaluation. When there is high probability of finding a sonographic correlate, targeted ultrasound followed by ultrasound-guided core needle biopsy should be considered before MRI-guided biopsy. Compared with MRI-guided biopsy, ultrasound-guided biopsy is less expensive and better tolerated by the patient. Ultrasound-guided biopsy is also technically easier if the suspicious finding is in the axilla or close to the chest wall. MRI-guided biopsy is generally recommended when there is low probability of accurately localizing the MRI finding with ultrasound (small lesion <10 mm, NME, lesion located in heterogeneous breast

tissue) or if no sonographic correlate is visible. It is important to remember that the absence of an ultrasound finding cannot obviate the need to biopsy a suspicious MRI finding.

PULSE SEQUENCES FOR MRI-GUIDED BIOPSY

After localizer sequences, pre- and postcontrast fat-suppressed images are performed in the sagittal or, less commonly, axial plane. A second postcontrast fat-suppressed image is obtained to confirm appropriate positioning of the coaxial sheath after the biopsy device is positioned but before sampling. Finally, after tissue sampling and biopsy clip placement, a third postcontrast fat-suppressed image is obtained to confirm the presence of biopsy site changes or the position of the biopsy marker clip.

APPROACH PLANNING

Planning the appropriate approach for MRI-guided biopsy requires careful review of the diagnostic MRI, including

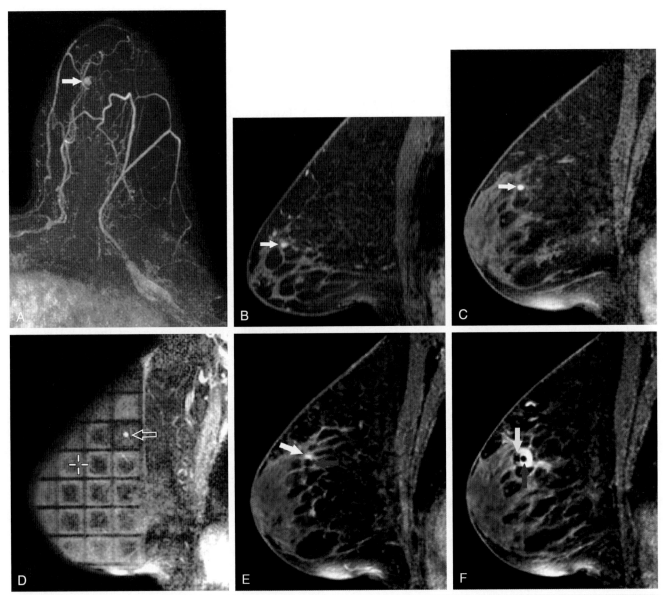

Fig. 8.19 Key steps in magnetic resonance imaging (MRI)-guided biopsy of a suspicious finding using manual targeting method. A 56-year-old woman with biopsy-proven right breast invasive ductal carcinoma (IDC) (not shown). Axial maximum-intensity projection (A) and postcontrast T1-weighted sagittal images (B) from the extent of disease MRI demonstrate a round mass with circumscribed margin and homogeneous internal enhancement in the contralateral left breast (*solid arrow*). Postcontrast sagittally acquired images during MRI-guided biopsy redemonstrate the round mass (C). A cursor is placed on this mass, and coordinates in antero-posterior, medio-lateral, and superior-inferior dimensions are recorded. The cursor is then propagated onto a sagittal slice at the level of the skin, fiducial marker (*open arrow*), and grid (D). Skin entry site relative to the fiducial marker, appropriate location in the tunneled needle guide, and the depth to which the introducer sheath should be advanced are then determined. After local anesthetics, the introducer sheath is inserted using a cutting introducer stylet to the appropriate depth. The inner stylet is then exchanged for a plastic obturator (*red arrow*). Subsequently, a sagittal sequence is obtained confirming location of the obturator, which should end in the targeted finding (E). Vacuum-assisted breast biopsy is then performed and a clip is placed at the site of biopsy. Finally, postbiopsy sagittal images (F) demonstrate the biopsy marker clip (*yellow arrow*), which appears as susceptibility artifact within the targeted mass. Coordinates of the biopsy marker clip is recorded and compared with the coordinates of the targeted lesion. Pathology revealed fibroadenoma, which is benign and concordant.

determination of lesion location (quadrant, clock position, depth) and identification of landmarks in the surrounding background parenchyma. MRI-guided biopsy is performed using a medial or lateral approach with preference for the shortest route to the lesion. Special considerations include compression thickness, distance from the skin, and feasibility of reaching the lesion with MRI guidance. In cases where the optimal approach is uncertain, the approach can be determined after the initial scan with grids placed on the medial and lateral sides of the breast.

Basic Steps of MRI-Guided Biopsy

The basic steps of MRI-guided biopsy are similar regardless of vendor, biopsy device, and platform (Fig. 8.19). Here is a summary of basic steps:

1. Position the patient in prone position with the breast containing the lesion of interest compressed using a grid
2. Place a fiducial marker (visible on T1-weighted images)
3. Obtain pre- and postcontrast sagittal T1-weighted images

4. Determine location of the lesion (box on the grid and depth)
5. Sterilize skin
6. Administer local anesthesia
7. Place a plastic needle guide (typically a plastic box with nine tunnels) into the appropriate grid box
8. Introduce outer component of the coaxial system to the appropriate depth using the inner cutting stylet
9. Remove the inner stylet and replace with a plastic obturator while keeping the coaxial sheath in place
10. Perform scan to confirm location of the coaxial sheath and obturator
11. Replace the obturator with the vacuum-assisted biopsy device
12. Obtain 6 to 12 samples while rotating the biopsy device to various clockface directions
13. Once sampling is complete, the biopsy site is irrigated and suctioned
14. Remove the biopsy device and place a biopsy marker clip through the coaxial sheath
15. Perform postbiopsy scan to confirm biopsy marker clip location
16. Release breast from compression and use manual compression to achieve hemostasis
17. Obtain two-view conventional mammogram to confirm clip location

Confirming biopsy marker clip location on mammography is important because a subsequent mammographically guided localization for surgery is much easier to perform if necessary.

RADIOLOGY-PATHOLOGY CONCORDANCE AND FOLLOW-UP

As for all breast biopsies, radiology-pathology concordance is important. MRI-guided biopsy has inherent challenges, as patients are often high risk, findings are often subtle or occult on mammography and ultrasound, and the lesion of interest is not visualized in real time as samples are obtained. Repeat biopsy should be considered if the lesion appears to be inadequately sampled or the histopathologic result is discordant with imaging findings. Follow-up imaging 6 to 12 months after biopsy should also be considered if there are concerns about adequate sampling even if the result is benign and concordant.

Occasionally, MRI-guided biopsy must be cancelled because the targeted lesion cannot be visualized at the time of biopsy. Although most of these findings are benign and represent fluctuating BPE, a short-term follow-up MRI in 3 to 6 months is generally recommended to exclude malignancy. Biopsy is indicated if the lesion persists or increases in size on subsequent MRI.

KEY POINTS

- Indications for breast magnetic resonance imaging (MRI)
  - Supplemental screening of women with >20% lifetime risk for breast cancer
  - Extent of disease assessment for known breast cancer
  - Evaluation of response to neoadjuvant therapy
  - Evaluation of silicone implant integrity
  - Evaluation of suspicious nipple discharge with otherwise negative workup
- High temporal and spatial resolution is crucial for characterization of lesions on MRI. Conventional clinical breast MRI includes a precontrast fluid-sensitive sequence and T1-weighted dynamic contrast-enhanced sequences consisting of precontrast, initial postcontrast, and at least one delayed postcontrast acquisitions.
- A systematic approach to interpreting breast MRI using Breast Imaging Reporting and Data System (BI-RADS) lexicon improves accuracy and clinical relevance of reporting.
- A BI-RADS assessment should be given for each breast. When multiple findings are present, the BI-RADS assessment hierarchy organizes findings from the most clinically actionable to the least: 5 > 4 > 0 > 6 > 3 > 2 > .
- A lesion on breast MRI is an enhancing finding that is unique and different from BPE. The BI-RADS lexicon describes three lesion types on breast MRI: focus, mass, and non-mass enhancement. Lesions can further be described based on morphology, internal enhancement characteristics, and enhancement kinetics. Among these features, morphology is the most important factor for distinguishing benign and malignant lesions.
- MRI-guided biopsy is recommended when there is low probability of accurately localizing an MRI finding with ultrasound (small lesion <10 mm, non-mass enhancement, lesion located in heterogeneous breast tissue) or if no sonographic correlate is visible. Absence of an ultrasound finding cannot obviate the need to biopsy a suspicious MRI finding.

Suggested Reading

Mann RM, Cho N, Moy L, Breast MRI: state of the art. *Radiology*. 2019;292(3):520–536.

Martaindale SR, Breast MR. Imaging: atlas of anatomy, physiology, pathophysiology, and breast imaging reporting and data systems lexicon. *Magn Reson Imaging Clin N Am*. 2018;26(2):179–190.

Sippo DA, Burk KS, Mercaldo SF, et al. Performance of screening breast MRI across women with different elevated breast cancer risk indications. *Radiology*. 2019;292(1):51–59.

DeMartini WB, Rahbar H. Breast magnetic resonance imaging technique at 1.5 T and 3 T: requirements for quality imaging and American College of Radiology accreditation. *Magn Reson Imaging Clin N Am*. 2013;21(3):475–482.

McGrath AL, Price ER, Eby PR, Rahbar H. MRI-guided breast interventions. *J Magn Reson Imaging*. 2017;46(3):631–645.

9 *Breast Pathology and Radiologic–Pathologic Correlation*

DEBBIE LEE BENNETT AND LINDA MOY

OVERVIEW *This chapter covers normal breast anatomy and correlation between imaging and pathology, including management of benign lesions, high-risk lesions, and malignancies.*

Knowledge of breast anatomy and pathology is critical for accurate image interpretation. Understanding the spectrum of benign and malignant pathologies allows radiologists to confidently identify abnormal findings, give a reasonable differential diagnosis, and assign an accurate probability of malignancy with appropriate management recommendations.

Careful radiologic–pathologic correlation is a critical component of image-guided breast biopsy. American College of Radiology (ACR) practice parameters for stereotactic, ultrasound-guided, and magnetic resonance imaging (MRI)-guided biopsies highlight the importance of determining concordance after receiving pathology results. Appropriate determination of radiologic–pathologic concordance and subsequent management hinges on radiologists' understanding of breast pathologies. If pathology results are felt to be discordant, repeat or excisional biopsy should be performed to prevent potential delays in cancer diagnosis. Further, although some pathologies may not be malignant, they may require further clinical management or surgical referral. This chapter provides a basic understanding of breast pathology and radiologic–pathologic correlation for radiologists.

Overview of Normal Breast Anatomy

ANATOMY

The anatomic borders of the breast are defined as the sternum (medial), mid-axillary line (lateral), second rib (superior), sixth to seventh rib (inferior), superficial fascia (anterior), and deep/pectoral fascia (posterior). The majority of the breast lies anterior to the pectoralis muscle; a portion lies anterior to the serratus anterior muscle. Because the upper outer quadrant of the breast has an extension into the axilla, known as the tail of Spence, this quadrant contains more breast tissue than other quadrants.

The breast is composed of skin, subcutaneous fat, fascia, parenchymal tissue, and the nipple-areolar complex (Fig. 9.1). The fascia envelops the breast parenchyma anteriorly and posteriorly. The parenchymal tissue is where breast pathologies arise, and consists of glandular tissue, stromal elements, fat, and suspensory (Cooper) ligaments, which travel through the breast parenchyma and insert in the dermis.

There is a branching system of ducts throughout the glandular tissue, which take milk from the acini where it is produced all the way to the nipple, where it is excreted during breast feeding. There are seven to nine lactiferous ducts, each of which open into an orifice in the nipple. Each lactiferous duct is connected to 15 to 20 lobes, each of which has several lobules. Within the lobules, terminal ducts are surrounded by acini; this forms the functional unit of the breast, known as the terminal ductal lobular unit (TDLU). The TDLU is generally 1 to 4 mm in diameter. The number of acini in each TDLU varies from about 11 in nulliparous women to about 80 acini during pregnancy and breast feeding. The ducts are lined by epithelium, which has an inner secretory epithelial cell layer and an outer myoepithelial cell layer. There is a continuous basement membrane along the course of the ductal epithelium. Stromal elements surround the glandular tissue and may be either interlobular or extralobular in location.

The areola consists of sebaceous, sweat, and accessory glands, which form Montgomery tubercles. Smooth muscle fibers are also present, which are responsible for nipple erection.

The arterial supply to the breast comes from the axillary artery branches (30%, mostly upper outer quadrant), internal mammary artery (60%, mostly medial and central breast), and lateral branches of the intercostal arteries. The venous drainage parallels the arterial supply and is also through axillary, internal mammary, and intercostal veins. The innervation of the breast is through the lateral cutaneous branches of the third through sixth intercostal nerves.

Lymphatic drainage of the breast parenchyma occurs through deep lymphatic vessels, which travel along the lactiferous ducts, mostly to ipsilateral axillary nodes (these are discussed in Chapter 17). Some deep lymphatic vessels in the medial breast also drain to internal mammary nodes. There is a superficial lymphatic plexus that drains the skin and nipple-areolar complex; this is known as Sappey plexus.

BREAST EMBRYOLOGY AND DEVELOPMENT

Breast development in utero follows a predictable pattern that begins early in fetal development and results in differentiation of lobules, acini, lactiferous/mammary ducts, nipple-areolar complex, and Montgomery glands by birth.

Anatomy of the Breast

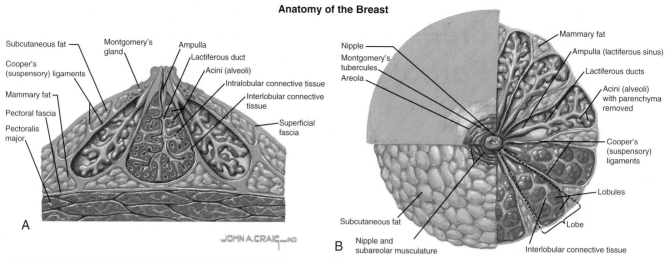

Fig. 9.1 Schematic of normal breast anatomy. Diagrams of breast in cross-sectional (A) and coronal plane (B) illustrating normal breast structures. (Netter medical illustration used with permission of Elsevier. All rights reserved.)

The ectodermal primitive milk streak develops between the axillae and groin during the fifth to sixth week of fetal development. Although most of the milk streak subsequently regresses, the thoracic portion does not. During the 12th week of fetal development, mesodermal ingrowth forms a breast bud, with formation of 16 to 24 secondary buds during the 12th week of fetal development. Differentiation then continues until birth. Under the influence of circulating maternal hormones, babies may have a breast bud under the nipple at birth, which can be asymmetric.

During early puberty, breast development occurs in response to hormonal changes; this stage of puberty is known as thelarche. Estrogen drives ductal development and progesterone leads to lobular development and epithelial differentiation. Alveolar buds form from the terminal ductules in the breast, forming type 1 breast lobules. There is also an increase in periductal connective tissue.

MENSTRUAL CYCLE AND MENOPAUSE

Hormonal changes throughout the menstrual cycle are also reflected in the breast tissue. During the luteal phase (day 15–28), there are increased progesterone levels, leading to dilation of the mammary ducts and differentiation of the epithelial cells into secretory cells. There is also increased blood flow to the breasts prior to the onset of menses, which can contribute to cyclical breast pain.

During menopause, the ductal, glandular, and stromal elements of the breast undergo involution and atresia and are gradually replaced with adipose tissue. Type 1 lobules again predominate in the breast.

Radiologic–Pathologic Correlation and Recommendations

The imaging appearance of masses and calcifications reflects their underlying pathophysiology. Analysis of the margins of a mass gives information about the biological nature of the mass. Infiltrative lesions, such as most cancers, have no sharp interface between normal and abnormal

---

Box 9.1   Factors Affecting Sensitivity of Core Needle Biopsy and Likelihood of Upgrade on Excision

Type of biopsy device (spring-loaded versus vacuum-assisted)
Needle gauge
Number of cores
Extent of lesion sampled
Specimen processing
Histopathologic analysis
Radiologic–pathologic correlation

---

tissue. This infiltrative appearance is associated with margin descriptors such as spiculated, indistinct, and angular. Infiltrative lesions and cancers may also be associated with surrounding desmoplastic response, leading to the imaging finding of architectural distortion. Benign masses, on the other hand, typically have "pushing borders" that are circumscribed, as there is no infiltration of benign tumor cells into adjacent tissue. Benign masses also commonly demonstrate parallel orientation, respecting the anatomic planes of the breast.

Similarly, analysis of the morphology and distribution of calcifications can guide the radiologist to the appropriate diagnosis and recommendation. Calcifications are often "casts" that form within an anatomic or pathologic space (e.g., within the lumen of a duct). Irregular calcifications are often associated with necrosis. Smooth calcifications are typically associated with a benign underlying process.

Radiologic–pathologic correlation is a critical component of breast biopsy procedures. The accuracy of core needle biopsy has been well established, with low false-negative rates ranging from 0.45% to 4.4%. Factors affecting the sensitivity of core needle biopsy include the type of biopsy device and gauge of biopsy needle (Box 9.1). Lower upgrade rates were reported for vacuum-assisted 9- to 11-gauge biopsy devices, compared with 14- to 18-gauge spring-loaded devices. Among pathologists, histologic analysis is also subjective for many lesions, with particular overlap in the appearance of high-risk and malignant lesions; this may also contribute to variable upgrade rates.

Given that many percutaneous biopsies are performed with imaging guidance, determination of concordance and subsequent management of benign, high-risk, and malignant pathology results are often the radiologist's responsibility. Concordant biopsies are those in which the pathology result adequately accounts for the imaging finding. Concordant biopsies may be concordant and benign (e.g., oval circumscribed mass with pathology showing fibroadenoma) or concordant and malignant (e.g., irregular spiculated mass with pathology showing invasive ductal carcinoma). Determination of concordance depends on careful assessment of the imaging features of the biopsied finding. In general, lower-suspicion findings (Breast Imaging Reporting and Data System [BI-RADS] 4 A and 4B) are likely to be considered concordant if a benign biopsy result is obtained. Cases in which the biopsy result shows only benign breast tissue without other pathologic process should be reviewed carefully; in some circumstances, this result may be deemed concordant (mammographic asymmetry, non-mass enhancement on MRI, possible hamartoma on ultrasound), and follow-up imaging should be performed.

The radiologist also takes into consideration the adequacy of lesion sampling, including number of samples taken, presence of targeted lesion on specimen radiograph if performed, postbiopsy appearance of lesion, and location of biopsy clip on postprocedure mammogram. Because the adequacy of sampling is best assessed by the physician performing the biopsy, ACR practice parameters for image-guided biopsies recommend that the physician performing the biopsy should be responsible for assessing concordance. Patients who have benign, concordant findings but are symptomatic may also be referred to a breast surgeon for clinical management.

Discordant biopsies are those in which the pathology result does not adequately explain the imaging findings. In general, a benign core needle biopsy result should be considered discordant if the prebiopsy level of suspicion was high and the abnormality was given a BI-RADS 5 assessment. Discordant pathology results should either be rebiopsied using imaging guidance or be referred for excisional biopsy. A malignancy rate of 24% has been reported in a combined series of both stereotactic and ultrasound-guided discordant core needle biopsies. A close working relationship among the radiologist, pathologist, and surgeon is important when there are questions about the concordance of imaging findings with the pathologic result. Surgical consultation should be recommended for patients who have discordant, high-risk, or malignant findings.

Appearance and Management of Benign Lesions

Many benign and concordant pathologies do not require clinical management unless symptomatic. Often these patients may return for annual screening mammography or short-interval follow-up imaging. However, some pathologies do require clinical management or excision. The radiologist performing the biopsy must understand

clinical management in order to ensure appropriate referral and care for the patient. The following is a description of benign pathologies that may be encountered in clinical breast imaging practice, with associated recommendations. Benign pathologies presenting most commonly as masses are described first (Boxes 9.2 and 9.3), followed by benign pathologies more often presenting as calcifications (Box 9.4).

BENIGN BREAST MASSES GENERALLY NOT REQUIRING ADDITIONAL MANAGEMENT

Many benign pathologies do not require surgical consultation or clinical management when concordant (see Box 9.2).

Fibroadenoma

Fibroadenomas are common benign masses that arise from proliferation of both the epithelial and stromal elements of the TDLU. This proliferation results in a confluence of lobules known as fibroadenomatoid nodules, which together form a fibroadenoma.

Fibroadenomas are the most common mass found in adolescents and younger women (10–30 years) and usually present as a palpable, slow-growing, painless mass (Fig. 9.2). They may also be incidentally found on screening mammography or ultrasound. They may be of any size; fibroadenomas over 5 cm in size are called giant fibroadenomas. Juvenile fibroadenomas are seen in patients younger than 20 years and typically grow rapidly. Fibroadenomas involute after menopause and may calcify, resulting in classic popcorn calcifications visible on mammography.

The typical imaging appearance of fibroadenoma is an oval mass with circumscribed margins, usually hypoechoic with parallel orientation on ultrasound. Fibroadenomas with these features may be assessed as probably benign (BI-RADS 3) and be followed with serial imaging to establish 2- or 3-year stability. If not all these imaging features are seen, biopsy should be recommended. If the mass has a

---

Box 9.2   Benign Concordant Masses Requiring No Additional Clinical Management (Unless Symptomatic or Enlarging)

Fibroadenoma
Lipoma
Hamartoma
Pseudoangiomatous stromal hyperplasia (PASH)
Intramammary lymph node
Fat necrosis
Fibrocystic change/cyst

Box 9.3   Benign Concordant Masses Usually Warranting Surgical Consultation (for Excision or Clinical Management)

Phyllodes tumor
Granular cell tumor
Desmoid tumor
Granulomatous mastitis

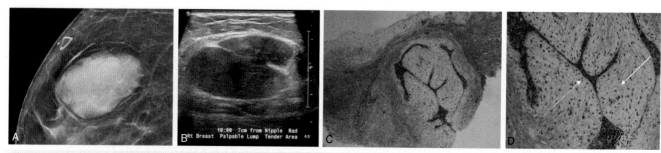

Fig. 9.2 Fibroadenoma. Mammogram (A) shows an oval, circumscribed, equal-density mass at site of palpable mass (triangle skin marker). Corresponding ultrasound (B) shows an oval, circumscribed, parallel, hypoechoic mass. Photomicrographs at 40× (C) and 100× (D) magnification show biphasic tumor with admixed stromal (*arrow*) and compressed glandular (*dashed arrow*) components. (Courtesy Kathryn Law, MD, St. Louis, MO.)

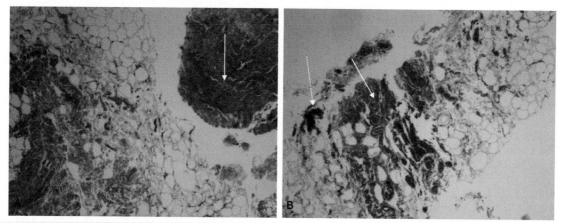

Fig. 9.3 Hamartoma. Photomicrographs at 40× magnification (A–B) demonstrate predominantly dense fibrotic tissue (*arrows*) and adipose tissue with rare, somewhat atrophic and disorganized ductal elements (*dashed arrow*). Breast hamartomas are benign tumor-like nodules of normal breast elements, often with one element predominating and lacking the structural organization of normal background breast tissue. (Courtesy Kathryn Law, MD, St. Louis, MO.)

growth rate of 20% or more over 6 months, biopsy should also be recommended to exclude phyllodes tumor. Histologic appearance of fibroadenomas is that of compressed glands within collagenous stroma.

No treatment is needed for fibroadenomas unless they are symptomatic or enlarging. However, excision should be recommended when pathology is indeterminate; if phyllodes tumor cannot be excluded on the basis of the limited core biopsy sample, the lesion may be called a "fibroepithelial lesion." Fibroadenomas do not confer significantly increased risk of breast cancer.

Lipoma

Lipomas are benign masses composed of bland adipose tissue. They may occur in any part of the body. Patients usually present with a soft, painless, mobile mass. Mammography shows a fat-containing circumscribed mass, correlating with a hyperechoic, circumscribed mass on ultrasound. Lesions with classic imaging features of lipoma can be assessed as benign (BI-RADS 2) and do not require biopsy. If biopsied, pathology shows an encapsulated mass with smooth borders, composed entirely of bland adipocytes. No treatment is needed unless the lipoma is bothersome to the patient, more commonly seen with larger masses. There is no association with breast cancer.

Hamartoma

Hamartomas are benign masses containing a combination of normal glandular, adipose, and stromal elements in a

disorganized structure. They are also called fibroadenolipomas. Patients typically present with a palpable, soft, mobile mass; hamartomas may also be found incidentally on imaging. Mammographic appearance of hamartoma is that of a partially fat-containing, circumscribed mass. They have been described as a "breast in a breast" appearance. Hamartomas with classic imaging features do not require biopsy.

Gross pathologic analysis of hamartomas demonstrates a smoothly marginated mass that contains glandular, adipose, and stromal elements within a pseudocapsule (Fig. 9.3). A diagnosis of hamartoma may not be able to be established from a core needle biopsy sample, as the appearance of the tissue within the hamartoma is so similar to normal breast tissue. Close correlation with the typical imaging appearance is needed in these cases. No management of hamartomas is required unless the patient is symptomatic. Hamartomas are not associated with increased risk of breast cancer.

Pseudoangiomatous Stromal Hyperplasia

Pseudoangiomatous stromal hyperplasia (PASH) is a benign proliferation of myofibroblasts that can mimic a vascular lesion on pathologic analysis, hence the term "pseudoangiomatous." PASH may present as a mammographic developing asymmetry or a mass and is generally not associated with calcifications. PASH is thought to be hormonally driven and is more common in premenopausal women and postmenopausal women on hormone replacement therapy. Because of the indeterminate appearance of PASH, biopsy is required for diagnosis.

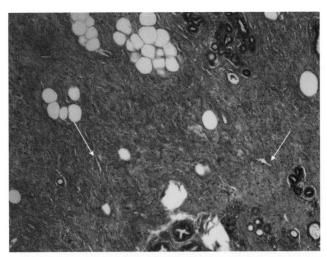

Fig. 9.4 Pseudoangiomatous stromal hyperplasia (PASH). Photomicrograph at 40× magnification shows slit-like spaces lined by spindled cells (*arrows*) in a background of dense stromal fibrosis; findings are characteristic of PASH. (Courtesy Kathryn Law, MD, St. Louis, MO.)

On pathologic analysis, a dense collagenous stroma is seen with myofibroblastic proliferation (Fig. 9.4). Because the myofibroblasts can mimic the endothelial cells of blood vessels, the main differential diagnosis for PASH is angiosarcoma. If definitive diagnosis of PASH cannot be established from core biopsy, excision should be recommended. PASH does not otherwise require surgical consultation unless the lesion continues to grow.

Intramammary Lymph Node

Lymph nodes are secondary lymphoid organs; they are responsible for lymph filtration and are sites of proliferation of B and T cells in response to foreign antigens. Lymph nodes are commonly seen in the axilla but may also be seen within the breast; these are known as intramammary lymph nodes. Intramammary lymph nodes are usually found in the upper outer quadrant, may be seen in other parts of the breast, and may present as a palpable finding. Lymph nodes that demonstrate a classically benign appearance as an oval, circumscribed mass with fatty notch on mammography and echogenic hilum on ultrasound do not require biopsy. If classic findings are not seen, however, biopsy should be considered.

Pathologic analysis of lymph nodes demonstrates an encapsulated mass with cortical (outer) and medullary (inner) components. The cortex consists of B-cell containing lymphoid follicles and the medulla consists of lymphoid tissue aggregates and lymphatic channels. Blood vessels enter and exit the lymph node through the hilum.

No management of benign intramammary lymph nodes is required. However, intramammary lymph nodes may be involved with the same pathologic processes as other lymph nodes (e.g., lymphoma, metastatic disease, benign systemic disease).

Fat Necrosis

Fat necrosis is a benign process in which an area of fat in the breast saponifies, or breaks down. This is commonly the result of blunt trauma or surgery; eliciting this history can be helpful in establishing the diagnosis. It is often an incidental finding on mammography. However, patients may also present with a palpable mass. The appearance of fat necrosis evolves over time. In the acute setting, a focal asymmetry may be seen mammographically, corresponding to an area of increased echogenicity with cystic spaces on ultrasound. Over time, an oil cyst may form, seen as a round, fat-density mass with circumscribed margins. The wall of the oil cyst typically develops rim calcifications over time. When classically benign findings of fat necrosis are seen, no further management is needed. However, given the variable imaging appearance, biopsy is sometimes required to confirm the diagnosis.

The pathologic appearance of fat necrosis also depends on the temporal course. Areas of hemorrhage may be seen the early phase. Over time, anucleated adipocytes, lipid-laden histiocytes, and multinucleated giant cells are seen. Fibrosis is typically seen later and may persist for years. No management is required for benign and concordant pathology of fat necrosis.

Fibrocystic Change

Fibrocystic change is a general term that refers to a spectrum of both nonproliferative and proliferative changes, often seen in conjunction with one another. Pathologies included under the nonproliferative category are cysts, apocrine metaplasia, and fibrosis. Patients with fibrocystic change may present with breast pain or palpable mass. Fibrocystic change may also present as calcifications, sometimes requiring stereotactic biopsy if not classically benign in appearance (Fig. 9.5).

Cysts are fluid-filled masses that are caused by fluid accumulation within terminal ducts. Cysts may be single or multiple and often fluctuate in size over time. Cysts are round or oval masses with circumscribed margins; simple cysts are anechoic on ultrasound. Definitively benign cysts do not require management unless symptomatic, in which case therapeutic cyst aspiration can be offered. If biopsied, a thin cyst wall lined by epithelial cells with adjacent fibrosis is often seen.

Apocrine metaplasia is often seen in the epithelial cells lining the cyst wall. Apocrine metaplasia refers to the transformation of normal breast epithelial cells to cells resembling apocrine sweat glands. This is a common, benign process and is not associated with increased risk of breast cancer.

Microscopic cysts may present as milk of calcium calcifications. Calcifications form within the cyst secretions and often layer on a lateral view mammogram. These calcifications are sometime composed of calcium oxalate crystals, which require polarized microscopy to visualize.

Nonproliferative fibrocystic changes are not associated with increased risk of breast cancer and do not require further management if concordant with imaging.

BENIGN MASSES THAT MAY WARRANT SURGICAL CONSULTATION

There are some benign breast masses for which surgical consultation should be considered, either for clinical management or excision (see Box 9.3).

Phyllodes Tumor

Phyllodes tumors are fibroepithelial lesions and are often benign. They differ from fibroadenomas in that they are

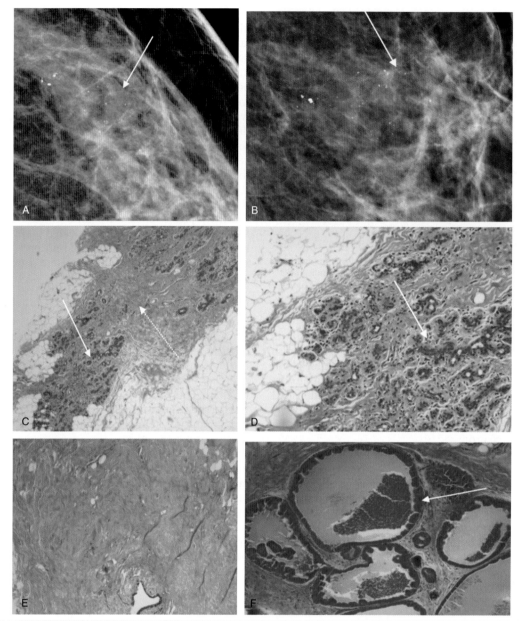

Fig. 9.5 Fibrocystic change. Magnification craniocaudal (CC) (A) and mediolateral (ML) (B) views of the left breast demonstrate scattered punctate and amorphous calcifications (*arrows*). Patient underwent stereotactic biopsy and benign fibrocystic changes were seen. Photomicrograph at 40× magnification (C) and 100× (D) show sclerosing adenosis involving the lobules, with a proliferation of glands (*arrows*) that are compressed by the surrounding stromal proliferation (*dashed arrow*). The lobular architecture is overall maintained. Photomicrograph at 40× (E) shows densely fibrotic stroma with little intervening adipose tissue, consistent with stromal fibrosis. Photomicrograph at 40× (F) shows cysts lined by epithelial cells showing apocrine metaplasia (*arrow*). (Courtesy Kathryn Law, MD, St. Louis, MO.)

faster growing, have potential for local recurrence, and may be malignant in approximately a quarter of cases. Like fibroadenomas, phyllodes tumors also reflect proliferation of both stromal and epithelial components of the TDLU, with relatively more stromal proliferation.

The median age of presentation is 45 and women tend to present with large, rapidly growing palpable masses. The clinical history of rapid growth can help distinguish these masses from fibroadenomas. Most phyllodes tumors are large on presentation (5 cm or greater). Phyllodes tumors have similar imaging characteristics to fibroadenomas and are generally circumscribed round or oval masses that are hypoechoic on ultrasound. Cystic spaces may be seen within larger tumors.

The pathologic appearance of phyllodes tumor shows proliferation of the cellular stroma into cystic spaces (Fig. 9.6). Because the configuration of these proliferations is leaf-shaped, the term *phyllodes* (Greek, meaning "leaf") was given to these tumors. Phyllodes tumors may be characterized as benign, borderline, and malignant. Malignant tumors are identified by highly cellular stroma, infiltrative borders of the tumor, marked atypia, and high mitotic rate.

Wide surgical excision is recommended for both benign and malignant phyllodes tumors, as both can be locally recurrent. Risk of local recurrence depends on the amount of normal breast tissue present at the margins of the

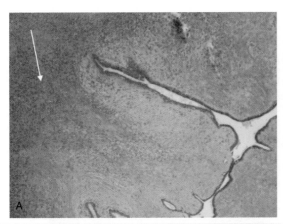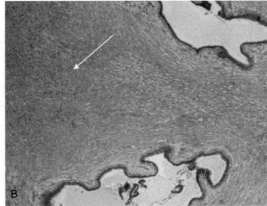

Fig. 9.6. Benign phyllodes tumor. Photomicrographs at 40× magnification (A–B) demonstrate increased stromal cellularity (*arrows*) and a leaf-like organization of epithelial and stromal elements, differentiating phyllodes tumor from fibroadenoma. (Courtesy Kathryn Law, MD, St. Louis, MO.)

resection. Approximately 25% of phyllodes tumors are malignant, and 20% of malignant phyllodes tumors metastasize. Metastases are usually hematogenously spread to the lung, liver, and bone.

Stromal Fibrosis

Stromal fibrosis is a benign proliferation of stromal tissue that results in obliteration of the acini and ducts. The resulting histologic appearance is of densely fibrotic fibrous tissue with little intervening adipose tissue. Stromal fibrosis may present as a mass, focal asymmetry, or architectural distortion and is often seen in association with other fibrocystic changes. The imaging findings are similar to malignancy, and biopsy should be recommended. Excision is not required for concordant results. However, surgical consultation or multidisciplinary review should be considered when there is uncertainty regarding concordance.

Granular Cell Tumor

Granular cell tumors are rare, benign masses that originate from Schwann cells, which are part of the peripheral nervous system. They typically present as a mass, which may either be palpable or found on a screening mammogram. They are more common medially, due to their perineural origin from the supraclavicular nerve. As there are no distinct features of granular cell tumors, biopsy is required as imaging features overlap with those of malignancy. Pathology demonstrates a smoothly bordered mass with polygonal cells that are similar in appearance to Schwann cells. Granular cell tumors are very rarely malignant (less than 2%). However, surgical consultation is recommended, as these tumors are usually treated with wide local excision to exclude malignancy. The recurrence rate is low and there is no associated increased risk of breast cancer.

Granulomatous Mastitis

Granulomatous mastitis is an idiopathic inflammatory condition affecting the breast parenchyma. Patients are typically premenopausal women, presenting with symptoms, including galactorrhea, pain, mass, and skin changes. Granulomatous mastitis is classically described as occurring within a few years of the patient's last pregnancy. Imaging findings may

be subtle and include focal asymmetry and mass with indistinct margins. Because the appearance overlaps with malignancy, biopsy is usually recommended. Pathology shows noncaseating granulomatous inflammation. Concurrent infection should be excluded, including tuberculosis or other bacteria. Patients should be referred for surgical consultation. Treatment protocols are not well established, but options include steroids, anti-inflammatory drugs, methotrexate, and in some cases surgical excision. Antibiotics are given if superimposed infection or abscess develops. The recurrence rate of granulomatous mastitis is high.

Diabetic Mastopathy

Diabetic mastopathy is a focal fibrotic process, thought to be caused by an autoimmune reaction to glycosylated proteins in the setting of long-standing hyperglycemia. Patients usually present with a hard mass. Many have a history of type 1 diabetes mellitus, often poorly controlled. Imaging may show a focal asymmetry or mass, usually without calcifications (Fig. 9.7). Biopsy should be performed because imaging features overlap with malignancy. Pathology shows lymphocytic infiltrates in perivascular, periductal, and perilobular distribution. Recurrences are common and can be worsened with surgery. Excision is therefore not routinely recommended if the diagnosis is established with core needle biopsy.

Desmoid Tumor

Desmoid tumors are rare, benign but infiltrative and locally aggressive proliferations of fibroblasts and myofibroblasts. They may arise from the breast parenchyma or from the pectoral fascia. They typically present as hard, palpable masses and are often associated with injury to the breast, including iatrogenic injury (e.g., surgery or implants). Desmoid tumors can be seen in the setting of Gardner syndrome and familial adenomatous polyposis syndrome. The imaging findings are nonspecific and overlap with malignancy; biopsy is therefore warranted. The pathologic appearance of desmoid tumor is that of an infiltrative mass with broad sheets of spindle cells, consistent with fibromatosis. Surgical referral is recommended for desmoid tumor as they are treated with wide local excision. Desmoid tumors recur in 20% to 30% of cases, but they do not metastasize. Radiation is sometimes needed in addition to surgery.

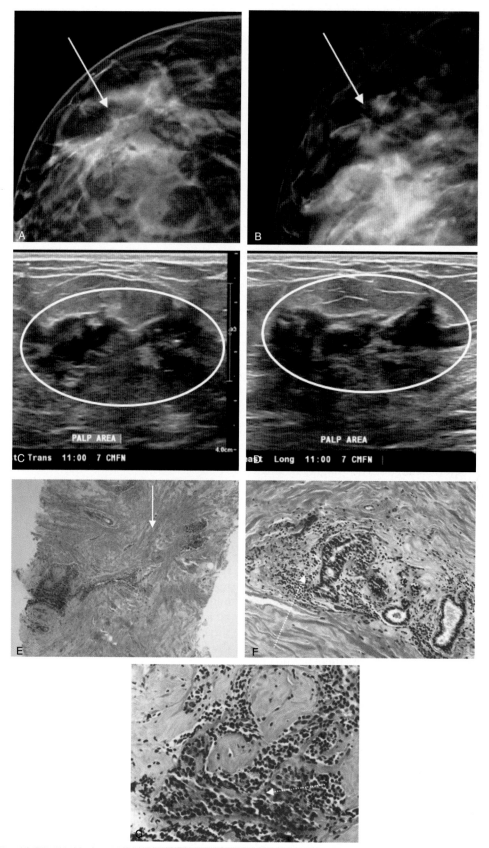

Fig. 9.7 Diabetic mastopathy. Craniocaudal (CC) (A) and mediolateral oblique (MLO) (B) tomosynthesis images of the right breast demonstrate an area of architectural distortion corresponding to site of palpable concern (*arrows*). Corresponding transverse (C) and longitudinal (D) ultrasound images show an irregular hypoechoic mass with angular margins (*circles*). Photomicrographs at 40× (E), 100× (F), and 200× (G) magnification show poorly defined areas of stromal fibrosis (*arrow*) and variable lymphocytic infiltrates (*dashed arrows*) that are generally lobulocentric but may also involve perivascular and periductal regions. These changes may obliterate the affected ducts and lobules. Appearance is typical for diabetic mastopathy. (Courtesy Kathryn Law, MD, St. Louis, MO.)

BENIGN CALCIFICATIONS

In addition to fat necrosis and fibrocystic changes that were described above, there are other common etiologies that do not require additional management when concordant (Box 9.4). In order to be deemed concordant, targeted calcifications must be present on the specimen radiograph and found at pathology.

Usual Ductal Hyperplasia

Usual ductal hyperplasia (UDH) is a benign proliferation of ductal epithelial cells. Although there is cellular overgrowth, the cells themselves look very close to normal; this distinguishes UDH from atypical ductal hyperplasia (see later). UDH is typically seen in association with other fibrocystic changes and can present as calcifications, or in association with cysts. UDH is not associated with significantly increased risk of breast cancer, and excision is not required.

Adenosis and Sclerosing Adenosis

Adenosis is a general term that refers to the benign proliferation of acini in the TDLU, which enlarges the lobule. Adenosis is commonly found in patients with fibrocystic changes. Sclerosing adenosis is a specific type of benign lobular proliferation that results in the formation of fibrous stromal tissue that compresses and distorts glandular tissue. Sclerosing adenosis may present as an irregular mass, architectural distortion, or calcifications (typically round, punctate, or amorphous). Because the imaging appearance is similar to that of cancer, biopsy is required to establish the diagnosis and close radiology-pathology correlation is needed to establish concordance. If results are concordant, excision is not required.

Columnar Cell Change and Columnar Cell Hyperplasia

Columnar cell lesions are proliferative lesions involving the lobular acini; these lesions are characterized by enlarged acini lined by epithelial cells with a columnar appearance, instead of their normal cuboidal shape (Fig. 9.8). The term

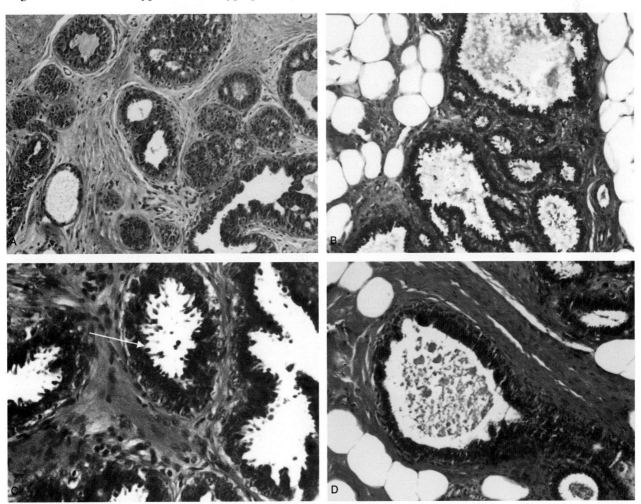

Fig. 9.8 Columnar cell lesions: columnar cell change (A, 100×), columnar cell hyperplasia (B, 100×), and flat epithelial atypia (C, 200×; D, 100×). Columnar cell lesions occur along a spectrum but all include dilated acini lined by cells with elongated nuclei and apical cytoplasmic snouts (*arrow*), often with intraluminal secretions. These lesions are separated by degree of hyperplasia and presence or absence of atypia in the lining cells. (Courtesy Kathryn Law, MD, St. Louis, MO.)

columnar cell change is used when the epithelial lining is one to two cell layers. If more cells layers are seen, the lesion is considered columnar cell hyperplasia. If atypia is seen, the lesion is considered flat epithelial atypia (see later). The dilated acini may have intraluminal secretions and calcifications; these lesions are therefore often found on stereotactic biopsy for calcifications. There is no associated increased risk of cancer and no additional management is needed.

High-Risk Lesions

Some pathologic entities diagnosed from core needle biopsy are considered high risk or borderline due either to the potential upgrade to malignancy at surgical excision or to an association with increased risk of subsequent cancer development. In some cases, the small volume of tissue from core needle biopsy may undersample the lesion and not accurately diagnose the entire abnormality. These pathologic lesions may require surgical excision for complete histologic analysis (Box 9.5).

The management of high-risk lesions is a controversial topic, with variability in clinical practice at different facilities and among different providers. The recommendation for surgical excision is based on retrospective studies examining the upgrade rate from core needle biopsy to surgical excision (Table 9.1). There is a wide range of upgrade rates, due to differences in study design, including year of study, whether the lesion was palpable, patient population, baseline breast cancer risk, size of biopsy device, qualifications of pathologist, and outcomes measured. There is a lack of consensus within the surgical community regarding which high-risk lesions require surgical excision. The 2016 American Society of Breast Surgeons consensus statement recommends against routine excision of all high-risk lesions and suggests that close follow-up may be appropriate for some patients with lower chance of upgrade, in the context of shared decision making (Table 9.2). Multidisciplinary review of radiologic–pathologic findings may reduce the number of excisional biopsies needed.

ATYPICAL DUCTAL HYPERPLASIA

Atypical ductal hyperplasia (ADH) is a term used to describe an intraductal proliferation of atypical ductal epithelial cells that have some, but not all, features of low-grade ductal carcinoma in situ (DCIS). ADH is histologically similar to DCIS but characterized by only partial involvement of less than two duct sites and measuring less than 2 mm in extent

---

Box 9.5   High-Risk Lesions Usually Warranting Surgical Consultation (for Excision or Clinical Management)

Atypical ductal hyperplasia
Lobular neoplasia (atypical lobular hyperplasia/lobular carcinoma in situ)
Flat epithelial atypia
Complex sclerosing lesion/radial scar
Papillary lesion, particularly if associated atypia
Mucocele-like lesion

Table 9.1   Upgrade Rates of High-Risk Lesions

Lesion	Range[a]
ADH	13%–56%
ALH	0%–67%
Classic LCIS	5%–60%
Pleomorphic LCIS	18%–30%
Flat epithelial atypia	5%–15%
Radial scar/complex sclerosing lesion	0%–40%
Benign intraductal papilloma	0%–33%
Atypical papilloma	67%

ADH, Atypical ductal hyperplasia; *ALH*, atypical lobular hyperplasia; *LCIS*, lobular carcinoma in situ.
[a]These wide ranges of upgrade rates highlight inconsistencies in retrospective study designs and outcomes measured. Hence, there controversy remains regarding which high-risk lesions require surgical excision.

Table 9.2   Surgical Management of Benign and High-Risk Lesions Diagnosed on Core Needle Biopsy (Adapted from American Society of Breast Surgeons 2016 Consensus Statement)

Lesion	Surgical Recommendation	Comments
ADH	Excise	Can observe small-volume ADH if completely excised on CNB in multidisciplinary setting
Lobular neoplasia (ALH/LCIS)	Excise or clinical and imaging observation	Excise if discordant, limited sampling, or other high-risk lesion in sample
Pleomorphic LCIS	Excise	
Flat epithelial atypia	Clinical and imaging observation	Excise if ADH present
Papillary lesions	Excise or clinical and imaging observation	Excise if palpable or atypia, follow if benign and incidental
Radial scar/complex sclerosing lesion	Excise	Can observe small, adequately sampled CSLs
Fibroadenoma	Clinical observation; Does not require routine excision	Excise if enlarging or patient preference
Fibroepithelial lesion with concern for phyllodes tumor	Excise	
Mucocele-like lesion	Excise or observation	Excise if atypia present; observe if benign and atypia at excision would not alter management
Desmoid tumor	Wide local excision	Local recurrence common
PASH	Clinical observation	Excise if enlarging

ADH, Atypical ductal hyperplasia; *ALH*, atypical lobular hyperplasia; *CSL*, complex sclerosing lesion; *CNB*, core needle biopsy; *LCIS*, lobular carcinoma in situ; *PASH*, pseudoangiomatous stromal hyperplasia.

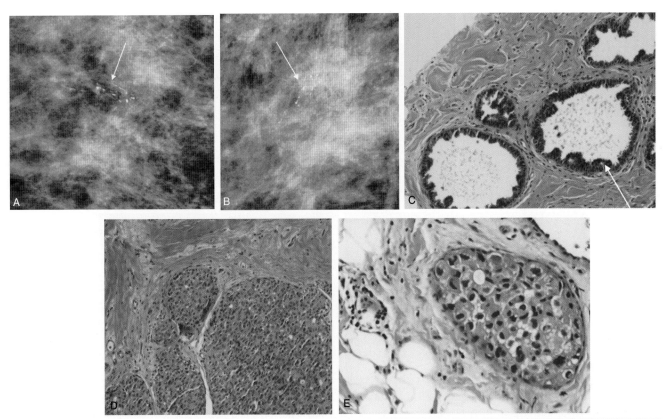

Fig. 9.9 Atypical ductal hyperplasia. Craniocaudal (CC) (A) and mediolateral (ML) (B) magnification views of the left breast demonstrate pleomorphic calcifications in a linear distribution (*arrows*). Patient underwent stereotactic biopsy. Photomicrograph at 100× (C) shows atypical ductal cells forming rigid arches and papillae (*arrow*), with overall involvement of less than two duct sites, measuring less than 2 mm. Photomicrographs are shown of usual ductal hyperplasia (D, 40×) and ductal carcinoma in situ (DCIS) (E, 200×) for comparison. (Courtesy Kathryn Law, MD, St. Louis, MO.)

(Fig. 9.9). ADH is most commonly found from stereotactic biopsy of calcifications.

Because of the extent-based criteria distinguishing ADH and DCIS, the small volume of tissue present in core needle biopsy limits the pathologist's ability to make an accurate diagnosis. The upgrade rate of ADH on core needle biopsy to malignancy on surgical excision ranges from 13% to 56%, with a mean upgrade rate of 23%. There is low concordance and reproducibility for distinguishing ADH from DCIS among pathologists.

Because of the high upgrade rate, there is consensus agreement that most cases of ADH should be excised when found on core biopsy. These patients should be referred for surgical excision. Factors that contribute to a higher upgrade rate include smaller-size (i.e., higher-gauge) biopsy needle, smaller proportion of calcifications/lesion sampled, and presence of fine linear branching calcifications. Upgrade rate is lower when three or fewer duct sites are involved and all mammographically visible calcifications are removed at biopsy. Consideration for observation with clinical and imaging surveillance may be made in context of multidisciplinary review.

The overall relative risk for subsequent development of cancer in women with a history of ADH is 3.1 to 4.7. In addition to annual screening mammography, the ACR recommends consideration of screening MRI for patients with history of ADH, particularly in the context of other risk factors.

LOBULAR NEOPLASIA (ATYPICAL LOBULAR HYPERPLASIA AND CLASSIC LOBULAR CARCINOMA IN SITU)

Lobular neoplasia is a general term for lesions with epithelial atypia involving the lobular portion of the TDLU. Lobular neoplasia includes both atypical lobular hyperplasia (ALH) and classic lobular carcinoma in situ (LCIS), which demonstrate similar histologic characteristics but are differentiated by extent of involvement. If less than half the acini in a lobular unit are distended with atypical proliferation, the term *ALH* is used. If more than half the acini are involved, the term *LCIS* is used. Lobular neoplasia is usually incidentally found on stereotactic biopsy samples performed for calcifications (Fig. 9.10). Although calcifications can be associated with lobular neoplasia, it is more often an incidental finding in the biopsy sample with no imaging correlate.

There is a wide range of reported upgrade rates for lobular neoplasia, ranging from 0% to 67% for ALH and 5% to 60% for LCIS. Older studies, in which lobular neoplasia was found on biopsies of palpable masses, have reported higher upgrade rates. Recent studies have demonstrated upgrade rates of less than 5% with small-volume lobular neoplasia, without presence of other high-risk lesions. Because of these recent data, excision is no longer routinely recommended for lobular neoplasia. However, surgical consultation should be still be considered for clinical management, including risk reduction strategies.

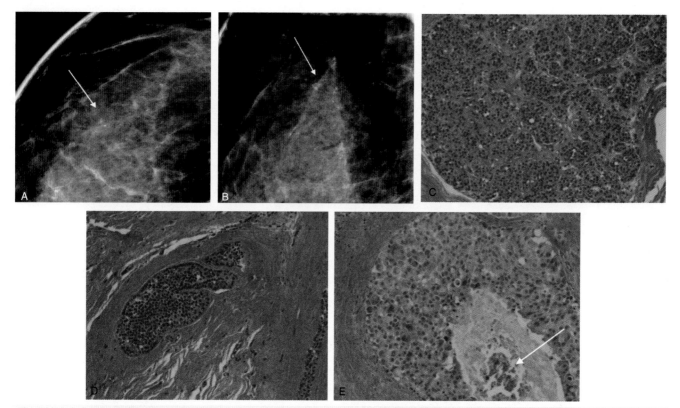

Fig. 9.10 Lobular neoplasia: atypical lobular hyperplasia (ALH), lobular carcinoma in situ (LCIS), and pleomorphic LCIS. Magnification craniocaudal (CC) (A) and mediolateral (ML) (B) views of the right breast demonstrate multiple groups of amorphous calcifications (*arrows*). Photomicrograph at 100× (C) shows atypical epithelial cells occupying less than half the acini in the lobular unit; this was described as atypical lobular hyperplasia. For comparison, photomicrograph at 100× magnification is shown of LCIS (D), where atypical epithelial cells occupy and expand the entire lobule. Photomicrograph at 200× (E) demonstrates pleomorphic LCIS with central necrosis and calcification (*arrow*). (Courtesy Kathryn Law, MD, St. Louis, MO.)

The relative risk of subsequent development of breast cancer for ALH and LCIS are approximately 4 and 10, respectively. Subsequent cancers may develop in both the contralateral or ipsilateral breast and may be either ductal or lobular carcinomas. Antiestrogen chemoprevention has been shown to reduce breast cancer risk in women with a history of LCIS. The NSABP P-1 trial showed a reduction in invasive breast cancers of 56% in women with LCIS who took tamoxifen. Raloxifene was also shown to be effective for risk reduction in the NSABP P-2 trial for postmenopausal women with a uterus (fewer endometrial cancers than tamoxifen). In addition to annual screening mammography, the ACR recommends consideration of screening MRI in women with history of LCIS.

PLEOMORPHIC LCIS

Pleomorphic LCIS is a distinct, more aggressive variant of LCIS that is characterized by greater nuclear polymorphism, central necrosis, and calcifications (see Fig. 9.10). It is considered an indolent, nonobligate precursor to invasive lobular carcinoma. Pleomorphic LCIS generally presents with calcifications.

Histologically, pleomorphic LCIS can be difficult to distinguish from DCIS. Immunohistochemical staining demonstrates loss of e-cadherin, a cellular adhesion protein.

There is a high upgrade rate of pleomorphic LCIS on core biopsy to DCIS or invasive carcinoma at excision, ranging from 18% to 30%. Surgical referral and excision are recommended for pleomorphic LCIS. Complete surgical excision is recommended for these cases.

FLAT EPITHELIAL ATYPIA

Flat epithelial atypia (FEA) is a columnar cell lesion in which enlarged acini show increased layers of monotonous columnar epithelial cells with low-grade cellular atypia. FEA exists on a spectrum with columnar cell change and columnar cell hyperplasia, which are distinguished by their lack of cellular atypia (see Fig. 9.8). FEA is a relatively new pathologic entity, established by the World Health Organization in 2003. FEA is most commonly found on stereotactic biopsy for calcifications.

FEA may be associated with ADH, low-grade DCIS, and lobular neoplasia; management is driven by these other pathologies if they are found in the sample. The upgrade rate for pure FEA on core biopsy to another atypia, DCIS, or invasive cancer on excision is 5% to 15%. Management is controversial, but the American Society of Breast Surgeons does not recommend excision for pure FEA.

COMPLEX SCLEROSING LESION/RADIAL SCAR

Complex sclerosing lesion and *radial scar* are both terms for a benign proliferative entity that contains a dense fibroelastotic core and stellate, entrapped ducts, and epithelial elements. In general, complex sclerosing lesions are termed radial scars if they are smaller than 1 cm in size. These may present with architectural distortion or as a spiculated mass and are more commonly found with digital breast tomosynthesis than two-dimensional (2D) mammography (Fig. 9.11). Biopsy is required as there is considerable imaging overlap with cancer.

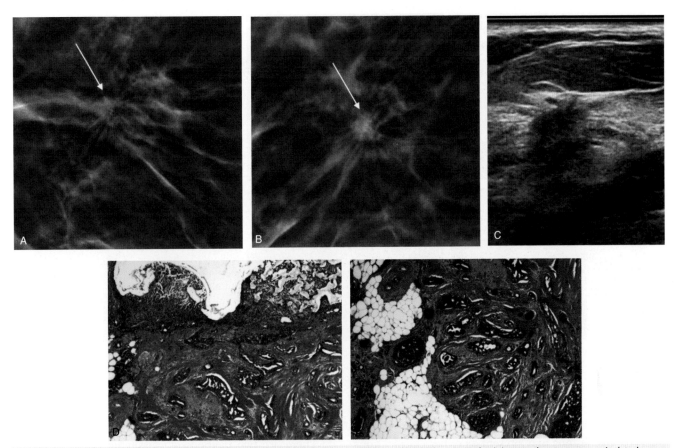

Fig. 9.11. Complex sclerosing lesion/radial scar. Spot craniocaudal (CC) (A) and mediolateral (ML) (B) tomosynthesis images demonstrate a spiculated mass with associated architectural distortion (*arrows*). Ultrasound (C) shows corresponding spiculated mass. Photomicrograph at 40× magnification (D–E) shows dense fibroelastotic core with entrapped ducts and epithelial elements, consistent with radial scar. (Courtesy Kathryn Law, MD, St. Louis, MO.)

Histologically, complex sclerosing lesions are distinguished from malignancy by the presence of benign epithelial and myoepithelial cells within the entrapped epithelial elements. Myoepithelial markers (such as p63 immunohistochemical stains) are used to distinguish complex sclerosing lesions from invasive carcinomas, particularly tubular carcinoma.

Complex sclerosing lesions may be associated with ADH, ALH, LCIS, and cancer. The reported upgrade rate to malignancy for pure complex sclerosing lesions/radial scars without atypia in most studies range from 0% to 12%, with one outlier study reporting a 40% upgrade. Upgrade rates are higher with smaller (larger-gauge) biopsy devices (14 gauge) and fewer core biopsy samples. Surgical excision is usually recommended for complex sclerosing lesions. However, imaging follow-up may be considered in cases of small radial scars (e.g., ≤5 mm) that were completely removed or adequately sampled with a large (i.e., smaller-gauge) core needle biopsy device. Excision is not recommended for microscopic radial scars incidentally found on histologic evaluation of another target lesion. Multidisciplinary radiologic–pathologic correlation may be helpful for avoiding unnecessary excision of radial scar.

PAPILLARY LESIONS

Papillary lesions refer to a group of ductal epithelial proliferations that are jointly characterized by the presence of a fibrovascular stalk. The group includes benign, atypical, and malignant lesions (Fig. 9.12). Papillary lesions may clinically present with nipple discharge, either clear or bloody, or with a palpable mass. Central papillomas, involving the more central ducts closer to the nipple, are more likely to be benign than peripheral papillomas. Peripheral papillomas are more likely to be incidentally detected on imaging and multiple. Ultrasound typically shows a solid or complex mass, which may be associated with a dilated duct. Vascularity may be seen within the fibrovascular stalk on Doppler imaging.

Because the epithelium of the papillary proliferation is the same as elsewhere in the breast, papillomas can be involved with the same pathologic processes affecting other ductal epithelial cells, such as ADH, DCIS, and benign ductal epithelial hyperplasia. Upgrade rates for papillomas without associated atypia are low, with most studies reporting a range of 0% to 13%, with one outlier study reporting a 33% upgrade. Management of solitary benign, concordant papillomas is controversial and varies among providers, but excision is often not performed. Atypical papillomas have a much higher upgrade rate, up to 67%. There is general consensus that atypical papillary lesions should be excised.

MUCOCELE-LIKE LESION

Mucocele-like lesions are rare benign lesions consisting of dilated epithelium-lined ducts that are distended with mucin. Mucin also extravasates into the adjacent stroma.

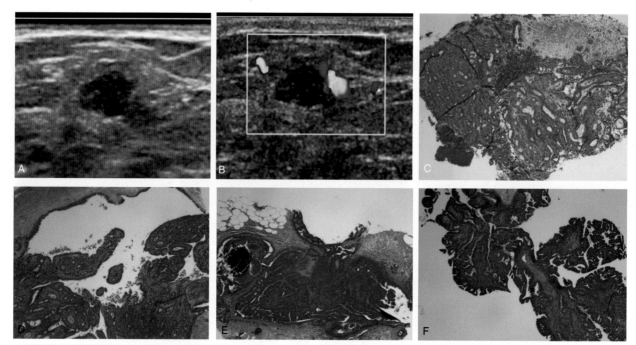

Fig. 9.12 Papillary neoplasms: benign intraductal papilloma, atypical papillary neoplasm. Grayscale (A) and color Doppler (B) ultrasound images demonstrate an irregular mass with feeding vessel. Photomicrographs at 40× magnification (C–D) show epithelial proliferation in papillary pattern, consistent with benign intraductal papilloma. Photomicrographs at 40× (E–F) show atypical ductal epithelial cells in similar papillary pattern; this is an atypical papillary lesion. (Courtesy Kathryn Law, MD, St. Louis, MO.)

Mucocele-like lesions may present as either calcifications or a mass. They are commonly associated with epithelial atypia and may also be associated with DCIS or mucinous carcinoma. Mucocele-like lesions with atypia on core needle biopsy should be excised to exclude cancer. Management of benign mucocele-like lesions without atypia is controversial and excision is not always recommended. However, if presence of atypia would change patient management (e.g., chemoprevention for risk reduction due to other risk factors), then excision should be considered, as many benign mucocele-like lesions are upgraded to atypia on excision.

Breast Malignancies

Malignant pathologies on core needle biopsy should be referred for surgical and oncologic consultation and treatment. Generally, breast cancer pathology is classified into two broad categories depending on whether the cancer is confined within ductal-lobular system (in situ) or not (invasive).

DUCTAL CARCINOMA IN SITU

DCIS refers to a malignant proliferation of cells arising from the ductal epithelium of the TDLU, which have not penetrated the basement membrane. DCIS accounts for 25% of new breast cancer diagnoses and has increased in incidence with screening mammography. Although DCIS may present with clinical signs and symptoms, it is more commonly diagnosed from identification of suspicious calcifications on screening mammography (Fig. 9.13).

There are two methods of classifying DCIS, one based on architectural pattern and one based on nuclear grade; neither is universally accepted. Histologically, DCIS may be classified as either comedocarcinoma (i.e., with comedonecrosis) or noncomedo type, which includes solid, cribriform, micropapillary, and papillary subtypes. Nuclear grade classification is low, intermediate, and high nuclear grade. In general, comedonecrosis and high-grade DCIS are associated with higher risk of recurrence.

Comedonecrosis refers to the presence of central necrosis in the duct lumen, which is associated with calcifications. These calcifications appear as "casts" within the ductal system and are seen as fine linear branching calcifications in a linear or segmental distribution, following ductal anatomy. These are typically seen in high-nuclear-grade DCIS. Amorphous grouped calcifications, in a lobular distribution, typically reflect lower-nuclear-grade DCIS and cribriform or micropapillary histologic subtypes.

DCIS is considered a nonobligate precursor to invasive ductal carcinoma. By definition, because DCIS has not penetrated the basement membrane, it cannot metastasize. Over time, DCIS can progress to invasive carcinoma by penetrating the basement membrane and invading the surrounding parenchyma. DCIS with microinvasion is defined as a focus of invasion through the basement membrane less than 1 mm in size. This is found in 5% to 10% of cases of DCIS and does have metastatic potential.

Current standard of care for DCIS is surgical excision with negative margins. There is an upgrade rate of 10% to 20% to invasive cancer at excision. Sentinel node biopsy is not routinely performed for pure DCIS. Adjuvant radiation therapy has been shown to decrease the risk of recurrence through multiple trials (NSABP B-17, EORTC, RTOG 9804).

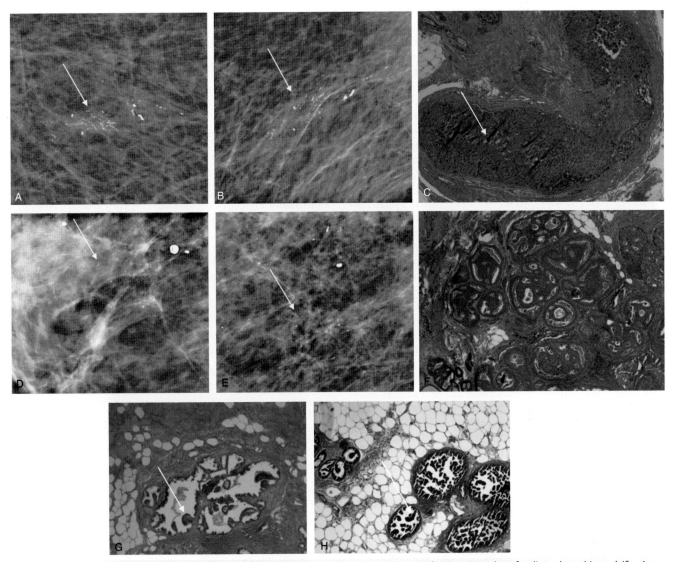

Fig. 9.13 Ductal carcinoma in situ (DCIS). Craniocaudal (CC) (A) and mediolateral (ML) (B) magnification views show fine linear branching calcifications in a segmental distribution (*arrows*). Photomicrograph at 40× (C) shows DCIS with comedonecrosis and calcifications (*arrow*). CC (D) and ML (E) magnification views show punctate and amorphous calcifications (*arrows*). Photomicrograph at 100× (F) shows cribriform DCIS. Photomicrographs at 100× are shown of papillary (G) and micropapillary (H) DCIS for comparison, showing papillary pattern of growth of DCIS (*arrows*). (Courtesy Kathryn Law, MD, St. Louis, MO.)

Endocrine therapy (tamoxifen) reduces the risk of future invasive breast cancer for patients with estrogen receptor (ER)-positive DCIS (NSABP B-24).

Given concerns about possible overtreatment of DCIS, there are clinical trials underway to determine whether less aggressive treatment for DCIS is feasible. There are three trials comparing active monitoring to standard treatment of low-risk DCIS that are ongoing (United States: COMET [Comparison of Operative versus Monitoring and Endocrine Therapy for Low Risk DCIS]), United Kingdom: LORIS [Low-Risk DCIS], European Organization for Research and Treatment of Cancer: LORD [Low Risk DCIS]).

MOLECULAR SUBTYPES OF BREAST CANCER

Routine pathologic evaluation of breast cancers includes reporting of ERs and progesterone receptors (PRs), which affect treatment options (e.g., antiestrogen hormone therapy) and are independent prognostic factors (e.g., better prognosis for ER+/PR+ cancers than ER−/PR− cancers). ER+ tumors are more likely to metastasize to bone; ER− tumors are more likely to metastasize to the brain and visceral organs.

Human epidermal growth factor receptor (HER2) status is important for tailored breast cancer treatment and prognosis. HER2 is involved in the regulation of cell growth; its overexpression leads to sustained cancer growth pathways (signaling, angiogenesis, cell division, and invasion). HER2 status is determined by immunohistochemical testing or fluorescent in situ hybridization assays (FISH). FISH is more accurate but not as widely available.

Breast cancers are classified into four groups according to their molecular subtype: luminal A, luminal B, HER2-enriched, and basal-like. The molecular subtype designation adds prognostic information regarding survival and response to treatment. Luminal cancers are characterized by expression of genes typical for breast glands; these are hormone receptor positive cancers (almost all are ER+). Luminal A cancers are low-grade with high levels of ER expression and low proliferation rates (low levels of the protein Ki-67); they are HER2−. Luminal A cancers have the best prognosis and respond to hormonal therapy. Luminal B cancers are higher grade, with lower hormone receptor expression and higher proliferation rates (high levels of Ki-67); these may be HER2+. They grow slightly faster than luminal A cancers and have slightly worse prognosis. HER2-enriched cancers are hormone-receptor negative (ER−/PR−) but overexpress the *HER2* gene (HER2+). HER2-enriched cancers have historically been associated with poor prognosis. However, specific HER2-targeted therapies (e.g., monoclonal antibodies such as trastuzumab and pertuzumab) have improved prognosis. Basal-like cancers are an aggressive tumor subtype that do not show overexpression of hormone receptors or HER2; in general, these are also known as triple-negative cancers (ER−, PR−, HER2−), although not all triple negative breast cancers (TNBCs) are basal-like. Basal-like cancers are named because of the expression of proteins that are usually seen in the basal/myoepithelial layer of the breast. Basal-like cancers and TNBCs have exceptionally high proliferation rates and poor prognosis. On imaging, they often demonstrate round or oval shape and may have circumscribed margins with "pushing borders." This cancer subtype tends to affect younger patients and has higher prevalence in women of African ancestry. Basal-like cancers usually respond to chemotherapy but have higher risk of recurrence within 5 years.

INVASIVE DUCTAL CARCINOMA NOT OTHERWISE SPECIFIED (IDC NOS)

Invasive ductal carcinoma is a proliferation of malignant cells arising from the ductal epithelium. It is also known as infiltrating ductal carcinoma and invasive carcinoma of no special type and accounts for approximately 90% of invasive breast cancers. IDC has a variable microscopic appearance, with tumor cells organized in sheets, clusters, cords, and solid patterns (Fig. 9.14). IDC may present with a clinical symptom (most commonly a palpable mass) or may first be detected by imaging. A common appearance is an irregular mass with indistinct or spiculated margins, which may

be associated with suspicious calcifications and/or architectural distortion. Standard treatment for IDC involves surgical excision with adjuvant radiation for lumpectomy. Decisions regarding endocrine therapy, HER2-directed therapy, and chemotherapy (neoadjuvant or adjuvant) are complex and depend on tumor characteristics and patient factors.

TUBULAR CARCINOMA

Tubular carcinoma is a low-grade subtype of IDC that is named for the well-differentiated tubular structures formed by tumor cells (Table 9.3). Tubular carcinomas account for approximately 2% of breast cancers. They often present as a slow-growing spiculated mass, often detected on screening mammography (Fig. 9.15). Pathology shows the tubular structures in a desmoplastic stroma, lined by a single layer of cells, with patent ductal lumen. There is no myoepithelial cell layer and no basement membrane, which distinguishes

Table 9.3   IDC Subtypes (Excluding IDC NOS)

Subtype	Common Appearance and Characteristics
Tubular carcinoma	Irregular spiculated mass
	Low-grade, slow-growing
	Excellent prognosis
Medullary carcinoma	Round or oval, circumscribed mass
	Often high-grade, but with less aggressive behavior
	Can be associated with *BRCA1*
	Prognosis is generally better than IDC NOS
Mucinous/colloid carcinoma	Round or oval, circumscribed mass
	Similar appearance to cyst on ultrasound but usually not entirely anechoic
	Very T2 bright with similar appearance to cyst on MRI, except usually with associated enhancement
	Pure mucinous carcinomas have a favorable prognosis
Papillary carcinoma (including intracystic)	Round or oval, circumscribed, solid or complex cystic and solid mass
	May be intraductal
	Prognosis is generally better than IDC NOS
	Prognosis for intracystic papillary carcinoma is excellent

IDC, Invasive ductal carcinoma; *IDC NOS*, invasive ductal carcinoma not otherwise specified.

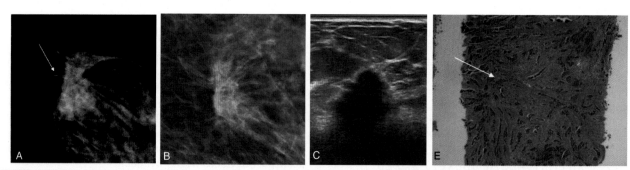

Fig. 9.14 Invasive ductal carcinoma (IDC) not otherwise specified. Magnification craniocaudal (CC) (A) and mediolateral (ML) (B) views of the left breast demonstrate a spiculated, irregular, high-density mass with associated fine linear branching calcifications (*arrow*). Ultrasound (C) shows corresponding irregular hypoechoic mass with spiculated margins and posterior acoustic shadowing. Photomicrograph at 40× magnification shows invasive ductal tumor cells throughout the biopsy sample (*arrow*). (Courtesy Kathryn Law, MD, St. Louis, MO.)

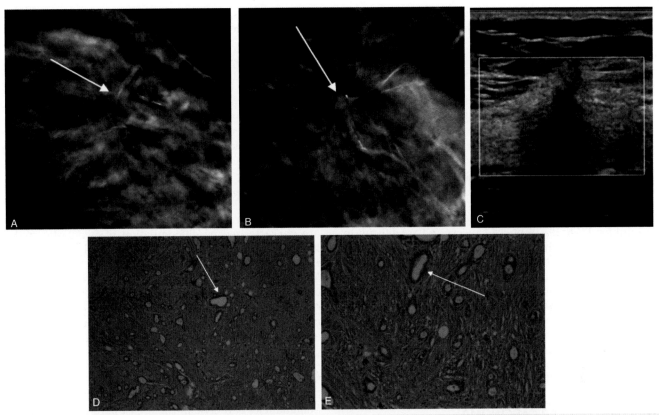

Fig. 9.15 Tubular carcinoma. Craniocaudal (CC) (A) and mediolateral (MLO) (B) tomosynthesis images of the left breast show a small spiculated mass with associated architectural distortion (*arrows*). Ultrasound (C) shows corresponding irregular mass with spiculated margins and posterior acoustic shadowing. Photomicrographs at 40× (D) and 100× (E) magnification show tumor cells forming tubular structures (*arrows*). (Courtesy Kathryn Law, MD, St. Louis, MO.)

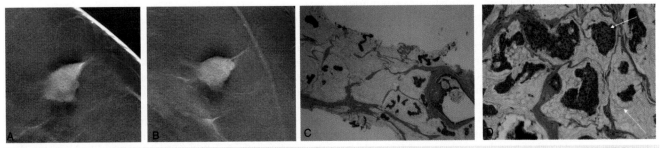

Fig. 9.16 Mucinous carcinoma. Craniocaudal (CC) (A) and mediolateral (ML) (B) tomosynthesis images show an irregular mass in the left breast. Photomicrographs at 40× (C) and 100× (D) show tumor cells (*arrow*) floating in lakes of mucin (*dashed arrow*). (Courtesy Kathryn Law, MD, St. Louis, MO.)

tubular carcinoma from sclerosing adenosis and complex sclerosing lesion, which may otherwise appear similar. Despite its suspicious morphology on imaging, the prognosis for tubular carcinoma is very good.

MEDULLARY CARCINOMA

Medullary carcinoma is a subtype of IDC that is named for its gross pathologic appearance of a soft, fleshy mass, similar to the medullary portion of the brainstem. Medullary carcinomas account for less than 2% of cancers and are often diagnosed in slightly younger women than IDC NOS. They can be associated with *BRCA1* mutations. Medullary carcinomas tend to present as round, circumscribed masses. Surrounding lymphoid infiltrate may be seen histologically.

Although tumor cells tend to be high-grade, their behavior is less aggressive, and prognosis of medullary carcinoma is better than that for IDC NOS unless atypical findings are seen.

MUCINOUS/COLLOID CARCINOMA

Mucinous and colloid carcinomas are interchangeable terms that describe a subtype of IDC consisting of tumor cells floating in lakes of mucin. These tumors account for less than 2% of cancers and often present as round, low-density masses with circumscribed margins (Fig. 9.16). They may be mistaken for cysts on ultrasound but are usually not entirely anechoic. Mucinous carcinomas demonstrate very high T2 signal on fluid-weighted MRI sequences similar to cysts but with enhancement on post-gadolinium images. Histologically, there is a solid tumor rim and mucinous central portion of the tumor, which contains malignant cells. There are two types of mucinous carcinoma, pure and mixed. Pure mucinous carcinoma is defined by at least 90% of the tumor demonstrating characteristic mucinous appearance. Mixed mucinous carcinoma demonstrates more imaging overlap with IDC NOS. Mucinous carcinomas, particularly pure mucinous carcinoma, have a favorable prognosis.

INVASIVE PAPILLARY CARCINOMA

Invasive papillary carcinomas are invasive ductal carcinomas showing exclusively papillary morphology. They account for 1% to 2% of breast cancers and are difficult to distinguish from benign papillomas on imaging. Patients generally present with similar symptoms, including nipple discharge or palpable mass. Papillary carcinomas tend to present in postmenopausal women. Imaging findings may show a round or oval mass, which may be intraductal. Biopsy is necessary to establish the diagnosis of malignancy. A distinct variant of papillary carcinoma is an intracystic papillary carcinoma, which appears as a circumscribed complex cystic and solid mass. Intracystic papillary carcinomas have an excellent prognosis.

INVASIVE LOBULAR CARCINOMA

Invasive lobular carcinoma (ILC) refers to the malignant proliferation of lobular epithelial cells. ILC reflects about 5% to 15% of invasive cancers. Tumor cells lack e-cadherin, a cellular adhesion protein, and therefore do not grow in a cohesive manner. Tumor cells spread single-file throughout the breast parenchyma; for this reason, ILC is more often mammographically occult than IDC. Imaging findings may include architectural distortion, spiculated mass, developing asymmetry or focal asymmetry (Fig. 9.17). Compared with IDC, ILC is more often multifocal, multicentric, and bilateral. Women with ILC have about a 20% increased risk of contralateral breast cancer.

Histologically, classic ILC demonstrates a concentric pattern of tumor cells around normal ducts and is low-to-intermediate grade. Other histologic variants of ILC include solid, alveolar, tubulolobular, and pleomorphic. Compared with IDC, ILC demonstrates more frequent metastases to

serosal surfaces, leptomeninges, gastrointestinal (GI) tract, and gynecologic organs.

ADENOID CYSTIC CARCINOMA

Adenoid cystic carcinoma is a rare primary breast malignancy that demonstrates histologic appearance similar to that of the salivary gland tumor. Adenoid cystic carcinomas may present as a palpable circumscribed mass, usually in subareolar location. Prognosis is good if completely resected.

METAPLASTIC CARCINOMA

Metaplastic carcinomas are a rare group of tumors that are characterized by differentiation of neoplastic epithelium into squamous and/or mesenchymal-appearing elements. They account for less than 1% of breast cancers. Metaplastic elements in these tumors may include spindle, chondroid, osseous, and rhabdomyoid cells. Metaplastic carcinomas typically present as larger masses and are more aggressive than other cancers. They are usually high-grade and more likely to metastasize.

Other Malignancies

Malignancies can arise in the breast parenchyma that are not of ductal or lobular origin. Per BI-RADS definitions, these are not "breast cancers" and would be classified as negative pathology results for purposes of the medical audit. Malignant phyllodes was described above. Other entities include lymphoma, metastasis to breast, and sarcoma.

LYMPHOMA

Lymphomas are cancers involving lymphocytes and can present on breast imaging studies as axillary lymphadenopathy. Primary or secondary breast lymphoma, involving the breast parenchyma, is rare and accounts for less than 1% of breast cancers. It is typically non-Hodgkin lymphoma, usually diffuse large B cell lymphoma. Breast lymphoma may present as a focal mass or as a diffuse process. Masses may be circumscribed, solitary or multiple, and of varying density. Treatment for breast lymphoma is with chemotherapy and radiation, not surgical excision.

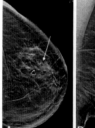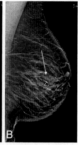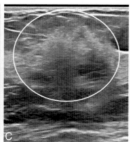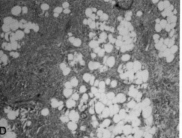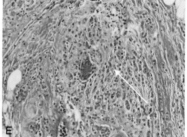

Fig. 9.17 Invasive lobular carcinoma (ILC). Craniocaudal (CC) (A) and lateromedial (LM) (B) synthetic mammograms show a vague focal asymmetry (*arrows*) associated with palpable finding, marked by triangle skin marker. Ultrasound (C) shows corresponding vague mass with indistinct margins and associated architectural distortion (*circle*). Photomicrograph at 40× (D) and 100× (E) show malignant lobular cells growing in a single-file and concentric pattern (*arrow*), typical for invasive lobular carcinoma. (Courtesy Kathryn Law, MD, St. Louis, MO.)

Breast implant–associated anaplastic large cell lymphoma (BIA-ALCL) is a rare T-cell subtype of non-Hodgkin lymphoma, which is more commonly seen in association with textured breast implants. Patients typically present with swelling and are found to have a fluid collection around the implant. Diagnosis occurs on average 7 to 10 years after implant placement. Diagnosis can be made via fine-needle aspiration of the peri-implant fluid collection, with testing of the fluid for CD30, a protein that is overexpressed in BIA-ALCL cells. Treatment involves removal of the implant, capsule, and any associated masses. Prognosis is generally good.

METASTASIS

Hematogenously spread metastatic disease may affect the breast and usually presents as multiple round, circumscribed, high-density masses. In the setting of known malignancy, the rule of multiplicity and bilaterality may not be appropriate to establish benignity. The most common cancers to metastasize to the breast are lymphoma, melanoma, rhabdomyosarcoma, lung, ovarian, renal cell, and cervical carcinomas.

SARCOMA

Breast sarcomas are rare malignancies that arise from the connective tissue elements of the breast. They include angiosarcoma, fibrosarcoma, osteosarcoma, and liposarcoma. Angiosarcoma is the most common breast sarcoma and may be either primary or secondary (related to previous radiation therapy). Angiosarcomas typically present as a painless mass or skin discoloration years after radiation. Pathology shows anastomosing vascular channels. Sarcomas require complete surgical excision and generally are associated with poor prognosis.

KEY POINTS

- Breast pathologies generally arise from the glandular tissue, stromal elements, and fat.
- Radiologic–pathologic correlation must be performed after all imaging guided breast biopsies.
- Assessment of concordance determines whether the pathology result adequately explains the imaging findings. Benign results for highly suspicious findings (BI-RADS 5) should generally be considered discordant, and either repeat biopsy or surgical excision should be recommended.
- High-risk lesions found on core needle biopsy should generally be referred for surgical consultation to determine further management.
- Although there is controversy regarding need for surgical excision versus observation of some benign and high-risk lesions, there is general consensus regarding the need for excision of atypical ductal hyperplasia (ADH), pleomorphic lobular carcinoma in situ (LCIS), atypical papillary lesions, complex sclerosing lesions, phyllodes tumor, and desmoid tumor.
- Breast cancers are classified as in situ or invasive. Ductal carcinoma in situ (DCIS) is a nonobligate precursor to invasive disease and is currently treated with surgical excision. Clinical trials are underway to determine whether low-risk DCIS can be safely observed.
- Invasive breast cancers are heterogeneous in their behavior and prognosis. Human epidermal growth factor receptor–positive (HER2+) and triple-negative cancers are more biologically aggressive than estrogen- and progesterone-positive (ER+/PR+) tumors.
- Subtypes of invasive ductal carcinoma (tubular, mucinous, medullary, papillary) often demonstrate characteristic imaging appearances. These subtypes tend to have a better prognosis than invasive ductal carcinoma not otherwise specified (IDC NOS).
- Cancers not of ductal or lobular origin, such as lymphoma, sarcoma, and metastatic disease, may also be found in the breast but are rare.

Suggested Readings

Neal L, Sandhu NP, Hieken TJ, et al. Diagnosis and management of benign, atypical, and indeterminate breast lesions detected on core needle biopsy. *Mayo Clin Proc.* 2014;89(4):536–547. https://doi.org/10.1016/j.mayocp.2014.02.004.

Liberman L, Drotman M, Morris EA, et al. Imaging-histologic discordance at percutaneous breast biopsy. *Cancer.* 2000;89(12):2538–2546. doi:10.1002/1097-0142(20001215)89:12<2538::aid-cncr4>3.0.co;2-#.

American Society of Breast Surgeons Consensus Guideline on Concordance Assessment of Image-Guided Breast Biopsies and Management of Borderline or High-Risk Lesions. 2016. Available at https://www.breastsurgeons.org/docs/statements/Consensus-Guideline-on-Concordance-Assessment-of-Image-Guided-Breast-Biopsies.pdf.

Georgian-Smith D, Lawton TJ. Variations in physician recommendations for surgery after diagnosis of a high-risk lesion on breast core needle biopsy. *AJR Am J Roentgenol.* 2012;198(2):256–263. https://doi.org/10.2214/AJR.11.7717. Review.

Irshad A, Ackerman SJ, Pope TL, Moses CK, Rumboldt T, Panzegrau B. Rare breast lesions: correlation of imaging and histologic features with WHO classification. *Radiographics.* 2008;28(5):1399–1414. https://doi.org/10.1148/rg.285075743.

Thomas PS. Diagnosis and management of high-risk breast lesions. *J Natl Compr Canc Netw.* 2018;16(11):1391–1396. https://doi.org/10.6004/jnccn.2018.7099.

Krishnamurthy S, Bevers T, Kuerer H, Yang WT. Multidisciplinary considerations in the management of high-risk breast lesions. *AJR Am J Roentgenol.* 2012;198(2):W132–W140. https://doi.org/10.2214/AJR.11.7799.

Morrow M, Schnitt SJ, Norton L. Current management of lesions associated with an increased risk of breast cancer. *Nat Rev Clin Oncol.* 2015;12(4):227–238. https://doi.org/10.1038/nrclinonc.2015.8.

Lewin AA, Mercado CL. Atypical ductal hyperplasia and lobular neoplasia: update and easing of guidelines. *AJR Am J Roentgenol.* 2020;214(2):265–275. https://doi.org/10.2214/AJR.19.21991.

Li CI, Uribe DJ, Daling JR. Clinical characteristics of different histologic types of breast cancer. *Br J Cancer.* 2005;93(9):1046–1052.

Tirada N, Aujero M, Khorjekar G, et al. Breast cancer tissue markers, genomic profiling, and other prognostic factors: a primer for radiologists. *Radiographics.* 2018;38(7):1902–1920. https://doi.org/10.1148/rg.2018180047.

Parikh U, Chhor CM, Mercado CL. Ductal carcinoma in situ: the whole truth. *AJR Am J Roentgenol.* 2018;210(2):246–255. https://doi.org/10.2214/AJR.17.18778.

Dieci MV, Orvieto E, Dominici M, Conte P, Guarneri V. Rare breast cancer subtypes: histological, molecular, and clinical peculiarities. *Oncologist.* 2014;19(8):805–813. https://doi.org/10.1634/theoncologist.2014-0108.

10 Breast Cancer Risk Assessment

DANA ATAYA, KIMBERLY FUNARO AND BETHANY L. NIELL

OVERVIEW | *This chapter discusses determining breast cancer risk, population subgroups at higher risk, and models to evaluate breast cancer risk.*

Early detection and treatment of breast cancer reduces breast cancer–related mortality. Evaluating and predicting an individual woman's risk of developing breast cancer are important for tailoring screening regimens and breast cancer prevention strategies in order to facilitate early detection. Knowledge of risk determination will help a radiologist communicate knowledgeably with patients and referring providers about breast cancer risk and screening strategies.

Definitions: Average Versus Higher-Than-Average Risk

Knowledge of a woman's risk is important in creating screening and prevention recommendations appropriate to the level of risk. In the United States, one in eight women will develop breast cancer during her lifetime, so an average-risk woman has an estimated lifetime risk of developing breast cancer of approximately 13% (1/8).[1] A woman is considered high risk if she has a 20% or greater lifetime risk of developing breast cancer.[2] Women with an estimated lifetime risk of developing breast cancer from 15% to less than 20% are at higher-than-average risk of developing breast cancer but do not meet the designated threshold of a 20% lifetime risk. Unlike the high-risk subgroup (that has well-defined screening guidelines), supplemental screening recommendations for this intermediate-risk subgroup lack consensus (Box 10.1).

The American College of Radiology (ACR) and Society of Breast Imaging (SBI) recommend that all women undergo a breast cancer risk assessment by age 30 to identify high-risk women who would benefit from supplemental screening.[3] A formal risk assessment, utilizing a risk assessment model, can be used to estimate an individual's lifetime risk of developing breast cancer (see section titled: Models for Risk Assessment").

Population Subgroups at Higher Risk

Certain population subgroups are widely recognized as carrying a 20% or greater lifetime risk of developing breast cancer without the use of a formal risk assessment model (Box 10.2).

GENETIC MUTATION CARRIERS AND HEREDITARY SYNDROMES

About 5% to 10% of women diagnosed with breast cancer have an associated genetic mutation.[4] The *BRCA1* and *BRCA2* mutations are the most widely recognized; however, the use of multigene panel testing in recent years has identified additional pathogenic variants associated with an increased risk of developing breast cancer.

The lifetime risk of developing breast cancer is 50% to 85% among *BRCA1* mutation carriers and approximately 45% among *BRCA2* mutation carriers. Because the *BRCA1* and *BRCA2* mutations are seen at a higher frequency in individuals with Ashkenazi Jewish ancestry, incorporation of ethnicity and race is important in a detailed risk assessment. Other, less common pathogenic variants include *TP53* (Li-Fraumeni syndrome; 85% lifetime risk), *PTEN* (Cowden and Bannayan-Riley-Ruvalcaba syndrome; 25%–85% lifetime risk), *STK11* (Peutz-Jeghers syndrome; 45%–50% lifetime risk), *PALB2* (interacts with *BRCA2*; 35% lifetime risk), *CDH1* (hereditary diffuse gastric cancer; 39%–52% lifetime risk), *ATM* (ataxia-telangiectasia; 33%–38% lifetime risk), *CHEK2* (28%–37% lifetime risk), and *NBN* (30% lifetime risk).[3,5] The National Comprehensive Cancer Network (NCCN) routinely updates its published guidelines on which genetic mutation carriers require early and more rigorous breast cancer screening.[6]

Box 10.1   Breast Cancer Risk: Definitions

- Average risk: ~13% estimated lifetime risk of developing breast cancer
- Higher-than-average risk:
  - High risk: 20% or greater estimated lifetime risk of developing breast cancer
  - Intermediate risk: 15% to <20% estimated lifetime risk of developing breast cancer

---

Box 10.2   Population Subgroups With High Risk of Developing Breast Cancer

- Disease-causing genetic mutations (such as *BRCA1, BRCA2, TP53, PTEN, STK11, PALB2, ATM, CHEK2, CDH1, NBN*) and hereditary syndromes associated with an increased risk of developing breast cancer
- First-degree relative with *BRCA* mutation (or any other autosomal dominant deleterious genetic mutation known to increase breast cancer risk) but the patient herself remains untested
- History of chest radiation therapy before age 30

CHEST/MANTLE RADIATION BEFORE AGE 30

Women who have been treated with chest or mantle radiation therapy before age 30 with a collective dose of ≥10 Gy are at a high risk for developing breast cancer. To put it in perspective, a Hodgkin lymphoma survivor receiving mantle radiation therapy at age 25 will have an estimated 20% to 25% risk of developing breast cancer by age 45,[7,8] similar to a *BRCA* mutation carrier.[9] Patients treated with chest radiation in the first and second decades of life and those receiving ≥20 Gy are at greatest risk for developing a breast malignancy.[3] As such, the American Cancer Society (ACS) and ACR recommend that women who have a history of chest radiation therapy before age 30 begin annual screening mammography at age 25 or 8 years after radiation therapy (whichever is later).[2,3] In addition, the ACS and ACR recommend annual supplemental screening with breast magnetic resonance imaging (MRI) beginning at age 25 to 30.[2,3]

FAMILY HISTORY OF BREAST CANCER

Important factors to consider during evaluation of a patient's family history include the number of family members with breast cancer, the number of maternal and paternal first- and second-degree relatives with breast cancer, and the age of the family members at diagnosis. The ACS therefore recommends the use of risk assessment models that incorporate significant family history in order to identify women with a high estimated lifetime risk of developing breast cancer who should undergo supplemental screening with breast MRI.[2,10] It is important to remember that the vast majority of women who develop breast cancer have no family history of breast cancer.[1,11]

PERSONAL HISTORY OF BREAST CANCER

It has long been recognized that women with a personal history of breast cancer are at risk for a second breast cancer or recurrence. For women diagnosed with breast cancer, the chance of locoregional recurrence within 10 years is about 15% to 19%, and the chance of breast cancer–related mortality within 15 years of the cancer diagnosis is approximately 21%.[3,12] In 2018, the ACR published guidelines recommending supplemental screening with breast MRI for women with a personal history of breast cancer diagnosed at or under age 50.[3] This recommendation was based on a risk modeling study that found that women diagnosed with breast cancer at or before age 50 (treated with breast-conserving therapy) have a 20% or higher lifetime risk for developing a new breast cancer.[13]

Additional Risk Factors for Breast Cancer

GENERAL RISK FACTORS

Gender and age are the strongest nonmodifiable risk factors for breast cancer. Women are 100 times more likely to develop breast cancer compared with men, and roughly 85% of breast cancer cases occur in women ages 50 and older. Approximately one-third of postmenopausal breast cancers are thought to be linked to modifiable risk factors. Postmenopausal obesity, use of hormonal replacement therapy, alcohol consumption, physical inactivity, and lack of breastfeeding are all recognized modifiable breast cancer risk factors.[1,14] Additional risk factors that affect a woman's lifetime exposure of breast tissue to estrogen include early menarche, late menopause, and nulliparity.[1]

LOBULAR NEOPLASIA AND ATYPICAL DUCTAL HYPERPLASIA

Diagnosis of lobular neoplasia, lobular carcinoma in situ (LCIS) or atypical lobular hyperplasia (ALH), confers an increased risk of developing breast cancer in both breasts. Women who have been diagnosed with lobular neoplasia have a 10% to 20% estimated lifetime risk of developing breast cancer.[15] Although the diagnosis of atypical ductal hyperplasia (ADH) has long been recognized as a risk factor for future breast cancer development, it is currently thought to confer a smaller degree of subsequent breast cancer risk compared with a diagnosis of LCIS. The relative risk for invasive breast cancer is approximately four-fold for women diagnosed with ADH or ALH, compared with up to 10-fold for women diagnosed with LCIS[16] (Table 10.1). Because of this, the ACR recommends annual screening mammography with consideration for annual supplemental screening with breast MRI in women with a history of atypia. In addition, women diagnosed with lobular neoplasia or ADH should discuss the role of chemoprevention with a breast specialist.

BREAST DENSITY

There has been increased attention on the impact of breast density on breast cancer risk and breast cancer screening. Dense breast tissue—defined as heterogeneously dense or extremely dense breast tissue—is an independent risk factor for the development of breast cancer. It is important to note that the relative risk depends on which groups are compared (see Table 10.1). For example, women with extremely dense breasts are four to six times more likely to develop breast cancer compared with women with fatty breast tissue. However, most women fall into the scattered and heterogeneously dense breast tissue categories. Compared with

Table 10.1 Relative Risk of Developing Subsequent Breast Cancer During a Woman's Lifetime

Risk Factor	Relative Risk
BRCA1 or *BRCA2* mutation	10–30
Family history: two first-degree relatives with breast cancer	3–4
LCIS on prior biopsy	8–10
Atypia on prior biopsy	4–5
Extremely dense versus fatty	4–6
Heterogeneously dense versus scattered	1.2–1.45
Extremely dense versus scattered	2

LCIS, Lobular carcinoma in situ.

women with scattered fibroglandular tissue, women with extremely dense breast tissue have a two fold increased risk of developing breast cancer.[17]

Moreover, it has long been recognized that dense breast tissue can limit the sensitivity of mammography by masking breast cancers.[3] The false-negative rate of mammography can be as high as 20% and can increase to nearly 50% in premenopausal women with dense breasts.[18] Given the masking effect of dense breast tissue and recognition of breast density as an independent risk factor for developing breast cancer, the ACR recommends supplemental screening with breast MRI for women with a personal history of breast cancer and dense breast tissue.[3]

In March 2019, the U.S. Food and Drug Administration (FDA) announced proposed changes to the Mammography Quality Standards Act (MQSA), including new mandatory reporting requirements on breast density within mammography reports and patient letters.[19] As of March 2020, 38 states have passed breast density laws. This represents a culmination of work initiated by multiple grassroots organizations aiming to educate women and the public on the implications of dense breast tissue on both breast cancer risk as well as missed and delayed breast cancer diagnoses.

However, much work remains to be done. Widespread education is necessary to reduce patient confusion about implications of breast density and supplemental screening, particularly as more women receive mammography reports with breast density language. Widespread education must also include primary care physicians and providers, as many may not feel well informed or prepared to answer patient questions about breast density and supplemental screening. The implementation of state legislation, reporting of breast density in patient mammography reports and widespread recognition of breast density as a risk factor has resulted in an increased demand for supplemental screening tools. Important questions arise: Do all women with dense breast tissue need supplemental screening? Which supplemental screening modality should be used? As nearly half of women in the United States have dense breast tissue, the answers to these questions impact a considerable number of women. Radiologists are poised to play a critical role in answering these questions and defining guidelines.

One major challenge with breast density assessment is the interobserver and intraobserver variability. Breast density has been traditionally assessed qualitatively by the interpreting radiologist via a global visual assessment. This qualitative assessment remains the most widely used method in determination of mammographic breast density. Although there is strong interobserver agreement when assessing fatty and extremely dense breast tissue, agreement is only slight-to-fair in making a decision between scattered fibroglandular and heterogeneously dense categories—the two density categories that encompass approximately 80% of women in the United States.

As density assessments vary depending on the interpreting radiologist and may be influenced by other factors (such as hormonal/endocrine therapy and weight loss), semiautomated and fully automated density software has been introduced to quantify breast density, in order to reduce inter- and intraobserver variability. Some of these methods utilize two-dimensional imaging and perform area-based measurements, while others use digital breast tomosynthesis (DBT) views to generate a more volumetric-based quantification. Quantifying breast density may increase reproducibility and provide measurements to incorporate into risk stratification models.[20]

BACKGROUND PARENCHYMAL ENHANCEMENT

Background parenchymal enhancement (BPE) is a term used to describe the volume and intensity of gadolinium enhancement within normal fibroglandular tissue on breast MRI.[21] BPE is visually assessed on the first postcontrast sequence on breast MRI and is assigned by the radiologist to one of the following categories: (1) minimal, (2) mild, (3) moderate, or (4) marked. It is important to recognize that BPE is not directly related to the amount of fibroglandular tissue present. For example, a patient with extremely dense breasts may demonstrate minimal BPE; conversely, a patient with scattered fibroglandular tissue may demonstrate moderate or marked BPE.[21] The degree, volume, and intensity of BPE can vary depending on the patient. BPE is known to be affected by hormonal levels. BPE can increase in the setting of hormone replacement therapy and may decrease in patients undergoing antiestrogenic therapy with aromatase inhibitors or selective estrogen receptor modulators (SERMs) such as tamoxifen.[22] Published data in recent years has identified BPE as a biomarker for breast cancer risk.[23–25] Elevated BPE levels—measured both qualitatively and quantitatively—are associated with greater risk of developing breast cancer in high-risk women. The impact of BPE on breast cancer risk continues to be an active area of study.

Models for Risk Assessment

In order to identify women at higher than average risk who may benefit from earlier annual screening mammography and supplemental screening, the ACR recommends all women be evaluated for breast cancer risk no later than age 30.[3]

A woman's risk is estimated using risk assessment models: statistical models that incorporate known breast cancer risk factors. Various models have different input parameters and different output. Some models predict the risk of invasive malignancy and/or ductal carcinoma in situ (DCIS) over various time horizons (5 years, 10 years, or lifetime), some models predict the risk of carrying a pathogenic genetic mutation, and some models do both. From the breast radiologist's standpoint, the purpose of the models is to stratify patients into risk categories in order to personalize screening and surveillance plans—such as identifying patients who meet criteria for high-risk screening breast MRI. The models can also help identify women who may benefit from primary chemoprevention or genetic evaluation.[26,27]

The performance of each model varies among individuals and across populations. Currently, risk models demonstrate only moderate accuracy in estimating an individual woman's risk.[28,29] The breast cancer risk assessment models are discussed in this section with key differences highlighted in Table 10.2.

Table 10.2 Key Differences Between Breast Cancer Risk Assessment Models

	Gail (BCRAT)	BRCAPRO	IBIS (Tyrer-Cuzick)	Claus	BOADICEA	BCSC
Endorsed by ACS for supplemental screening MRI		✓	✓	✓	✓	
Endorsed by NCCN for chemoprevention	✓					
Calculates risk of both invasive and in situ cancer			✓	✓	✓	
Includes breast density			✓ (version 8)		✓ (2019 version)	✓
Calculates risk of carrying genetic mutation	✓	✓			✓	

ACS, American Cancer Society; *MRI*, magnetic resonance imaging; *NCCN*, National Comprehensive Cancer Network.

GAIL MODEL

Originally developed in 1989 and later modified in 1999, the modified Gail model or Breast Cancer Risk Assessment Tool (BCRAT) primarily focuses on a woman's medical and reproductive history and only includes family history in first-degree female relatives.[30,31] The modified Gail model calculates a patient's risk of developing invasive breast cancer over various time intervals. Although initially validated in white women, the modified Gail model has been subsequently investigated in Black/African American, Asian and Pacific Islander, and Hispanic women.[31,32] This model should not be used in women with a personal history of breast cancer (invasive or DCIS), LCIS, prior chest radiation, or a known genetic mutation. The ACS does not recommend the Gail model to identify women who should undergo supplemental screening with breast MRI due to limited family history input.[2,10] The NCCN endorses using the Gail model for identifying women who would benefit from chemoprevention (5-year risk of 1.67% or greater).[33,34]

BRCAPRO

The BRCAPRO model assesses the probability of carrying a *BRCA* mutation as well as the risk for developing an invasive breast cancer.[35] The model includes data from affected and unaffected family members, allowing for a more comprehensive family history. As such, the ACS endorses use of this model for identifying women who would benefit from supplemental breast MRI screening.[2,10] BRCAPRO does not include nonhereditary risk factors (e.g., chest radiation, prior history of high-risk lesions) or non-*BRCA* gene mutations and would therefore likely underestimate risk in those subpopulations.[29]

IBIS (TYRER-CUZICK)

The IBIS model, also known as the Tyrer-Cuzick model, assesses a patient's risk of developing breast cancer and predicts the risk of a pathogenic mutation. The model outputs 5-year, 10-year, and lifetime risks for developing invasive as well as in situ breast cancer. Of all the risk assessment models, this is the most comprehensive model and includes a wide variety of both personal risk factors and detailed family history (breast and ovarian cancers).[36] Input parameters include age, height, weight, age at menarche, menopausal status, obstetric history, hormone replacement therapy usage, pathology from prior breast biopsies, and Ashkenazi Jewish descent.[26,36] The newest version, version 8, also includes breast density.[37] The ACS endorses use of this model for assessing screening breast MRI eligibility.[2,10]

CLAUS

The Claus model incorporates family history of breast and ovarian cancer and calculates risk for both invasive and in situ breast cancers.[38,39] Because it includes breast cancer family history from first- and second-degree relatives, the ACS considers the Claus model appropriate to determine breast MRI screening eligibility.[2] Disadvantages of the Claus model include lack of nonhereditary risk factors as well as exclusion of known genetic mutations.[29]

BOADICEA

The Breast and Ovarian Analysis of Disease and Carrier Estimation Algorithm (BOADICEA) is also endorsed by the ACS for risk assessment for supplemental screening with breast MRI.[2] This model incorporates a detailed pedigree and includes *BRCA* mutations and polygenetic factors.[40] Lifetime risk for developing invasive and in situ cancer is calculated, as well as the probability of carrying a deleterious genetic mutation. A prior limitation of the BOADICEA model was lack of inclusion of nonhereditary risk factors, thus underestimating risk in those women.[26] In 2019, BOADICEA was updated to incorporate additional risk factors, including mammographic density.[41]

BREAST CANCER SURVEILLANCE CONSORTIUM

Developed in 2008, the Breast Cancer Surveillance Consortium (BCSC) risk calculator was the first model to incorporate mammographic density into risk assessment.[42] In addition to including breast density and first-degree female relative breast cancer history, the model also extensively incorporates pathology from benign breast biopsies, including high-risk lesions.[43] The BCSC model outputs 5-year and 10-year risk estimates for developing an invasive breast cancer but does not calculate estimated lifetime risk. Therefore this model is not currently used to determine eligibility for supplemental screening breast MRI.

KEY POINTS

- All women should undergo a breast cancer risk assessment by age 30.
- Risk assessments can identify women at a higher-than-average risk for breast cancer and inform supplemental screening recommendations.

Suggested Readings

1. Monticciolo DL, et al. Breast cancer screening for average-risk women: recommendations from the ACR commission on breast imaging. *J Am Coll Radiol.* 2017;14(9):1137–1143.

2. Monticciolo DL, et al. Breast cancer screening in women at higher-than-average risk: recommendations from the ACR. *J Am Coll Radiol*. 2018;15(3 Pt A):408–414.

References

1. American Cancer Society (ACS). Breast Cancer Facts & Figures 2019–2020. Accessed: March 26, 2020; Available from: https://www.cancer.org/content/dam/cancer-org/research/cancer-facts-and-statistics/breast-cancer-facts-and-figures/breast-cancer-facts-and-figures-2019-2020.pdf.

2. Saslow D, et al. American Cancer Society guidelines for breast screening with MRI as an adjunct to mammography. *CA Cancer J Clin*. 2007;57(2):75–89.

3. Monticciolo DL, et al. Breast cancer screening in women at higher-than-average risk: recommendations from the ACR. *J Am Coll Radiol*. 2018;15(3 Pt A):408–414.

4. Claus EB, et al. The genetic attributable risk of breast and ovarian cancer. *Cancer*. 1996;77(11):2318–2324.

5. Nguyen J, T M, Beyond BRCA: Review of hereditary syndromes predisposing to breast cancer. *J Breast Imaging (JBI)*. 2019;1(2):84–91.

6. National Comprehensive Cancer Network (NCCN). Genetic/Familial High-Risk Assessment: Breast, Ovarian, and Pancreatic (Version 2.2022). Accessed: February 7, 2022. Available from: DOI: 10.6004/jnccn.2021.0001.

7. Travis LB, et al. Cumulative absolute breast cancer risk for young women treated for Hodgkin lymphoma. *J Natl Cancer Inst*. 2005;97(19):1428–1437.

8. Mulder RL, et al. Recommendations for breast cancer surveillance for female survivors of childhood, adolescent, and young adult cancer given chest radiation: a report from the International Late Effects of Childhood Cancer Guideline Harmonization Group. *Lancet Oncol*. 2013;14(13):e621–e629.

9. Metcalfe K, et al. Family history of cancer and cancer risks in women with BRCA1 or BRCA2 mutations. *J Natl Cancer Inst*. 2010;102(24):1874–1878.

10. Smith RA, Cokkinides V, Brawley OW. Cancer screening in the United States, 2012: a review of current American Cancer Society guidelines and current issues in cancer screening. *CA Cancer J Clin*. 2012;62(2):129–142.

11. Shiyanbola OO, et al. Emerging trends in family history of breast cancer and associated risk. *Cancer Epidemiol Biomarkers Prev*. 2017;26(12):1753–1760.

12. Early Breast Cancer Trialists' Collaborative G, et al. Effect of radiotherapy after breast-conserving surgery on 10-year recurrence and 15-year breast cancer death: meta-analysis of individual patient data for 10, 801 women in 17 randomised trials. *Lancet*. 2011;378(9804):1707–1716.

13. Punglia RS, Hassett MJ. Using lifetime risk estimates to recommend magnetic resonance imaging screening for breast cancer survivors. *J Clin Oncol*. 2010;28(27):4108–4110.

14. Tamimi RM, et al. Population attributable risk of modifiable and non-modifiable breast cancer risk factors in postmenopausal breast cancer. *Am J Epidemiol*. 2016;184(12):884–893.

15. Arpino G, Laucirica R, Elledge RM. Premalignant and in situ breast disease: biology and clinical implications. *Ann Intern Med*. 2005;143(6):446–457.

16. Dupont WD, Page DL. Risk factors for breast cancer in women with proliferative breast disease. *N Engl J Med*. 1985;312(3):146–151.

17. Cummings SR, et al. Prevention of breast cancer in postmenopausal women: approaches to estimating and reducing risk. *J Natl Cancer Inst*. 2009;101(6):384–398.

18. Kolb TM, Lichy J, Newhouse JH. Comparison of the performance of screening mammography, physical examination, and breast US and evaluation of factors that influence them: an analysis of 27,825 patient evaluations. *Radiology*. 2002;225(1):165–175.

19. Department of Health and Human Services, Food and Drug Administration (FDA). Mammography Quality Standards Act: A Proposed Rule. 21 CFR Part 900. Accessed: March 25, 2020.; Available from: https://www.govinfo.gov/content/pkg/FR-2019-03-28/pdf/2019-05803.pdf.

20. Destounis SV, Santacroce A, Arieno A. Update on breast density, risk estimation, and supplemental screening. *AJR Am J Roentgenol*. 2020;214(2):296–305.

21. Morris EA, C C, Lee CH, et al. ACR BI-RADS® Magnetic Resonance Imaging. In: *ACR BI-RADS® Atlas, Breast Imaging Reporting and Data System*. Reston, VA: American College of Radiology; 2013.

22. Liao GJ, et al. Background parenchymal enhancement on breast MRI: A comprehensive review. *J Magn Reson Imaging*. 2019.

23. Dontchos BN, et al. Are qualitative assessments of background parenchymal enhancement, amount of fibroglandular tissue on MR images, and mammographic density associated with breast cancer risk? *Radiology*. 2015;276(2):371–380.

24. King V, et al. Background parenchymal enhancement at breast MR imaging and breast cancer risk. *Radiology*. 2011;260(1):50–60.

25. Telegrafo M, et al. Breast MRI background parenchymal enhancement (BPE) correlates with the risk of breast cancer. *Magn Reson Imaging*. 2016;34(2):173–176.

26. Barke LD, Freivogel ME. Breast cancer risk assessment models and high-risk screening. *Radiol Clin North Am*. 2017;55(3):457–474.

27. Lee CS, Sickles EA, Moy L. Risk stratification for screening mammography: benefits and harms. *AJR Am J Roentgenol*. 2019;212(2):250–258.

28. Meads C, Ahmed I, Riley RD. A systematic review of breast cancer incidence risk prediction models with meta-analysis of their performance. *Breast Cancer Res Treat*. 2012;132(2):365–377.

29. Amir E, et al. Assessing women at high risk of breast cancer: a review of risk assessment models. *J Natl Cancer Inst*. 2010;102(10):680–691.

30. Gail MH, et al. Projecting individualized probabilities of developing breast cancer for white females who are being examined annually. *J Natl Cancer Inst*. 1989;81(24):1879–1886.

31. Costantino JP, et al. Validation studies for models projecting the risk of invasive and total breast cancer incidence. *J Natl Cancer Inst*. 1999;91(18):1541–1548.

32. Banegas MP, et al. Projecting individualized absolute invasive breast cancer risk in US Hispanic women. *J Natl Cancer Inst*. 2017;109(2).

33. Fisher B, et al. Tamoxifen for prevention of breast cancer: report of the National Surgical Adjuvant Breast and Bowel Project P-1 Study. *J Natl Cancer Inst*. 1998;90(18):1371–1388.

34. National Comprehensive Cancer Network (NCCN). Breast Cancer Risk Reduction. Version 2.2022. Accessed: February 7, 2022.; Available from: https://doi.org/10.6004/jnccn.2021.0001.

35. Parmigiani G, Berry D, Aguilar O. Determining carrier probabilities for breast cancer-susceptibility genes BRCA1 and BRCA2. *Am J Hum Genet*. 1998;62(1):145–158.

36. Tyrer J, Duffy SW, Cuzick J. A breast cancer prediction model incorporating familial and personal risk factors. *Stat Med*. 2004;23(7):1111–1130.

37. Brentnall AR, et al. lA case-control study to add volumetric or clinical mammographic density into the Tyrer-Cuzick breast cancer risk model. *J Breast Imaging*. 2019;1(2):99–106.

38. Claus EB, Risch N, Thompson WD. The calculation of breast cancer risk for women with a first degree family history of ovarian cancer. *Breast Cancer Res Treat*. 1993;28(2):115–120.

39. Claus EB, Risch N, Thompson WD. Autosomal dominant inheritance of early-onset breast cancer. Implications for risk prediction. *Cancer*. 1994;73(3):643–651.

40. Antoniou AC, et al. The BOADICEA model of genetic susceptibility to breast and ovarian cancer. *Br J Cancer*. 2004;91(8):1580–1590.

41. Lee A, et al. BOADICEA: a comprehensive breast cancer risk prediction model incorporating genetic and nongenetic risk factors. *Genet Med*. 2019;21(8):1708–1718.

42. Tice JA, et al. Using clinical factors and mammographic breast density to estimate breast cancer risk: development and validation of a new predictive model. *Ann Intern Med*. 2008;148(5):337–347.

43. Tice JA, et al. Breast density and benign breast disease: risk assessment to identify women at high risk of breast cancer. *J Clin Oncol*. 2015;33(28):3137–3143.

11 Breast Cancer Screening Guidelines and Supplemental Screening

DANA ATAYA, KIMBERLY FUNARO AND BETHANY L. NIELL

OVERVIEW *This chapter discusses screening guidelines for women at average risk and elevated risk, and supplemental screening tools beyond full-field digital mammography (FFDM).*

Breast cancer is the most commonly diagnosed nonskin cancer and is the second leading cause of cancer death in women in the United States. For the year 2020, the American Cancer Society estimated 268,600 new cases of invasive breast cancer and over 41,000 deaths from breast cancer.[1] Knowledge of screening guidelines and supplemental imaging tools will help you—the radiologist—communicate knowledgeably with patients and the referring providers about breast cancer screening strategies.

Breast Cancer Screening Guidelines

If breast cancer is diagnosed and treated when localized to the breast, the 5-year relative survival rate is 99%. However, 5-year relative survival drops to 27% when distant metastatic disease is present at the time of diagnosis.[2] Mammographic screening results in early detection of breast cancer, and early detection of breast cancer saves lives. Multiple randomized control trials (RCTs), observational studies, and service screening studies have demonstrated that regular screening mammography decreases breast cancer mortality, as described in Chapter 12.

Despite this, continued controversy and confusion persists in the media, public, and medical community with respect to screening mammography recommendations. Disagreement in mammography screening guidelines can be boiled down to three main disputed factors: (1) which published studies are analyzed and how that subset of data is interpreted; (2) what benefits and risks are incorporated; and (3) how the benefits and risks are weighed. Despite differences in screening mammography recommendations, annual screening mammography beginning at age 40 saves the most lives, confers the greatest reduction in breast cancer mortality, and results in the largest increase in life-years gained from screening. Please also refer to Chapter 12 for additional reading on screening mammography. This section will review and discuss the various guidelines pertaining to screening mammography.

SCREENING GUIDELINES FOR AVERAGE-RISK WOMEN

In this section, we will review the screening mammography recommendations from various organizations, which are summarized in Fig. 11.1.

ACR, SBI, ASBrS, NCCN, and NCBC

The American College of Radiology (ACR) recommends annual screening mammography for average-risk women beginning at age 40, with no specific age limit to stop screening as long as a woman is in good health.[3-7] The American Society of Breast Surgeons (ASBrS), the National Comprehensive Cancer Network (NCCN), the National Consortium of Breast Centers (NCBC), and the Society of Breast Imaging (SBI) also recommend annual screening mammography beginning at age 40, for as long as a woman is healthy.

American Cancer Society

The American Cancer Society (ACS) guidelines recommend that average-risk women have the option to begin annual screening at 40 to 44 years (qualified recommendation), strongly recommend regular screening by age 45, and recommend cessation of screening if a woman's life expectancy is less than 10 years.[7] For screening intervals, the ACS strongly recommends annual mammography for women 45 to 54 years old, and either annual or biennial screening in women 55 years and older (qualified recommendation).[8] The ACS acknowledges that there is a clear benefit to annual screening mammography beginning at age 40 but qualifies recommendations due to uncertainty about how each individual woman might balance the benefits and risks of screening.

USPSTF, AAFP, and ACP

The United States Preventive Services Task Force (USPSTF) recommends screening average-risk women biennially (every 2 years) from ages 50 to 74 years (Grade B: moderate certainty that the net benefit is moderate to substantial).[9] The USPSTF guidelines state that beginning screening before age 50 should be individualized (Grade C: balance of benefits and harms is close with small net benefit).[9]

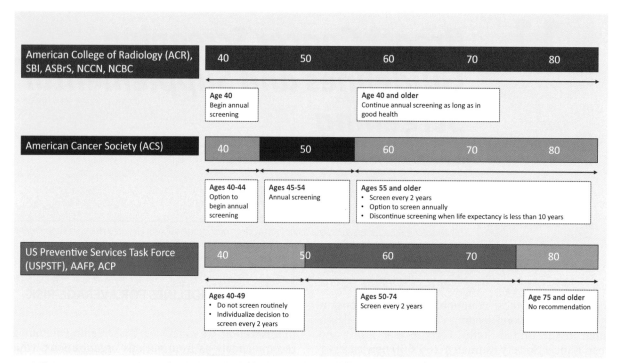

Fig. 11.1 Differences in mammography screening recommendations for average risk women.

Table 11.1   ACR Guidelines for Screening Women at Higher-Than-Average Risk

Indication	Mammographic Interval	Breast MRI Interval
Estimated lifetime risk ≥20%	Annual, starting at age 30	Annual, starting at age 25–30
Genetic mutation carriers and their untested first degree relatives	Annual, starting at age 30	Annual, starting at age 25–30
Chest radiation before age 30	Annual, starting at age 25 or 8 years after radiation, whichever is later	Annual, starting at age 25–30
Personal Hx of breast cancer diagnosed ≤ age 50	Annual	Annual
Personal Hx of breast cancer and dense breast tissue	Annual	Annual
History of atypia or LCIS	Annual	Consider annual MRI, especially if other risk factors present

ACR, American College of Radiology; *LCIS*, lobular carcinoma in situ; *MRI*, magnetic resonance imaging.

The USPSTF considers evidence as insufficient for offering screening guidelines to women older than 75 years. These screening guidelines are supported by the American Academy of Family Physicians (AAFP) and the American College of Physicians (ACP).

Despite differences in screening mammography recommendations, all guidelines agree on several points:

1. Annual mammography beginning at age 40 saves the most lives.
2. Patients should discuss benefits and risks of screening with a health care provider so that they can make an informed decision.
3. All women should have a choice to begin screening at age 40 and a choice to decide when to stop screening.

SCREENING GUIDELINES FOR HIGHER-THAN-AVERAGE-RISK WOMEN

Women at a higher risk for developing breast cancer benefit from earlier and more intensive screening. The ACR, ACS, and ASBrS have all issued screening guidelines for high-risk women. Table 11.1 summarizes the ACR guidelines for screening women at higher-than average risk. The ACR recommends that high-risk women begin annual screening mammography at age 30; however, high-risk women who have received chest radiation before 30 years of age should begin annual screening mammography at age 25 or 8 years after radiation (whichever is later).[10] The ACR, ACS, and ASBrS all recommend supplemental screening with breast magnetic resonance imaging (MRI) for women with a ≥20% lifetime risk of developing breast cancer. The ACR recommends initiation of supplemental breast MRI screening for high-risk women at 25 to 30 years of age.[10]

Supplemental Screening

Although mammography has been validated by multiple RCTs and meta-analyses to reduce breast cancer mortality via early detection, it has limitations. The sensitivity of mammography ranges from 25% to 59% in higher risk women.[10,11] Moreover, about 20% of all breast cancers are interval cancers—cancers that present symptomatically within 12 months of a negative mammogram.[12–14] Because of the limitations in mammography, other supplemental imaging modalities have been pursued to increase cancer detection and decrease the frequency of interval cancers. With the recent adoption of breast density legislation across the United States, more women and their referring providers might seek information on supplemental screening modalities. Further work is needed to provide affordable, effective, and efficient supplemental breast imaging tools. This section will review currently available supplemental screening options.

INCREMENTAL CANCER DETECTION RATE PER MODALITY

Cancer detection rate (CDR) is defined as the number of cancers detected at imaging per 1000 examinations performed.[15] Screening with full-field digital mammography (FFDM) detects approximately 5 cancers per 1000 examinations.[16,17] Supplemental screening with digital breast tomosynthesis (DBT) will find an additional 1 to 2 cancers per 1000 examinations performed (incremental CDR of 1–2),[18–21] whole breast ultrasound an additional 2 to 4 cancers per 1000 (incremental CDR of 2–4),[22–24] and breast MRI will find approximately 15 to 30 additional cancers per 1000 prevalent breast MRI examinations (incremental CDR of 15–30).[25–30] These reported ranges of incremental CDR per modality include women at both average and higher-than-average risk. It is important to note that incremental CDR is expected to vary by risk group since the underlying prevalence of breast cancer varies across risk groups. For example, supplemental screening with breast MRI has a higher incremental CDR in women with *BRCA* mutations compared with women at average risk or women with a family history of breast cancer and no known genetic mutation.[27–31] Furthermore, incremental CDR will differ for baseline (prevalent) and subsequent (incident) supplemental screening rounds.[30] Table 11.2 displays incremental CDR by modality.

DIGITAL BREAST TOMOSYNTHESIS

DBT has been rapidly adopted into clinical practices since FDA approval in 2011. Multiple studies have demonstrated the increased sensitivity and specificity of DBT compared FFDM alone. Specifically, the use of DBT results in a reduction in false-positive recalls of approximately 15% to 30% compared with FFDM alone.[18–21] The reduction in recall rates seen with DBT is found to be particularly notable for baseline mammograms, patients with dense breast tissue, and women under age 50.[32,33] DBT finds 1 to 2 additional cancers per 1000 examinations[18–21] (Fig. 11.2; see Table 11.2).

Although published studies in average-risk women report an incremental CDR of 1 to 2 cancers per 1000 examinations with the use of DBT, there is limited data regarding comparative DBT versus FFDM performance in high-risk women. One study evaluating over 2000 high-risk women found no statistically significant difference in DBT CDR between average-risk and high-risk women, although this finding may be secondary, at least in part, to the small sample size.[34] Nonetheless, DBT has widely replaced FFDM as the primary mammographic screening tool for both average-risk and higher-than-average-risk women, due to published data demonstrating lower recall rates and higher incremental CDR. The ACR appropriateness criteria—guidelines routinely updated to provide the most current evidence-based recommendations for imaging or treatment of a specific clinical scenario—classify both DBT and FFDM as appropriate for screening in average-risk and higher-than-average risk populations (Box 11.1).[35]

Table 11.2 Incremental Cancer Detection Rate (CDR) Per Modality Across Risk Groups

Modality	CDR (per 1000)
Mammography	3–5
+DBT	+1–2
+US	+2–4
+MRI	+15–30

DBT, Digital breast tomosynthesis; *MRI,* magnetic resonance imaging; *US,* ultrasound.

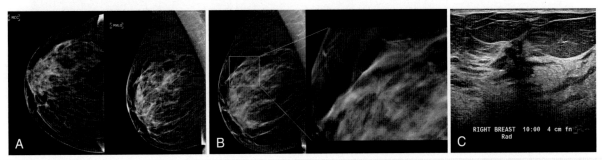

Fig. 11.2 Digital breast tomosynthesis (DBT). (A) Right breast full-field digital mammography (FFDM) views from a FFDM/DBT screening examination are negative. (B) Selected mediolateral oblique (MLO) DBT slice demonstrates an area of architectural distortion in the upper outer right breast. (C) Targeted ultrasound demonstrates an irregular hypoechoic mass, correlating with the distortion seen at DBT. Biopsy yielded invasive ductal carcinoma.

Dose is a consideration with DBT. Although the radiation dose with combined FFDM/DBT examinations is below the MQSA limit of 3 mGy per acquisition, there is over a two fold increase (approximately 2.25) when comparing FFDM/DBT with DBT alone. The use of synthetic mammography (SM)—where data from the tomosynthesis acquisition is synthesized to create a "two-dimensional" view—can obviate the need for a separate FFDM exposure and thereby reduce average glandular dose (AGD) by 39%.[36] Studies evaluating the performance of SM/DBT to FFDM/DBT have found similar sensitivity, specificity, CDR, and diagnostic accuracy.[36-40] Despite this—and although many practices with DBT have SM capability—SM has not yet widely replaced FFDM in the clinical setting.

SCREENING BREAST ULTRASOUND

Published studies have demonstrated that supplemental screening with breast ultrasound finds additional breast cancers over mammography alone. The ACRIN 6666 trial—a landmark prospective multicenter breast imaging trial evaluating women at an elevated risk for developing breast cancer—found an incremental CDR of 4.3 per 1000 with supplemental screening ultrasound following negative FFDM.[22] Importantly, the cancers identified sonographically tended to be small invasive cancers that were node negative (Fig. 11.3). Supplemental screening ultrasound in women whose only risk was dense breast tissue shows an incremental CDR of 2.3 to 4.0 per 1000 (see Table 11.2).[24,41]

However, supplemental screening with breast ultrasound results in increased false positives and a markedly lower positive predictive value (PPV) for biopsy compared with mammography and MRI. In the ACRIN 6666 trial, the PPV2 for ultrasound-only findings was 8.9% (compared with the PPV of mammography at 22.6%).[22] However, other more recent studies have demonstrated improved PPV with increasing reader experience and availability of prior examinations.[41,42] In addition to lower PPV, screening with breast ultrasound also increases short-term follow-up recommendations (8.6% for ultrasound versus 2.2% for mammography).[22] In patients screened with annual mammography and supplemental breast MRI, do not perform screening breast ultrasound in addition. Screening ultrasound can substantially increase false positives without incremental cancer detection in patients who are being screened with mammography and breast MRI.[11,43,44]

Whole-breast screening ultrasound can be performed via a handheld technique or via automated breast ultrasound. Handheld whole-breast screening ultrasound is operator dependent and labor intensive. In contrast, automated breast ultrasound can decouple the imaging acquisition and interpretation experience (thereby addressing limitations with operator dependence and labor intensity) but is associated with concerns regarding incomplete breast coverage in patients with larger breasts (Box 11.2).

BREAST MAGNETIC RESONANCE IMAGING

Breast MRI has higher sensitivity (90%–100%) than mammography.[1,44-48] This enhanced sensitivity is attributable to the contrast-enhanced component of breast MRI, which captures the neoangiogenesis of breast cancers. As such, the performance of breast MRI is not hindered by breast density. Comparatively, anatomically based techniques (such as mammography, DBT, and ultrasound) have a lower sensitivity. The average sensitivity of mammography

---

Box 11.1   Digital Breast Tomosynthesis (DBT)

- Indications: widespread replacement of FFDM as screening tool for both average and higher-than-average-risk patients
- Pros: decreased recall rate, increased CDR
- Cons: increased radiation dose (reduced with use of SM/DBT)

CDR, Cancer detection rate; *FFDM,* full-field digital mammography; *SM,* synthetic mammography.

Box 11.2   Screening Breast Ultrasound

- Indications: high-risk women who have absolute or relative contraindications to breast MRI; average or intermediate-risk women who desire supplemental screening
- Pros: increased CDR
- Cons: low PPV

CDR, Cancer detection rate; *MRI,* magnetic resonance imaging; *PPV,* positive predictive value.

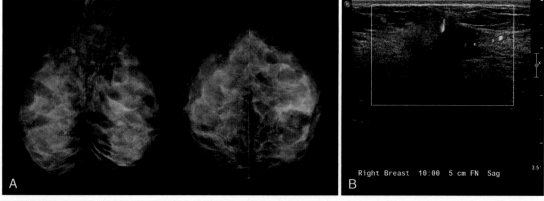

Fig. 11.3 Screening breast ultrasound. (A) Full-field digital mammography (FFDM) screening mammogram demonstrates extremely dense breast tissue and no mammographic abnormality. (B) Supplemental screening breast ultrasound found an irregular hypoechoic mass in the right breast. Biopsy yielded invasive ductal carcinoma.

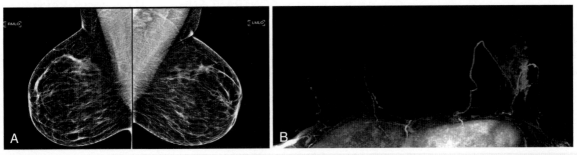

Fig. 11.4 Screening breast magnetic resonance imaging (MRI). (A) Mediolateral oblique (MLO) images from a negative full-field digital mammography/digital breast tomosynthesis (FFDM/DBT) screening examination demonstrate scattered fibroglandular breast tissue. (B) Maximum intensity projection (MIP) image from supplemental screening breast MRI demonstrates segmental non-mass enhancement in the left breast. Biopsy yielded invasive ductal carcinoma and ductal carcinoma in situ (DCIS).

alone can be as low as 33%, with the combined sensitivity of mammography and ultrasound reported at 48%.[46] Although the reported incremental CDR of screening breast MRI ranges from 8 to 67 per 1000 examinations, many studies have shown that breast MRI can detect about 15 to 30 additional cancers per 1000 examinations performed in women with negative FFDM[25–27,29,30,49] (see Table 11.2). The high incremental CDR observed with MRI is irrespective of breast density and menopausal status[50] (Fig. 11.4).

The reported specificity of breast MRI ranges from 81% to 97%. Comparatively, the specificity of mammography is reported as 93% to 97%.[11,43,51–53] Although breast MRI has been historically criticized for its lower specificity, recent publications demonstrate the PPV of biopsies performed (PPV3) of breast MRI to be similar to mammography.[25,54] More importantly, breast MRI preferentially detects more invasive cancers and intermediate and high-grade ductal carcinoma in situ (DCIS), which are more likely to be biologically significant.[27,55] In addition, the DENSE trial showed that the use of supplemental MRI screening in women with extremely dense breast tissue resulted in significantly fewer interval cancers than mammography alone.[56]

The negative predictive value (NPV) of breast MRI is also exceedingly high, reported as 97% to 100%.[57–59] This means that when no abnormality or abnormal enhancement is detected on breast MRI, the likelihood of a breast malignancy is remarkably low. The few malignancies missed by breast MRI are typically low-grade DCIS lesions.[60,61]

Limitations of breast MRI screening include the increased cost of breast MRI and the longer examination time (compared with mammography and ultrasound). Additionally, patients with metallic implants/devices and patients with extreme claustrophobia may not be able to undergo MRI screening. Finally, patients require an intravenous (IV) and injection of a gadolinium-based contrast agent. Contrast reactions to gadolinium agents are rare but do occur. In addition, gadolinium deposition in the brain has been reported in patients who have undergone multiple contrast-enhanced MRI examinations. A recent study evaluating 25 healthy women who had undergone multiple screening breast MRI examinations (mean gadolinium dose of 129 mL) found no gadolinium deposition within the brain using 3 T MRI.[62] The frequency and clinical significance of gadolinium deposition requires further research.

Supplemental Breast MRI Screening in High-Risk Women

Supplemental screening with breast MRI increases early detection of predominantly invasive, node-negative breast cancers in high-risk patients.[63] The ACR, ACS, and ASBrS all recommend supplemental screening with breast MRI for women with a ≥20% lifetime risk of developing breast cancer, carriers of BRCA and other deleterious genetic mutations that increase breast cancer risk, first-degree relatives of women with those deleterious genetic mutations (with autosomal dominant inheritance) who remain untested themselves, and women who have received chest radiation between ages 10 and 30.[10,63] Per ACR guidelines, initiation of supplemental breast MRI screening for high-risk women should begin at 25 to 30 years of age.[10] (See Screening Guidelines for Higher-Than-Average-Risk Women and Table 11.1).

Supplemental Breast MRI Screening in Average-Risk Women

There are no existing guidelines on screening breast MRI in average-risk women. However, with the widespread implementation of breast density legislation across the United States, efforts have been made to offer effective, efficient, and economical supplemental breast imaging tools. Abbreviated Breast MRI (AB-MRI) is one tool offered by some breast imaging centers. Although AB-MRI protocols may vary slightly per institution, only the most essential MRI sequences are included (typically, at least a T1W pre-contrast and one T1W postcontrast sequence). This allows for a reduction in imaging time, interpretation time, and cost. Studies evaluating AB-MRI demonstrate comparable diagnostic accuracy and CDRs when comparing AB-MRI to a full MRI protocol.[64–67]

The recently published results from the EA-1141 trial comparing abbreviated breast MRI (AB-MRI) to DBT confirm the superior sensitivity and CDR of breast MRI (95.7%; 15.2/1000) compared with DBT (39.1%; 6.2/1000) in women with dense breast tissue as their sole risk factor, with no statistically significant difference in PPV.[28] The majority of cancers detected by AB-MRI in the study were invasive breast cancers (invasive CDR of 11.8/1000 AB-MRI versus 4.8/1000 DBT).[28]

Specific limitations in widespread implementation of AB-MRI include accessibility and capacity restrictions. Although AB-MRI uses the same equipment utilized for a full MRI protocol, more MRI units at additional centers would be needed in order to offer widespread AB-MRI screening to a significantly larger number of women. In addition, although AB-MRI is a fraction of the cost of a full MRI protocol, it is currently an out-of-pocket expense for patients (Box 11.3).

MOLECULAR BREAST IMAGING

Molecular breast imaging (MBI) requires an IV injection of a radiopharmaceutical agent (technetium-99m sestamibi) followed by imaging with a dedicated breast-specific gamma camera. Similar to breast MRI, MBI is able to capture the neoangiogenesis of tumors and therefore has high sensitivity and an increased incremental CDR (iCDR) for breast cancers measuring over 1 cm in size (95% sensitivity and 8.8 iCDR).[68-71] Studies evaluating MBI as a supplemental screening tool in women with dense breast tissue report an incremental CDR of 7 to 9 per 1000 examinations.[70,71] The sensitivity of MBI is lower for DCIS and invasive cancers measuring less than 1 cm (84%–88%).[68] In women with a higher-than-average risk of breast cancer, the incremental CDR of MBI was comparable to breast MRI when a higher activity radiopharmaceutical dose was used.[72] Similar to MRI, MBI is not hindered by breast density.[10] However, MBI results in whole-body radiation exposure, which limits its widespread use in the screening setting (Box 11.4).

Box 11.3   Screening Breast MRI

- Indications: high-risk women; average- or intermediate-risk women who desire supplemental screening
- Pros: highest CDR and sensitivity, high NPV
- Cons: cost, IV injection needed

CDR, Cancer detection rate; *IV*, intravenous; *MRI*, magnetic resonance imaging; *NPV*, negative predictive value.

Box 11.4   Molecular Breast Imaging

- Indications: consider as an alternative to breast MRI in high-risk women with contraindications to MRI; average- or intermediate-risk women who desire supplemental screening
- Pros: comparable sensitivity and CDR to MRI for invasive cancers ≥1 cm
- Cons: whole-body radiation exposure, dedicated breast-specific cameras needed, IV injection needed

CDR, Cancer detection rate; *IV*, intravenous; *MRI*, magnetic resonance imaging.

CONTRAST-ENHANCED MAMMOGRAPHY

Contrast-enhanced mammography (CEM)—also known as contrast-enhanced spectral mammography (CESM) or contrast-enhanced digital mammography (CEDM)—is a dual-energy mammography technique obtained after IV injection of iodinated contrast. Iodinated contrast administration is similar to computed tomography; a power injector is used for a flow rate of 3 mL/second, using a 300 to 370 mg/mL iodine concentration at 1.5 mL/kg body weight (typically 90–150 mL total). After a delay of at least 90 seconds, the patient is positioned in the conventional fashion for full-field mammographic views. Two images of each breast are then obtained—dual-energy image pairs in each projection. After image acquisition, weighted subtraction is performed where nonenhancing tissue is eliminated and enhancement (iodine) is displayed.

Similar to contrast-enhanced breast MRI and MBI, CEM captures tumor neoangiogenesis (Fig. 11.5). As would be predicted, CEM shows increased sensitivity, specificity, and accuracy in a diagnostic setting compared with digital mammography alone.[73,74] Screening with CEM in a higher-than-average-risk population has a sensitivity of 87.5% (versus 50% with digital mammography alone), and a CDR of 15.5 per 1000 examinations in one recently published study.[75] Additional studies comparing CEM and contrast-enhanced breast MRI have found similar sensitivities with variable specificities and accuracy.[76-80] More prospective studies are needed to evaluate the performance of CEM in comparison with MRI.

The advantages of CEM as a supplemental screening tool include the lower cost and shorter examination time compared with breast MRI. Limitations of CEM include the workflow and contrast screening process. An IV and injection of an iodinated contrast agent is required. As such, a contrast screening process must be in place to evaluate renal function and review contrast allergy history. Adverse reactions to contrast media are more commonly encountered with iodinated contrast compared with gadolinium-based agents.[81]

The European Society of Breast Imaging (EUSOBI) recommendations state that CEM can be considered as an alternative to breast MRI for women with contraindications to breast MRI (such as an MRI-unsafe device or extreme claustrophobia). Unlike breast MRI, only one time point is typically obtained with CEM (and therefore kinetic data are not routinely acquired during CEM for lesion characterization). In addition, the radiation dose of CEM is approximately 1.2 to 1.8 times that of FFDM (Box 11.5).[82]

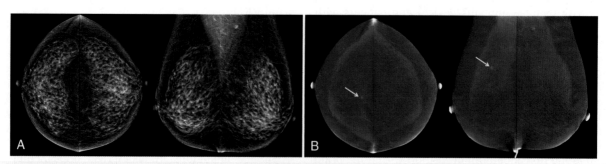

Fig. 11.5 Contrast-enhanced mammography (CEM). (A) Low-energy images demonstrate heterogeneously dense breast tissue and no mammographic abnormality. (B) Recombined images from the CEM examination demonstrate a small enhancing mass in the right breast (*arrows*). The mass was identified and sampled under sonographic guidance; biopsy yielded invasive ductal carcinoma.

Box 11.5   Contrast-Enhanced Mammography

■ Indications: consider as an alternative to breast MRI in high-risk women with contraindications to MRI; average- or intermediate-risk women who desire supplemental screening

■ Pros: comparable sensitivity to MRI, lower cost, shorter examination time

■ Cons: IV injection needed, higher radiation dose

IV, Intravenous; *MRI*, magnetic resonance imaging.

KEY POINTS

- Average-risk women: The American College of Radiology (ACR) recommends annual screening mammography beginning at age 40 because it saves the most lives. The American Cancer Society (ACS), United States Preventive Services Task Force (USPSTF), and other professional organizations recommend different regimens.
- Higher-than-average-risk women: The ACR recommends annual screening mammography beginning at age 30 and annual breast magnetic resonance imaging (MRI) beginning at age 25–30.
- The ACR and ACS recommend annual mammography and supplemental screening magnetic resonance imaging (MRI) in women with:
  - Disease-causing genetic mutation(s) (e.g., *BRCA1, BRCA2, TP53, PTEN*) or hereditary syndromes associated with an increased risk for developing breast cancer
  - First-degree relative who carries a deleterious genetic mutation that increases breast cancer risk and is transmitted in an autosomal dominant inheritance pattern, if the patient herself remains untested
  - History of prior chest radiation therapy before age 30
  - 20% or greater estimated lifetime risk of developing breast cancer
- For women with personal histories of breast cancer and dense breast tissue, or those diagnosed ≤50 years, annual surveillance breast MRI in addition to annual mammography is recommended by the ACR.
- For women with personal histories of breast cancer diagnosed ≥50 years with nondense breast tissue, and women with a personal history of atypical ductal hyperplasia (ADH), atypical lobular hyperplasia (ALH), or lobular carcinoma in situ (LCIS), the ACR suggests that supplemental screening breast MRI should be considered.
- Digital breast tomosynthesis (DBT) decreases recall rates, increases cancer detection rate (CDR), and is widely used for screening in average and higher-than-average-risk populations.
- Screening breast ultrasound increases CDR at the cost of a lower positive predictive value (PPV) compared with mammography and can be considered for women with dense breasts or other risk factors who do not meet criteria for supplemental screening with breast MRI.
- Breast MRI has high sensitivity, CDR, and negative predictive value (NPV) and finds additional breast cancers in both higher-than-average-risk and average-risk populations compared with mammography alone or mammography combined with supplemental screening ultrasound.

References

1. American Cancer Society (ACS). *Breast Cancer Facts & Figures 2019-2020.* Accessed: March 26, 2020; Available from: https://www.cancer.org/content/dam/cancer-org/research/cancer-facts-and-statistics/breast-cancer-facts-and-figures/breast-cancer-facts-and-figures-2019-2020.pdf.
2. Cancer Stat Facts: Female Breast Cancer. National Cancer Institute (NIH) Surveillance, Epidemiology, and End Results Program (SEER). 2019; Available from: https://seer.cancer.gov/statfacts/html/breast.html.
3. Tabar L, et al. Swedish two-county trial: impact of mammographic screening on breast cancer mortality during 3 decades. *Radiology.* 2011;260(3):658–663.
4. Shapiro S, et al. Ten- to fourteen-year effect of screening on breast cancer mortality. *J Natl Cancer Inst.* 1982;69(2):349–355.
5. Broeders M, et al. The impact of mammographic screening on breast cancer mortality in Europe: a review of observational studies. *J Med Screen.* 2012;19(Suppl 1):14–25.
6. Coldman A, et al. Pan-Canadian study of mammography screening and mortality from breast cancer. *J Natl Cancer Inst.* 2014;106(11).
7. Monticciolo DL, et al. Breast Cancer Screening for Average-Risk Women: Recommendations From the ACR Commission on Breast Imaging. *J Am Coll Radiol.* 2017;14(9):1137–1143.
8. Oeffinger KC, et al. Breast cancer screening for women at average risk: 2015 guideline update from the American Cancer Society. *JAMA.* 2015;314(15):1599–1614.
9. Siu AL, Force USPST. Screening for breast cancer: U.S. preventive services task force recommendation statement. *Ann Intern Med.* 2016;164(4):279–296.
10. Monticciolo DL, et al. Breast cancer screening in women at higher-than-average risk: recommendations from the ACR. *J Am Coll Radiol.* 2018;15(3 Pt A):408–414.
11. Kuhl CK, et al. Mammography, breast ultrasound, and magnetic resonance imaging for surveillance of women at high familial risk for breast cancer. *J Clin Oncol.* 2005;23(33):8469–8476.
12. Houssami N, Hunter K. The epidemiology, radiology and biological characteristics of interval breast cancers in population mammography screening. *NPJ Breast Cancer.* 2017;3:12.
13. Gilliland FD, et al. Biologic characteristics of interval and screen-detected breast cancers. *J Natl Cancer Inst.* 2000;92(9):743–749.
14. Kolb TM, Lichy J, Newhouse JH. Comparison of the performance of screening mammography, physical examination, and breast US and evaluation of factors that influence them: an analysis of 27,825 patient evaluations. *Radiology.* 2002;225(1):165–175.
15. Sickles E, D'Orsi CJ. ACR BI-RADS® Follow-up and Outcome Monitoring. In: ACR BI-RADS® *Atlas, Breast Imaging Reporting and Data System.* Reston, VA: American College of Radiology; 2013.
16. Lehman CD, et al. National Performance Benchmarks for Modern Screening Digital Mammography: Update from the Breast Cancer Surveillance Consortium. *Radiology.* 2017;283(1):49–58.
17. Grabler P, et al. Recall and cancer detection rates for screening mammography: finding the sweet spot. *AJR Am J Roentgenol.* 2017;208(1):208–213.
18. Friedewald SM, et al. Breast cancer screening using tomosynthesis in combination with digital mammography. *JAMA.* 2014;311(24):2499–2507.
19. Lourenco AP, et al. Changes in recall type and patient treatment following implementation of screening digital breast tomosynthesis. *Radiology.* 2015;274(2):337–342.
20. Ciatto S, et al. Integration of 3D digital mammography with tomosynthesis for population breast-cancer screening (STORM): a prospective comparison study. *Lancet Oncol.* 2013;14(7):583–589.
21. Greenberg JS, et al. Clinical performance metrics of 3D digital breast tomosynthesis compared with 2D digital mammography for breast cancer screening in community practice. *AJR Am J Roentgenol.* 2014;203(3):687–693.
22. Berg WA, et al. Combined screening with ultrasound and mammography vs mammography alone in women at elevated risk of breast cancer. *JAMA.* 2008;299(18):2151–2163.
23. Weigert J, Steenbergen S. The connecticut experiment: the role of ultrasound in the screening of women with dense breasts. *Breast J.* 2012;18(6):517–522.
24. Weigert J, Steenbergen S. The connecticut experiments second year: ultrasound in the screening of women with dense breasts. *Breast J.* 2015;21(2):175–180.

25. Niell BL, et al. Auditing a breast MRI practice: performance measures for screening and diagnostic breast MRI. *J Am Coll Radiol.* 2014;11(9):883–889.

26. Lehman CD. Role of MRI in screening women at high risk for breast cancer. *J Magn Reson Imaging.* 2006;24(5):964–970.

27. Kuhl CK, et al. Supplemental breast MR imaging screening of women with average risk of breast cancer. *Radiology.* 2017;283(2):361–370.

28. Comstock CE, et al. Comparison of Abbreviated Breast MRI vs Digital Breast Tomosynthesis for Breast Cancer Detection Among Women With Dense Breasts Undergoing Screening. *JAMA.* 2020;323(8):746–756.

29. D'Orsi CJ, S.E., Mendelson EB, Morris EA, et al. *ACR BI-RADS® Atlas, Breast Imaging Reporting and Data System.* Reston, VA: American College of Radiology; 2013.

30. Baltzer P, et al. Diffusion-weighted imaging of the breast-a consensus and mission statement from the EUSOBI International Breast Diffusion-Weighted Imaging working group. *Eur Radiol.* 2020;30(3):1436–1450.

31. Sippo DA, et al. Performance of screening breast MRI across women with different elevated breast cancer risk indications. *Radiology.* 2019;292(1):51–59.

32. Sharpe RE, Jr. et al. Increased cancer detection rate and variations in the recall rate resulting from implementation of 3D digital breast tomosynthesis into a population-based screening program. *Radiology.* 2016;278(3):698–706.

33. McDonald ES, et al. Baseline screening mammography: performance of full-field digital mammography versus digital breast tomosynthesis. *AJR Am J Roentgenol.* 2015;205(5):1143–1148.

34. Haas BM, et al. Comparison of tomosynthesis plus digital mammography and digital mammography alone for breast cancer screening. *Radiology.* 2013;269(3):694–700.

35. Expert Panel on Breast I, et al. ACR Appropriateness Criteria((R)) Breast Cancer Screening. *J Am Coll Radiol.* 2017;14(11S):S383–S390.

36. Zuckerman SP, et al. Implementation of synthesized two-dimensional mammography in a population-based digital breast tomosynthesis screening program. *Radiology.* 2016;281(3):730–736.

37. Gilbert FJ, et al. Accuracy of Digital Breast Tomosynthesis for Depicting Breast Cancer Subgroups in a UK Retrospective Reading Study (TOMMY Trial). *Radiology.* 2015;277(3):697–706.

38. Zuley ML, et al. Comparison of two-dimensional synthesized mammograms versus original digital mammograms alone and in combination with tomosynthesis images. *Radiology.* 2014;271(3):664–671.

39. Skaane P, et al. Two-view digital breast tomosynthesis screening with synthetically reconstructed projection images: comparison with digital breast tomosynthesis with full-field digital mammographic images. *Radiology.* 2014;271(3):655–663.

40. Aujero MP, et al. Clinical performance of synthesized two-dimensional mammography combined with tomosynthesis in a large screening population. *Radiology.* 2017;283(1):70–76.

41. Weigert JM. The connecticut experiment; the third installment: 4 years of screening women with dense breasts with bilateral ultrasound. *Breast J.* 2017;23(1):34–39.

42. Tagliafico AS, et al. Adjunct screening with tomosynthesis or ultrasound in women with mammography-negative dense breasts: interim report of a prospective comparative trial. *J Clin Oncol.* 2016;34(16):1882–1888.

43. Kriege M, et al. Efficacy of MRI and mammography for breast-cancer screening in women with a familial or genetic predisposition. *N Engl J Med.* 2004;351(5):427–437.

44. Riedl CC, et al. Triple-modality screening trial for familial breast cancer underlines the importance of magnetic resonance imaging and questions the role of mammography and ultrasound regardless of patient mutation status, age, and breast density. *J Clin Oncol.* 2015;33(10):1128–1135.

45. Sardanelli F, et al. Multicenter surveillance of women at high genetic breast cancer risk using mammography, ultrasonography, and contrast-enhanced magnetic resonance imaging (the high breast cancer risk Italian 1 study): final results. *Invest Radiol.* 2011;46(2):94–105.

46. Kuhl C, et al. Prospective multicenter cohort study to refine management recommendations for women at elevated familial risk of breast cancer: the EVA trial. *J Clin Oncol.* 2010;28(9):1450–1457.

47. Lehman CD, et al. Screening women at high risk for breast cancer with mammography and magnetic resonance imaging. *Cancer.* 2005;103(9):1898–1905.

48. Morris EA, et al. MRI of occult breast carcinoma in a high-risk population. *AJR Am J Roentgenol.* 2003;181(3):619–626.

49. Berg WA, et al. Detection of breast cancer with addition of annual screening ultrasound or a single screening MRI to mammography in women with elevated breast cancer risk. *JAMA.* 2012;307(13):1394–1404.

50. Lehman CD, et al. MRI evaluation of the contralateral breast in women with recently diagnosed breast cancer. *N Engl J Med.* 2007;356(13):1295–1303.

51. Leach MO, et al. Screening with magnetic resonance imaging and mammography of a UK population at high familial risk of breast cancer: a prospective multicentre cohort study (MARIBS). *Lancet.* 2005;365(9473):1769–1778.

52. Hagen AI, et al. Sensitivity of MRI versus conventional screening in the diagnosis of BRCA-associated breast cancer in a national prospective series. *Breast.* 2007;16(4):367–374.

53. Warner E, et al. Surveillance of BRCA1 and BRCA2 mutation carriers with magnetic resonance imaging, ultrasound, mammography, and clinical breast examination. *JAMA.* 2004;292(11):1317–1325.

54. Kuhl CK, et al. Not all false positive diagnoses are equal: On the prognostic implications of false-positive diagnoses made in breast MRI versus in mammography / digital tomosynthesis screening. *Breast Cancer Res.* 2018;20(1):13.

55. Sung JS, et al. Breast cancers detected at screening MR imaging and mammography in patients at high risk: method of detection reflects tumor histopathologic results. *Radiology.* 2016;280(3):716–722.

56. Bakker MF, et al. Supplemental MRI screening for women with extremely dense breast tissue. *N Engl J Med.* 2019;381(22):2091–2102.

57. Giess CS, et al. Clinical utility of breast MRI in the diagnosis of malignancy after inconclusive or equivocal mammographic diagnostic evaluation. *AJR Am J Roentgenol.* 2017;208(6):1378–1385.

58. Niell BL, et al. Utility of breast MRI for further evaluation of equivocal findings on digital breast tomosynthesis. *AJR Am J Roentgenol.* 2018;211(5):1171–1178.

59. Debruhl ND, et al. MRI evaluation of the contralateral breast in women with recently diagnosed breast cancer: 2-year follow-up. *Journal of Breast Imaging.* 2019;2(1):50–55.

60. Baltzer PAT, et al. Is breast MRI a helpful additional diagnostic test in suspicious mammographic microcalcifications? *Magn Reson Imaging.* 2018;46:70–74.

61. Strobel K, et al. Assessment of BI-RADS category 4 lesions detected with screening mammography and screening US: utility of MR imaging. *Radiology.* 2015;274(2):343–351.

62. Bennani-Baiti B, et al. Evaluation of 3.0-T MRI brain signal after exposure to gadoterate meglumine in women with high breast cancer risk and screening breast MRI. *Radiology.* 2019;293(3):523–530.

63. Saslow D, et al. American Cancer Society guidelines for breast screening with MRI as an adjunct to mammography. *CA Cancer J Clin.* 2007;57(2):75–89.

64. Kuhl CK, et al. Abbreviated breast magnetic resonance imaging (MRI): first postcontrast subtracted images and maximum-intensity projection-a novel approach to breast cancer screening with MRI. *J Clin Oncol.* 2014;32(22):2304–2310.

65. Mango VL, et al. Abbreviated protocol for breast MRI: are multiple sequences needed for cancer detection? *Eur J Radiol.* 2015;84(1):65–70.

66. Panigrahi B, et al. An abbreviated protocol for high-risk screening breast magnetic resonance imaging: impact on performance metrics and BI-RADS assessment. *Acad Radiol.* 2017;24(9):1132–1138.

67. Strahle DA, et al. Systematic development of an abbreviated protocol for screening breast magnetic resonance imaging. *Breast Cancer Res Treat.* 2017;162(2):283–295.

68. Sun Y, et al. Clinical usefulness of breast-specific gamma imaging as an adjunct modality to mammography for diagnosis of breast cancer: a systemic review and meta-analysis. *Eur J Nucl Med Mol Imaging.* 2013;40(3):450–463.

69. Kim BS, Moon BI, Cha ES. A comparative study of breast-specific gamma imaging with the conventional imaging modality in breast cancer patients with dense breasts. *Ann Nucl Med.* 2012;26(10):823–829.

70. Rhodes DJ, et al. Journal club: molecular breast imaging at reduced radiation dose for supplemental screening in mammographically dense breasts. *AJR Am J Roentgenol.* 2015;204(2):241–251.

71. Shermis RB, et al. Supplemental breast cancer screening with molecular breast imaging for women with dense breast tissue. *AJR Am J Roentgenol.* 2016;207(2):450–457.

72. Brem RF, et al. Breast-specific gamma-imaging for the detection of mammographically occult breast cancer in women at increased risk. *J Nucl Med.* 2016;57(5):678–684.

73. Cheung YC, et al. Diagnostic performance of dual-energy contrast-enhanced subtracted mammography in dense breasts compared to mammography alone: interobserver blind-reading analysis. *Eur Radiol.* 2014;24(10):2394–2403.

74. Lobbes MB, et al. Contrast-enhanced spectral mammography in patients referred from the breast cancer screening programme. *Eur Radiol.* 2014;24(7):1668–1676.

75. Sung JS, et al. Performance of dual-energy contrast-enhanced digital mammography for screening women at increased risk of breast cancer. *Radiology.* 2019;293(1):81–88.

76. Jochelson MS, et al. Comparison of screening CEDM and MRI for women at increased risk for breast cancer: A pilot study. *Eur J Radiol.* 2017;97:37–43.

77. Jochelson MS, et al. Bilateral contrast-enhanced dual-energy digital mammography: feasibility and comparison with conventional digital mammography and MR imaging in women with known breast carcinoma. *Radiology.* 2013;266(3):743–751.

78. Luczynska E, et al. Comparison between breast MRI and contrast-enhanced spectral mammography. *Med Sci Monit.* 2015;21:1358–1367.

79. Chou CP, et al. Clinical evaluation of contrast-enhanced digital mammography and contrast enhanced tomosynthesis-Comparison to contrast-enhanced breast MRI. *Eur J Radiol.* 2015;84(12):2501–2508.

80. Zhu X, et al. Diagnostic value of contrast-enhanced spectral mammography for screening breast cancer: systematic review and meta-analysis. *Clin Breast Cancer.* 2018;18(5):e985–e995.

81. American College of Radiology. ACR manual on contrast media; Available at: https://www.acr.org/Clinical-Resources/Contrast-Manual.

82. Phillips J, et al. Comparative Dose of Contrast-Enhanced Spectral Mammography (CESM), Digital Mammography, and Digital Breast Tomosynthesis. *AJR Am J Roentgenol.* 2018;211(4):839–846.

Suggested Readings

Bakker MF, et al. Supplemental MRI Screening for Women with Extremely Dense Breast Tissue. *N Engl J Med.* 2019;381(22):2091–2102.

Berg WA, et al. Detection of breast cancer with addition of annual screening ultrasound or a single screening MRI to mammography in women with elevated breast cancer risk. *JAMA.* 2012;307(13):1394–1404.

Comstock CE, et al. Comparison of abbreviated breast MRI vs digital breast tomosynthesis for breast cancer detection among women with dense breasts undergoing screening. *JAMA.* 2020;323(8):746–756.

Friedewald SM, et al. Breast cancer screening using tomosynthesis in combination with digital mammography. *JAMA.* 2014;311(24):2499–2507.

Kuhl CK, et al. Supplemental breast MR imaging screening of women with average risk of breast cancer. *Radiology.* 2017;283(2):361–370.

Mann RM, Kuhl CK, Moy L. Contrast-enhanced MRI for breast cancer screening. *J Magn Reson Imaging.* 2019;50(2):377–390.

Monticciolo DL, et al. Breast Cancer Screening for Average-Risk Women: Recommendations From the ACR Commission on Breast Imaging. *J Am Coll Radiol.* 2017;14(9):1137–1143.

Monticciolo DL, et al. Breast cancer screening in women at higher-than-average risk: recommendations from the ACR. *J Am Coll Radiol.* 2018;15(3 Pt A):408–414.

Organized Approach to Screening Mammography

BONNIE N. JOE

OVERVIEW *This chapter will review the science behind screening mammography including a summary of different screening guidelines and discussion of controversies surrounding screening recommendations. The second part of this chapter will review how to systematically approach screening mammography interpretation.*

Why Perform Screening Mammography? (Screening Evidence)

HISTORICAL PERSPECTIVE

Before there was mammography or any breast imaging, breast cancers presented when they became clinically apparent, for example as a large palpable mass. Diagnosis was based on surgical excision, and many benign lesions were excised. With screening mammography, breast cancers are detected at an earlier stage before they are clinically apparent resulting in improved survival, less invasive therapy, and lower morbidity.

SCREENING MAMMOGRAPHY REDUCES BREAST CANCER MORTALITY

Screening mammography has been proven to reduce breast cancer mortality in multiple randomized controlled trials. These trials included women aged 40 to 69, with an overall mortality benefit of approximately 20% across all trials as shown in Fig. 12.1. Randomized controlled trial data is considered the strongest screening evidence to prove benefit of screening mammography but will necessarily underestimate the magnitude of benefit of screening mammography due to noncompliance and contamination. First, it is important to understand that the randomized controlled trials randomized invitation to screening, not the screening examination itself. In other words, half the study participants

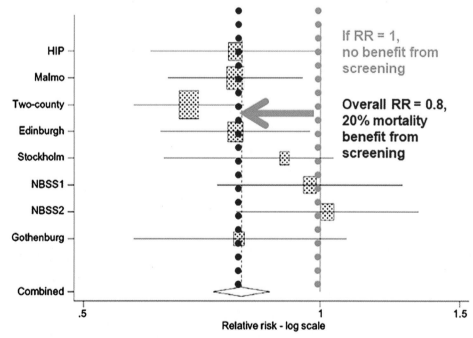

Fig. 12.1 Summary of eight randomized controlled trials in women aged 40–69. A relative-risk of 1 means there is no benefit from screening mammography. The combined results of these randomized controlled trials show a relative risk of 0.8 indicating an overall 20% mortality benefit of screening mammography. The NBSS (Canadian) screening trials were outliers as the only trials to not show a benefit from screening mammography, and many critics have called for these trials to be discounted citing problems with randomization (palpable lumps and disproportionate number of advanced cancers in the screening arm) and substandard mammography image quality (direct x-ray instead of screen-film mammography) for 4 of 5 years of the trial. *HIP*, Health Insurance Plan; *NBSS*, National Breast Screening Study; *RR*, relative risk. (Adapted from Smith RA, Duffy SW, Gabe R, Tabar L, Yen AM, Chen TH, The randomized trials of breast cancer screening: what have we learned? *Radiol Clin North Am* 42:793–806, 2004.)

were sent a letter inviting the woman to attend screening while the other half did not receive an invitation letter.

Noncompliance occurs when a woman ignores the invitation letter and does not get screened. If this woman unfortunately later dies of breast cancer, she is still counted in the screening arm.

Contamination occurs when a woman who did not receive an invitation letter seeks screening mammography on her own. If the woman's life is subsequently saved through early detection of a breast cancer, she is still counted in the control or no screening arm.

Thus while randomized controlled trials rigorously prove the life-saving benefit of screening mammography, they necessarily underestimate the magnitude of mortality benefit due to noncompliance and contamination (Box 12.1).

Service screening experience has demonstrated an approximately 40% breast cancer mortality reduction with screening mammography. As an example, the Canadian service screening experience is summarized in Fig. 12.2. Service screening experience provides a more accurate estimate of the magnitude of benefit of screening mammography because it reflects real-world experience, includes larger patient populations, and includes modern screening technology such as digital mammography (Box 12.2). Note that the randomized controlled trials did not include any digital mammography, only (now obsolete) analog mammography. Fig. 12.3 illustrates the evolution of mammography technology.

Box 12.1   Randomized Controlled Trials Underestimate Screening Benefit Due to Contamination and Noncompliance

- Trials randomized *invitation* to screen versus *no invitation* to screen (not the same as randomizing who gets mammography)
- Contamination: Person in "no invitation" group gets screened and life is saved by early detection of breast cancer.
- Noncompliance: Person in "invitation to screen" group does not get screened and dies of breast cancer.

Box 12.2   Service Screening Experience (Observational Studies)

- Reflect actual clinical practice and more current practice
- Include larger populations
- More accurately reflect the magnitude of benefit of screening mammography

---

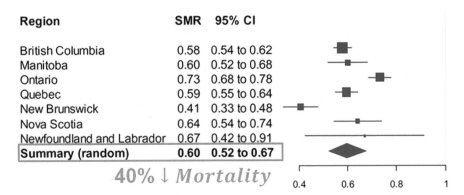

Region	SMR	95% CI
British Columbia	0.58	0.54 to 0.62
Manitoba	0.60	0.52 to 0.68
Ontario	0.73	0.68 to 0.78
Quebec	0.59	0.55 to 0.64
New Brunswick	0.41	0.33 to 0.48
Nova Scotia	0.64	0.54 to 0.74
Newfoundland and Labrador	0.67	0.42 to 0.91
Summary (random)	**0.60**	**0.52 to 0.67**

40% ↓ *Mortality*

Fig. 12.2 Summary of service screening experience in Canada showing overall 40% mortality reduction among women screened with mammography. Service screening reflects real-world experience using screening mammography, includes a larger number of patients, and includes current technology such as digital mammography. *CI*, confidence interval; *SMR*, standardized mortality ratio (Adapted from Coldman A, et al. Pan-Canadian study of mammography screening and mortality from breast cancer. *J Natl Cancer Inst* 106(11), 2014.)

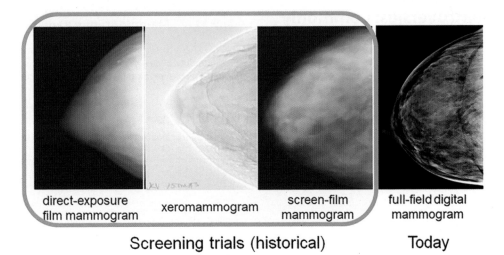

direct-exposure film mammogram   xeromammogram   screen-film mammogram   full-field digital mammogram

Screening trials (historical)   **Today**

Fig. 12.3 Craniocaudal views of extremely dense breasts illustrating the evolution of two-dimensional mammography technology. Note that the randomized controlled screening trials only included analog technology (*circled*). (Adapted from Joe BN, Sickles EA: The evolution of breast imaging: past to present. *Radiology* 273: S23–S44, 2014.)

Screening Guidelines

While organizations agree that screening mammography saves lives, they disagree on what ages to screen and frequency of screening. Hence, there are currently three major guidelines for screening average risk women. Please refer to Chapter 10: Breast Cancer Risk Assessment and Chapter 11: Breast Cancer Screening Guidelines and Supplemental Screening for discussion of screening for patients at higher than average risk and additional discussion of screening guidelines. The American College of Radiology (ACR) recommends annual screening starting at age 40 in order to save the most lives. These recommendations are supported by the National Comprehensive Cancer Network, the Society of Breast Imaging, and other organizations placing emphasis on early detection of breast cancer. The U.S. Preventive Services Task Force (USPSTF) guidelines recommend biennial screening starting at age 50 and ending at age 74, placing emphasis on reducing benign-outcome recalls and biopsies and with significantly lower mortality benefit (23% for biennial screening compared with nearly 40% mortality benefit for annual screening starting at age 40). The American Cancer Society guidelines are a hybrid of annual and biennial screening recommending annual screening between the ages of 45 and 54 and then biennial screening from 55 to 79. These guidelines result in a mortality benefit in between that of the ACR and the USPSTF.

Table 12.1 compares these different screening strategies in terms of number of mammograms, lives saved, and life years gained. This comparison of differing screening strategies comes from the Cancer Intervention and Surveillance Modeling Network (CISNET) models. The CISNET models used the original randomized controlled trial data to model outcomes for different screening strategies. CISNET models were considered by the USPSTF in the development of their 2009 and 2016 (current) screening recommendations.

All organizations agree the most lives are saved with annual screening starting at age 40. The American Cancer Society guidelines note that the majority of American women would choose to screen annually at age 40. The decision to screen and what guideline to follow is ultimately a woman's choice based on shared decision making. All guidelines allow women to screen annually starting at age 40.

Screening Controversies: Commonly Cited Screening "Harms" (Risks)

Much of the controversy surrounding when to start screening and at what interval is due to cited "harms" or risks of screening. Although the word *harm* is often used, this term is pejorative, meaning that it implies more substantial adverse outcomes than most women would think. A more appropriate term to use is *risk*, analogous to the terminology for adverse outcomes used during the informed consent process. For example, when consenting for a breast biopsy we discuss the risks versus benefits of a procedure with the patient, not the harms versus benefits.

The four most commonly cited risks ("harms") of mammography screening are radiation, benign-outcome recalls and biopsies, patient anxiety, and overdiagnosis. As will be discussed in the subsequent sections, none of these risks are substantial.

RADIATION

We are all exposed to natural background radiation. Our annual background dose is approximately 3 mSv per year at sea level. People living at higher elevations are exposed to slightly more background radiation. For a standard two-view screening mammogram, the radiation dose is equivalent to approximately 2 months of natural background radiation at sea level. Hence, radiation risk from mammography is classified in the "minimal" risk range, and it is generally accepted that the potential benefits of screening mammography far outweigh any potential risk of dying of breast cancer due to radiation exposure from mammography (Box 12.3).

BENIGN-OUTCOME RECALLS AND BIOPSIES (FALSE POSITIVES)

An abnormal screening mammogram (Breast Imaging Reporting and Data System [BI-RADS] 0: incomplete) that is ultimately resolved as negative (BI-RADS 1) or benign (BI-RADS 2) at diagnostic imaging is considered a false positive. A benign biopsy is another example of a false positive. In the United States, out of 100 women screened, approximately 10 women will be recalled from screening for additional diagnostic evaluation consisting of additional mammographic views and/or breast ultrasound. Often, the diagnostic evaluation provides reassurance to the patient,

---

Box 12.3	Mammography Radiation Risk

- Equivalent to ~2 months natural background radiation for bilateral two-view mammogram
- Benefits of screening far outweigh negligible radiation risks

---

Table 12.1 Comparison of Three Screening Strategies for Average-Risk Women

Screening Strategy	No. of Examinations[a]	Pecent Mortality Reduction	Breast Cancer Deaths Averted[a]	LYG[a]	NNS per Death Averted	NNS per LYG
A40–84	36,500	39.6%	11.9	189	84	5.3
H45–79	19,846	30.8%	9.25	149	108	6.7
B50–74	11,066	23.2%	6.95	110	144	9.1

Arleo EK, Hendrick RE, Helvie MA, Sickles EA. Comparison of recommendations for screening mammography using CISNET models. *Cancer* Oct 1;123(19):3673–3680, 2017.
The most lives are saved and the most life years are gained with annual screening from 40 to 84.
A40–84, American College of Radiology recommendation for annual screening from 40 to 84; *H45–79*, American Cancer Society hybrid strategy of annual screening from 45 to 54, then biennial screening from 55 to 79; *B50–74*, U.S. Preventive Services Task Force recommendation for biennial screening from 50 to 74. All organizations agree the most lives are saved with annual screening. All screening guidelines allow screening starting at age 40; *LYG*, life years gained; *NNS*, number needed to screen.
[a]Per 1000 women screened. Based on mean values of six 2009 CISNET models.

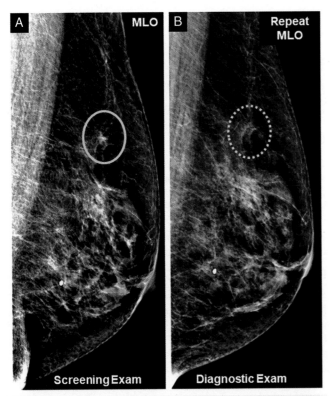

Fig. 12.4 Example of false positive at screening. Asymmetry seen on screening mammography examination, visible only on the mediolateral oblique (MLO) view (*circle*) and not on the craniocaudal view (not shown). Examination was interpreted as BI-RADS 0: Incomplete with a recommendation for additional imaging evaluation. Repeat MLO view at time of diagnostic examination resolves the asymmetry as superimposition of normal breast structures (*dotted circle*). Final assessment of BI-RADS 1: Negative with recommendation to return to annual screening.

for example in the case of an asymmetry resolved as superimposition (Fig. 12.4), and the patient's anxiety is relieved (see Chapter 1).

One to two patients out of the original 100 women screened may be recommended to undergo a breast biopsy. Breast biopsies are minimally invasive, well-tolerated outpatient procedures with few contraindications. See Chapter 7 for further discussion of breast interventions. Breast biopsy is recommended for BI-RADS 4 (suspicious) and BI-RADS 5 (highly suggestive of malignancy lesions).

The majority of breast biopsies are benign and considered false-positive biopsies. But it is important to recognize that about one-quarter to one-third of breast biopsies are true positives, meaning cancer is diagnosed.

PATIENT ANXIETY

Although false positives result in patient anxiety and inconvenience, 86% of women in the United States view recall from screening as an acceptable tradeoff to detect cancer early (Ganott et al. 2006.) Importantly, patient anxiety is temporary and generally relieved once diagnostic workup and/or biopsy results prove benign. If a cancer is diagnosed, then the patient can be directed toward appropriate management and treatment. Box 12.4 summarizes key points regarding false positives.

Box 12.4 Mammography False Positives

- 1-in-10 chance of benign-outcome recall from screening.
- 1–2 per 100 recommended for biopsy.
- One-quarter to one-third of biopsies result in cancer diagnosis.
- 86% of women view recall as an acceptable trade-off for earlier breast cancer diagnosis (Ganott et al. 2006).
- Anxiety from false positive is usually eliminated as soon as further evaluation shows no cancer.

Box 12.5 Overdiagnosis

- Overdiagnosis means finding a cancer that will not kill the patient.
- Magnitude is estimated, not measured.
- Estimates vary widely: >20% due to lack of adjustment or ≤10% with adjustment for confounding factors.
- No impact of age at first screening on overdiagnosis: Overdiagnosed cancer is still found whether screening starts at age 40 or age 50.
- No impact of screening interval on overdiagnosis: The overdiagnosed cancer will be found on the annual screen or on the screening examination performed 2 years later.

OVERDIAGNOSIS

Overdiagnosis refers to diagnosing a breast cancer that will not kill the patient. In other words, the patient dies with the disease, not from the disease. Overdiagnosis cannot be measured, it can only be estimated, and reported estimates vary widely depending on whether adjustments are made for confounding factors. Estimates of overdiagnosis that account for confounding factors range from 5% to 10% and likely involve lower grades of ductal carcinoma in situ (DCIS).

Note that the amount of overdiagnosis is not impacted by starting age for screening or screening interval. By definition, an overdiagnosed cancer does not kill the patient. If an overdiagnosed cancer is found in a person starting screening at age 40, the same overdiagnosed cancer will be found 10 years later should this person instead defer screening until age 50. Basically, the overdiagnosed cancer will be found at time of the first screening examination. Similarly, screening interval has no impact on the amount of overdiagnosis. If an overdiagnosed cancer is found on an annual screening examination, that same overdiagnosed cancer would be found a year later at the biennial examination should the person skip a year or choose every-other-year screening. The only way to avoid overdiagnosis is to not screen at all, and all organizations agree that screening is beneficial to reduce mortality from breast cancer.

Thus overdiagnosis should not be a factor in choosing among different screening guidelines (Box 12.5).

ADDITIONAL BENEFITS OF SCREENING MAMMOGRAPHY

Given the emphasis placed by the USPSTF on risks ("harms"), it is curious that the USPSTF does not acknowledge several benefits of mammography screening other than reduced breast cancer mortality. First, the USPSTF considers the benefit of reduced breast cancer mortality as only avoiding the misery of a prolonged breast cancer death without factoring in the added benefit of extended years of life. The USPSTF also ignores the benefits of less morbidity from cancer treatment (less extensive surgery, less frequent and less intensive chemotherapy) and the ability to diagnose high-risk breast lesions (e.g., lobular carcinoma in situ and atypical hyperplasia thereby facilitating chemoprevention treatment), all of which are acknowledged benefits of screening mammography. Finally, the USPSTF, in recommending less intensive screening guidelines, does not factor in the risk of denying people the several benefits that more intensive screening would provide.

RISK-BASED SCREENING

The USPSTF guidelines recommend women start screening in their 40s based on their future risk of developing breast cancer. The problem with this approach is the lack of a reliable means of determining which women are at such low risk as to safely defer screening until age 50. About 75% to 80% of breast cancers are diagnosed in women without known risk factors other than being of female gender. Of women diagnosed with breast cancer between the ages of 40 and 49, 80% of women had no family history (Neal et al. 2018) and 75% of women had neither very strong family history nor extremely dense breasts (Price et al. 2015) (Box 12.6).

For persons at higher than average risk, earlier screening mammography and supplemental screening with magnetic resonance imaging (MRI) are recommended. See Chapters 10 and 11 for information on risk assessment and screening recommendations for patients at higher than average risk. Also see Chapter 5 for additional information on screening breast ultrasound and Chapter 8 for additional information on screening breast MRI.

BREAST CANCER INCIDENCE BY RACE

Screening strategies that delay the age at which screening starts may disadvantage minority populations. Analysis of U.S. cancer registry data show differences in age distributions of breast cancer by race. For African American, Asian, and Hispanic populations, breast cancer incidence peaks in the mid-40s. For Caucasian population peak incidence is later, in the 60s. (Stapleton, Oseni et al. 2018). Following USPSTF guidelines to begin screening at age 50 would

---

miss the peak incidence of breast cancer for these minority groups, potentially contributing to health disparities.

How to Interpret Screening Mammography by Following a Systematic Approach

GENERAL APPROACH

This section will provide a general approach to reviewing screening mammography examinations. It will not go over details of specific mammographic findings, BI-RADS assessment, or management, which have been covered in earlier chapters. The focus of this section is to present a structured approach to enhance a radiologist's search for abnormalities and to avoid interpretive pitfalls.

Perform "Overview" and "Close-In" Visual Searches

Screening mammography is performed in asymptomatic patients. Fortunately, the majority of screening mammograms are normal and straightforward to pass as negative (BI-RADS 1) or benign (BI-RADS 2). When reviewing a screening mammography examination, it is important to use both overview (whole examination with priors, whole image) and close-in (pixel-to-pixel or "full resolution") visual searches to look for abnormalities. Create a set display protocol or "hanging protocol" on the review workstation such that all screening examinations will be presented in a consistent format. The goal is to facilitate the search for abnormalities and minimize wasted time and attention on manual image manipulation. One example of an overview display with prior examinations is shown in Fig. 12.5. Overview displays are useful to look for obvious masses and asymmetries. Comparison with priors facilitates detection of interval change (recall) as well as long-term stability (no recall). Close-in ("full-resolution") review is required to detect subtle findings such as microcalcifications or subtle architectural distortion. For historical perspective, in the days of analog film mammography, this close-in review was performed with a magnifying glass.

Look for a Second Lesion

If you see an obvious lesion, it is a good practice to actively look for a second lesion. This strategy is used to avoid the common interpretative pitfall "satisfaction of search," often nicknamed "SOS" to highlight its importance. The first lesion you see may often be an obvious benign finding, and the second lesion is the cancer. Fig. 12.6 illustrates these pitfalls of satisfaction of search and not performing close-in or full-resolution (1:1 resolution) image search.

Annotate and Describe Location of Findings to Help the Next Radiologist

Annotate findings on the screening image(s) and provide quadrant location of findings in the screening report to ensure the correct lesions are evaluated at time of diagnostic imaging and that all sites of concern are evaluated. This is particularly important as screening findings may be subtle and the diagnostic examination is often performed at a separate appointment by a different radiologist.

Box 12.6	**Problems With Risk-Based Screening in 40–49 Age Group**

Limiting screening based on family history or breast density would miss the great majority of breast cancers of patients diagnosed with breast cancer between ages 40 and 49.

- 80% of cancer patients had no family history.[a]
- ~75% of cancer patients had neither very strong Fam Hx nor extremely dense breasts.[b]

[a] Neal et al. 2018.
[b] Price et al. 2015.

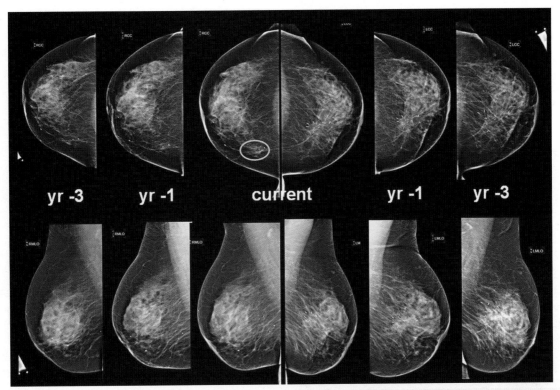

Fig. 12.5 Overview display of screening mammography examination with two prior comparisons (yr–1 is 1 year prior and yr–3 is 3 years prior to current study). The arrangement of images allows for ease of comparisons of like views and enhances detection of interval change. There is a developing asymmetry in the inner right breast seen on craniocaudal view (*circle*) for which patient was recalled (BI-RADS 0 incomplete for right breast). Left breast surgical scar and clips from prior breast conservation surgery for breast cancer appears stable (BI-RADS 2 benign for left breast). After subsequent diagnostic workup and breast biopsy, patient was diagnosed with invasive ductal carcinoma of the right breast.

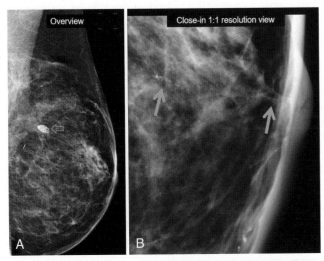

Fig. 12.6 (A) Overview of left mediolateral oblique image from screening examination in a patient with remote history of left breast cancer shows postsurgical changes of architectural distortion, surgical clip, and fat necrosis calcifications (*open arrow*). (B) On close-in 1:1 resolution view, subtle linear calcifications (*arrows*) are seen extending toward the nipple. These calcifications would have been missed if only reviewing the overview image or if search pattern stopped after noting the obvious postsurgical changes on the overview screen (satisfaction of search [SOS] error). Subsequent pathology showed intermediate- to high-grade ductal carcinoma in situ and invasive ductal cancer.

Box 12.7 General Approach to Screening Mammography Interpretation

- Use a consistent display protocol ("hanging protocol") for screening examinations.
- Use both overview and close-in visual searches (look twice).
  - First look is an overall search for obvious findings.
  - Second look is at full resolution (1:1 resolution) for subtle findings.
- If you see an obvious lesion, actively search for a second lesion to combat satisfaction of search (SOS).
- Annotate and describe location of your findings (ensures correct lesion is evaluated at time of diagnostic imaging).

Box 12.7 summarizes the general approach to screening mammography interpretation.

PERCEPTION AIDS FOR SCREENING MAMMOGRAPHY INTERPRETATION

The goal of screening mammography interpretation is to identify (perceive) an abnormality. Characterization of the abnormality occurs at the time of diagnostic imaging (see Chapter 13). Several strategies can be employed to improve your ability to perceive abnormalities at screening mammography (Box 12.8).

Box 12.8   Perception Aids for Screening Mammography Interpretation

- View right and left images "back-to-back" like mirror images.
- Concentrate on whitest areas of images.
- Search for one calcification or tiny artifact.
- Compare with two prior examinations.
- Interpret in batches without distractions.

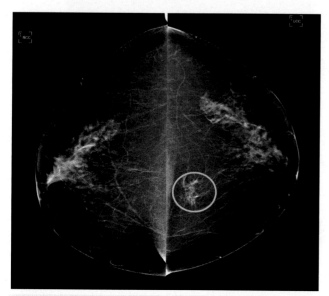

Fig. 12.7 Example of back-to-back display of right and left craniocaudal (CC) views from a screening mammogram. This display is designed to aid perception of right-left differences as our brains naturally look for symmetry. An asymmetry is readily identified in the inner left breast on CC view, posterior third depth (*circle*). This finding subsequently proved to be an invasive ductal carcinoma.

View Right and Left Images "Back-to-Back" as if They Were Mirror Images

Our eyes and brains naturally look for symmetry. Viewing right and left breast images "back-to-back" like mirror images allows easy right-left comparison and will highlight asymmetries and masses. Fig. 12.7 shows an example of an asymmetry seen in the inner breast on left craniocaudal (CC) view, which subsequently proved to be an invasive ductal carcinoma.

Concentrate on the Whitest Areas of the Image

Cancers tend to be less compressible than surrounding normal breast tissue and thus will appear whiter or denser on a mammogram. Concentrating on the whitest areas of the image will enhance detection of potential cancer. Fig. 12.8 illustrates a case of invasive lobular carcinoma presenting as a one-view asymmetry at screening and detectable by searching for the whitest area of the image.

Search for One Calcification or Tiny Artifact

At the end of each normal examination, make sure you have found at least one calcification or tiny white dot. If unsure, review the examination again. This strategy is a way to check yourself and ensure you are still concentrating during a batch screening readout, for instance if it is later in the day or if you are interpreting a large volume of

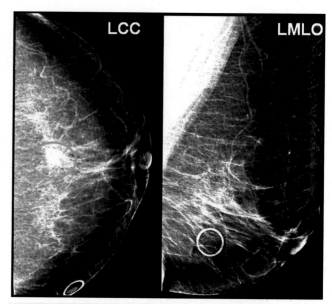

Fig. 12.8 Concentrate on whitest areas of image to improve perception of abnormalities. The whitest area of the left craniocaudal (CC) view from screening mammogram is an asymmetry (*circle*) that was not seen on the mediolateral oblique (MLO) view but which ultimately proved to be an invasive lobular carcinoma in this 62-year-old patient. Skin lesion marked by open circle markers on CC and MLO views.

examinations. Finding a small calcification or tiny artifact ensures you are concentrating on fine details and able to perceive subtle mammographic findings.

Compare With Two Prior Examinations

Comparison with more than one prior examination reduces recall rate and improves detection of subtle changes over time. Fig. 12.5 illustrates detection of a subtle developing asymmetry at screening, which proved to be an invasive ductal cancer after diagnostic evaluation and biopsy.

Interpret in Batches Without Distractions

Avoiding distractions makes common sense as this allows better concentration on the images, which improves detection of lesions. Batch interpretation is also more time efficient. Hence, the majority of screening examinations are interpreted "off-line" in batch mode and patients receive their results after they have left the mammography facility. Per the Mammography Quality Standards Act (MQSA), all patients are required by law to receive a lay letter with their mammogram results within 30 days of their examination. See the dedicated chapter on MQSA (Chapter 20) for further details regarding mammography regulations. Many practices interpret screening examinations within 24 hours, and some facilities offer same-day immediate interpretation of screening examinations. Benefits of immediate interpretation include reduced patient anxiety and shortened wait times for diagnostic evaluation.

Box 12.8 summarizes strategies for improving detection/ perception of lesions at screening mammography.

KEY POINTS

- Annual screening saves the most lives. The American College of Radiology recommends annual screening mammography starting at age 40 for average-risk women.

- Anxiety due to recall from screening mammography is temporary and resolves as soon as additional workup proves benign. Women usually titrate the timing of additional workup to their level of anxiety (those who are more anxious seek and obtain additional workup sooner than women who are less anxious).
- Radiation risk from screening mammography is minimal. Estimated radiation dose for a bilateral two-view mammogram is equivalent to 2 months of natural background radiation at sea level.
- Overdiagnosis should not be a factor in deciding when to start screening and how frequently to screen. Age to start screening and choice of screening interval have no impact on overdiagnosis.
- Limiting screening based on family history or breast density would miss the majority of mammographically detectable breast cancers in women aged 40 to 49.
- The goal of screening mammography is lesion detection. Lesion characterization occurs during diagnostic mammography.
- Look at images twice: first look is an overview search for masses and asymmetries and second look is a full (1:1) resolution search for microcalcifications and subtle distortion.
- Search for a second lesion after detection of an obvious lesion to avoid pitfall of satisfaction of search (SOS).
- Strategies to improve perception include concentrating on the whitest areas of the image, comparison with multiple prior examinations, and batch interpretation without distractions.

Suggested Readings

Arleo EK, Hendrick RE, Helvie MA, Sickles EA. Comparison of recommendations for screening mammography using CISNET models. *Cancer.* 2017;123(19):3673–3680.

Coldman A, Phillips N, Wilson C, et al. Pan-Canadian Study of Mammography Screening and Mortality from Breast Cancer. *JNCI: J Natl Cancer Inst.* 2014;106(11). dju261.

Ganott MA, Sumkin JH, King JL, et al. Screening mammography: do women prefer a higher recall rate given the possibility of earlier detection of cancer? *Radiology.* 2006;238(3):793–800.

Joe BN, Sickles EA. The evolution of breast imaging: past to present. *Radiology.* 2014;273(2 Suppl):S23–S44.

Mandelblatt JS, Cronin KA, Bailey S, et al. Effects of mammography screening under different screening schedules: model estimates of potential benefits and harms. *Ann Intern Med.* 2009;151:738–747.

Oeffinger KC, Fontham ET, Etzioni R, et al. Breast cancer screening for women at average risk: 2015 guideline update from the American Cancer Society. *JAMA.* 2015;314:1599–1614.

Price ER, Joe BN, Sickles EA. The developing asymmetry: revisiting a perceptual and diagnostic challenge. *Radiology.* 2015;274(3):642–651.

Siu AL. U.S. Preventive Services Task Force. Screening for breast cancer: U.S. Preventive Services Task Force recommendation statement. *Ann Intern Med.* 2016;164:279–296.

Smith RA, Duffy SW, Gabe R, Tabar L, Yen AM, Chen TH. The randomized trials of breast cancer screening: what have we learned? *Radiol Clin North Am.* 2004;42(5):793–806.

Tabar L, Yen MF, Vitak B, Chen HH, Smith RA, Duffy SW. Mammography service screening and mortality in breast cancer patients: 20-year follow-up before and after introduction of screening. *Lancet.* 2003;361:1405–1410.

13 Organized Approach to Diagnostic Imaging

KIMBERLY M. RAY

OVERVIEW | *This chapter outlines a systematic approach to the diagnostic evaluation of noncalcified findings identified at screening mammography, including masses and asymmetries. Modalities discussed include mammography, tomosynthesis, and ultrasound.*

For asymptomatic patients, the purpose of the diagnostic workup is to further evaluate potential abnormalities identified at screening mammography. Specific objectives include the following: confirmation that a finding is real, lesion localization, and lesion characterization.

Triangulation

DESCRIBING THE LOCATION OF FINDINGS IN THE BREAST

In order to describe the location of a finding in the breast, the convention of the clockface is used. The o'clock position of a finding is based on its position when an observer is facing the patient. For example, a finding in the lateral aspect of the right breast would be at the 9 o'clock position, whereas a lateral lesion in the left breast would be at the 3 o'clock position. In addition to the clockface, it is also important to specify the distance of a finding from the nipple in centimeters. These conventions are also observed when describing clinical breast examination findings such as palpable lumps. These rules facilitate clear and precise communication between radiologists and clinicians.

TRIANGULATION WITH TWO-DIMENSIONAL MAMMOGRAPHY

Once a finding has been determined to represent a true space-occupying lesion, it needs to be precisely localized in order to facilitate targeted ultrasound as well as biopsy. For findings that are visible on the standard craniocaudal (CC) and mediolateral oblique (MLO) screening views, it is helpful to be able to predict the location on a true lateral projection. As a general rule, lateral lesions will fall and medial lesions will rise as one goes from the MLO to true lateral projection. However, there are exceptions to this rule. A more reliable approach has been described by Sickles, as illustrated in Fig. 13.1. By lining up the CC and MLO projections, one can predict the location on the mediolateral (ML) view.

LESION LOCALIZATION WITH TOMOSYNTHESIS

A major advantage of tomosynthesis is that a lesion seen on a single projection can be localized based on its position

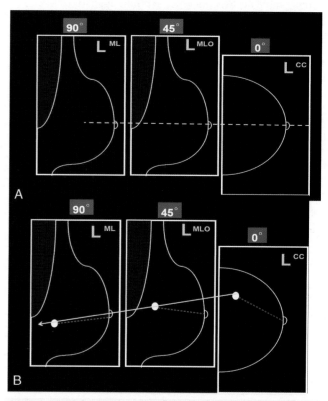

Fig. 13.1 Prediction of lesion location on the lateral projection using standard craniocaudal (CC) and mediolateral oblique (MLO) views. (A) Line up views progressing in obliquity from 0 degrees CC to 45 degrees MLO to 90 degrees. Mediolateral (ML) views with the nipples pointing in the same direction and positioned at the same level. Images should be equidistant from each other. (B) Draw a line connecting the lesion on the CC and MLO views, extending the line to the ML view. The lesion will be located along this line on the ML view, at the same distance from the nipple as on the other views (*blue dotted line*).

within the image stack, thus simplifying the diagnostic workup. The total number of images in the stack can be roughly divided between the halves of the breast. By convention, slice 1 is located on the detector side. Thus for the CC projection, slice 1 would be located at the bottom of the breast. For example, if there are 50 slices in a CC image stack, then a lesion located within slices 1 to 24 should be within the lower half of the breast. Slice 25 would be the central slice and a lesion within slices 26 to 50 should be within the upper half of the breast. In reality, lesion localization is not so precise since the nipple is not always at the center of the stack and there may be more slices on one side of the nipple or the other. Nevertheless, approximate lesion location can be inferred from its position within the stack.

Additional information regarding digital breast tomosynthesis is covered in Chapter 6: Basics of Digital Breast Tomosynthesis.

Supplemental Mammographic Views

The standard views obtained at screening mammography consist of CC and MLO views. Additional views that may be obtained in the diagnostic setting are:

- **True lateral projection:** The true lateral projection is obtained with the x-ray beam at a 90-degree angle to the vertical axis. In contrast to the MLO view, which is obtained at a 45-degree angle, the true lateral view is orthogonal to the CC view. As such, the lateral projection allows us to more precisely localize findings in the vertical axis.
- The lateral projection may be obtained either as a **mediolateral (ML) view**, in which the lateral aspect of the breast is placed against the detector, or **lateromedial (LM) view**, in which the medial aspect of the breast is placed against the detector. To minimize geometric unsharpness, the ML projection should be obtained for findings in the lateral half of the breast, whereas the LM view is preferable for findings in the medial breast.
- **Exaggerated craniocaudal lateral (XCCL) or exaggerated craniocaudal medial (XCCM) projections:** The XCCL and XCCM views are obtained to visualize findings in the far lateral or far medial aspect of the breast, respectively, areas that may be excluded on the CC view. These views are obtained by turning the patient laterally or medially in the CC projection so that either the lateral or medial half of the breast is positioned over the detector.
- **Cleavage view (CV):** This is an alternative to the XCCM view that may be helpful for visualizing far medial findings. In the CV view, the opposite breast is also placed on the detector and partially included in the field of view in the CC projection.
- **Axillary tail (AT) view:** In this view the axillary tail of the breast is imaged in isolation without inclusion of the remainder of the breast. The superolateral aspect of the breast is placed against the detector and the x-ray beam angle is intermediate between the MLO and ML views (approximately 60–80 degrees).
- **Tangential (TAN) view:** For lesions that are superficial, a view taken with the x-ray beam in tangent to the skin over the area of interest will project the lesion against the subcutaneous fat, improving visualization. Tangential views will also demonstrate whether a lesion is arising within the skin itself.
- **Caudocranial view or from below CC (FBCC) view:** The detector is placed against the top of the breast and compression is applied from below. In a conventional CC

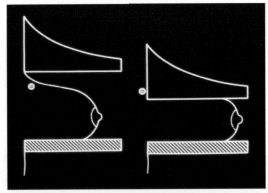

Fig. 13.2 When the compression paddle is lowered on a conventional craniocaudal (CC) view, a deep lesion in the upper breast near the chest wall may be excluded from view. Obtaining a caudocranial or from below CC view prevents this occurrence by pinning the upper breast against the detector while applying the compression paddle to the more mobile lower portion of the breast.

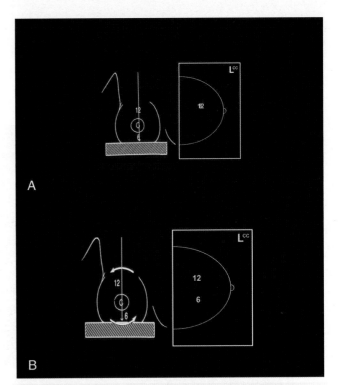

Fig. 13.3 (A) Tissue structures at the 12 o'clock and 6 o'clock positions are superimposed on the craniocaudal (CC) projection. (B) A rolled CC view separates the overlapping structures and resolves the summation artifact.

view, the relatively immobile tissue of the upper breast near the chest wall may slip out from underneath the compression paddle as it is lowered; thus a deep lesion in the upper breast may be excluded from view (Fig. 13.2). The FBCC view prevents this occurrence by pinning the upper breast against the detector while applying the compression paddle to the more mobile lower portion of the breast. The FBCC view is thus helpful for imaging lesions high up along the chest wall.

- **Rolled views (RL, RM, RI, RS):** These views are obtained by rolling the halves of the breast in opposite directions (Fig. 13.3). For example, in the CC projection, the top of the breast may be rolled laterally and the bottom rolled medially (CCRL view) or vice versa (CCRM). In the lateral projection, the lateral half of the breast can be rolled either superiorly (MLRS or LMRS) or inferiorly (MLRI or LMRI). Rolled views can help separate overlapping tissue structures and resolve summation artifacts. Rolled views can also help localize a true lesion. For instance, if a lesion seen on the CC projection moves

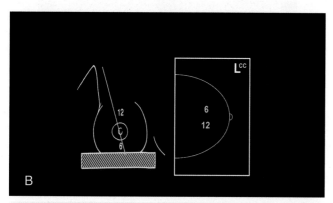

Fig. 13.4 A shallow oblique view resolves structures that overlap on the craniocaudal (CC) projection at the 12 o'clock and 6 o'clock positions.

laterally when the top of the breast is rolled laterally, then the lesion must be in the upper portion of the breast; if it moves medially, then it is inferior; and if it does not move, then it is central.

- **Shallow oblique views:** The obliquity of the x-ray beam is varied slightly (5–10 degrees) from the standard view in order to resolve overlapping tissue (Fig. 13.4).
- **Step oblique views:** These views are helpful for evaluating persistent one view asymmetries. Step obliques may help determine whether the asymmetry is real as well as to localize it on the orthogonal view. Images are obtained at 15-degree increments, beginning from the view in which the finding was originally seen and proceeding toward the view in which the finding was not seen (Fig. 13.5). Smaller (e.g., 10-degree) or larger (30-degree) increments may be used for problem solving.
- **Spot compression view:** A smaller compression paddle is used to compress only a portion of the breast so that greater pressure can be applied to that area than with whole breast compression. Spot compression spreads out overlapping tissue structures and brings lesions of interest closer to the detector, reducing geometric unsharpness.

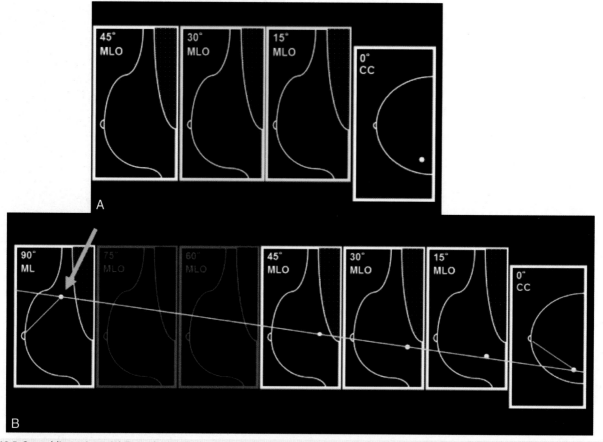

Fig. 13.5 Step oblique views. (A) To evaluate a lesion seen on the 0-degree craniocaudal (CC) view, but not on the 45-degree mediolateral oblique (MLO) view, first obtain two MLO views at 15 and 30 degrees of obliquity (shown in yellow). (B) Draw a line connecting the lesion on the 0-degree CC, 15-degree MLO, and 30-degree MLO views, extending the line to the 45-degree MLO view. The lesion will be located along this line on the 45-degree MLO view. (C) Once the lesion is identified on the 45-degree MLO view, its position (green arrow) on the 90-degree mediolateral (ML) view can be predicted by lining up the CC, MLO, and ML views as shown in Fig. 13.1. If necessary, additional intermediate steps at 60 and 75 degrees of obliquity (shown in gray) can be obtained to assist in localization.

- **Magnification:** Magnification is achieved by using a small focal spot and elevating the breast off the detector with a magnification stand, thus bringing the lesion of interest closer to the focal spot. Because of divergence of the x-ray beam, the lesion is projected over a greater number of pixels, resulting in a higher spatial resolution image and improved signal-to-noise ratio. Magnification can be performed with or without spot compression. Note that magnification can only be performed with two-dimensional (2D) mammography as it is not compatible with currently available tomosynthesis systems.

Diagnostic Workup of Masses

The workup of a mass identified at 2D screening mammography (Fig. 13.6) includes a true lateral view to more precisely localize the mass. In addition, spot compression views with or without magnification in CC and true lateral projections are obtained to further evaluate its shape and margin characteristics (Fig. 13.7). If there are associated microcalcifications, spot magnification views are necessary to evaluate their morphology and extent.

An exception to the above rule would be the identification of an oval mass that appears relatively well circumscribed at screening mammography. In this instance it would be appropriate to start with ultrasound as such a finding may represent a cyst. The finding of a simple cyst would obviate the need for additional mammographic views. However, if a solid mass is identified at ultrasound, then spot compression views may be obtained for further characterization.

If screening was performed with tomosynthesis, then it may also be appropriate to proceed directly to ultrasound in most cases, as shape and margin characteristics are often depicted more clearly at tomosynthesis than with conventional 2D spot compression views. However, 2D spot

Figure 12-6. Diagnostic Algorithm for Masses at mammography

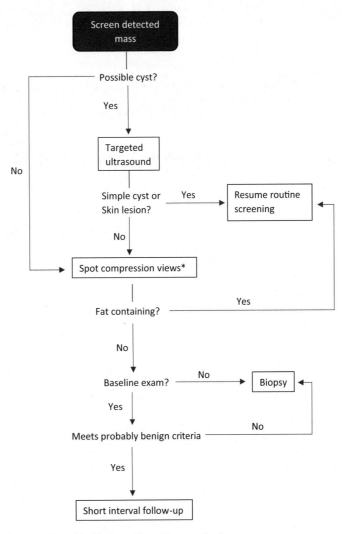

*Spot compression views may be omitted in the setting of tomosynthesis.

Fig. 13.6 Diagnostic algorithm for workup of masses at mammography.

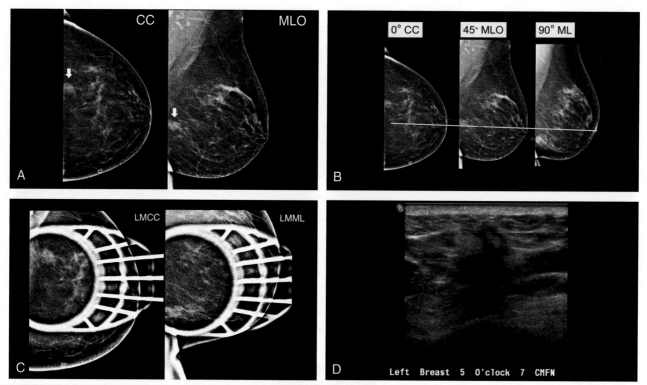

Fig. 13.7 (A) Mass identified at screening mammography on craniocaudal (CC) and mediolateral oblique (MLO) views of left breast. (B) At the time of diagnostic workup, a true lateral view was obtained. The CC, MLO, and true lateral views are lined up in sequence with the nipples at the same level (*yellow line*). A line (*red dotted line*) is drawn through the mass on CC and MLO views to predict its location on the true lateral view (red circle). The mass triangulates to the lower outer quadrant. (C) Spot compression magnification views obtained in the CC and true lateral projections demonstrate an irregular mass with indistinct margins. (D) Targeted ultrasound of the left breast demonstrates a corresponding irregular hypoechoic mass with angular margins and posterior shadowing in the lower outer quadrant at the 5 o'clock position, 7 cm from the nipple. Mammographic and sonographic features are suspicious for malignancy.

magnification views should be obtained if associated microcalcifications are present.

Besides the finding of a simple cyst on ultrasound, there are a limited number of other imaging features of masses that are considered typically benign. A lesion that is arising within the dermis such as a sebaceous cyst is considered benign, as primary breast cancer does not arise within the skin. Fat containing masses, including lipomas, oil cysts/fat necrosis, hamartomas, lymph nodes, and galactoceles are considered benign. Note, however, that small amounts of intralesional fat may be demonstrated at tomosynthesis within malignant masses. Therefore masses with suspicious shape and margin features at tomosynthesis should undergo biopsy despite the presence of intralesional fat.

The management of a mass should always be based on the most suspicious features present, whether at diagnostic mammography, tomosynthesis, or ultrasound. The presence of some benign features should not dissuade one from biopsy of a mass with any suspicious features.

A mass may be considered probably benign and given a BI-RADS 3 assessment if it is oval in shape with circumscribed margins (>75% circumscribed) and lacks suspicious features at ultrasound. It is important to recognize that these criteria only apply to masses identified on a baseline examination after a full diagnostic evaluation. If a mass with probably benign features is either new or enlarging,

then it should be considered inherently suspicious and biopsied.

Workup of Asymmetries

The diagnostic algorithm for breast asymmetries varies depending on the specific category of asymmetry. Approximately 80% of one view asymmetries will represent summation artifacts rather than true lesions. The remaining varieties of asymmetries typically represent true space-occupying lesions with varying likelihood of malignancy.

ASYMMETRY (ONE-VIEW) WORKUP

Because an asymmetry is likely to represent summation artifact, it is critical to establish whether or not it is real before attempting to localize it in another projection or proceeding to ultrasound (Fig. 13.8). The initial workup of an asymmetry should focus on varying the view on which it was originally seen. The simplest approach is to repeat that view since many asymmetries will resolve with a simple repeat (Fig. 13.9). A spot compression view of the asymmetry in the projection in which it was seen may also help resolve overlapping tissue structures. If the finding resolves after these views are obtained, then a negative assessment is appropriate and the patient may return to routine

Figure 12-8. Diagnostic Algorithm for Workup of One-View Asymmetry

§May omit spot compression views if tomosynthesis is performed.

*Choose the projection on which asymmetry was seen.

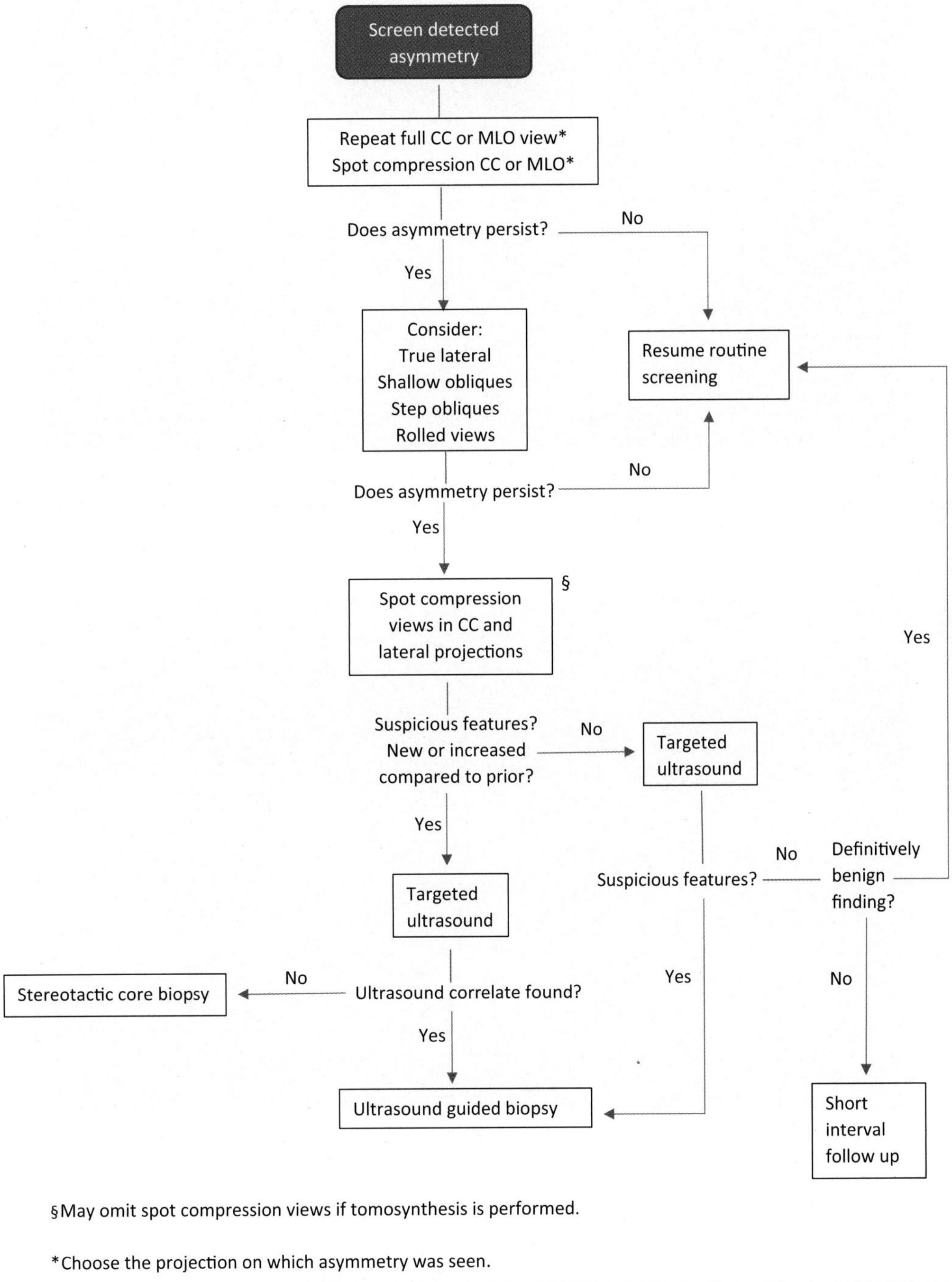

Fig. 13.8 Diagnostic algorithm for workup of one-view asymmetry.

screening. If the asymmetry persists on the views described above, then one may obtain a true lateral view as well as spot compression view in the lateral projection to fully characterize and localize the finding prior to proceeding to ultrasound.

Shallow Obliques

If the finding partially dissipates but fails to completely resolve on the above views, one may try to slightly alter the obliquity of the x-ray beam to resolve tissue overlap. Shallow oblique views may be obtained at ± 5 to 10 degrees from the projection on which the asymmetry was seen. Shallow oblique views are preferable to more extreme changes in the projection angle since the asymmetry could be obscured by overlapping tissue if the angle is altered too much. In that case, one might falsely assume that the asymmetry resolved, whereas it was merely obscured by overlapping tissue.

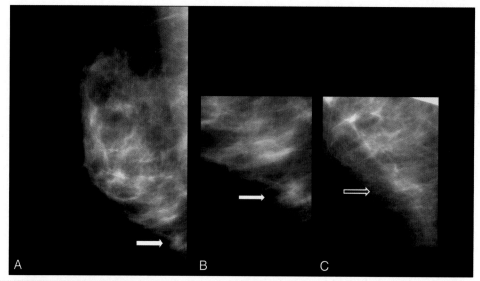

Fig. 13.9 (A) An asymmetry (*solid white arrow*) is identified in the inferior aspect of the right breast on the screening mediolateral oblique (MLO) view only, shown enlarged in (B). The asymmetry resolves on the repeat MLO view of the right breast (C) obtained at the time of recall. Area of the previously noted asymmetry (*open white arrow*) has been enlarged.

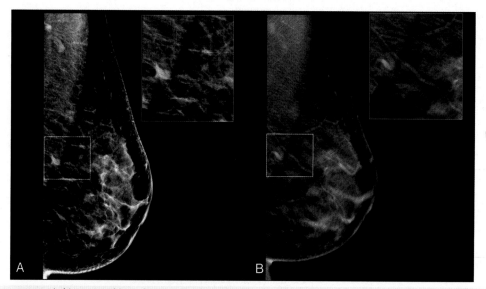

Fig. 13.10 (A) An asymmetry (*white rectangle*) on the two-dimensional (2D) screening mediolateral oblique (MLO) view overlapping the pectoralis muscle is shown to correspond to a normal blood vessel (*white rectangle*) on the screening tomosynthesis images (B) obtained during the same compression of the breast. Tomosynthesis averts recall of the patient for diagnostic workup.

Rolled Views

An alternative approach is to manually alter the relationship of the breast tissue structures by rolling the halves of the breast in opposite directions. Rolled views should be obtained in the projection in which the asymmetry was originally seen to determine whether the finding was due to overlapping tissue. Care must be taken not to roll the finding into a position that overlaps with dense tissue as a true lesion could thus be obscured. If the asymmetry persists on rolled views, the direction of its movement can predict its location on the orthogonal view. For instance, a lesion in the upper breast that is seen on the CC view only should move laterally if the top of the breast is rolled laterally on a rolled CC view.

Tomosynthesis

Asymmetries are much less likely to be recalled at screening with tomosynthesis due to the inherent ability of this technique to resolve overlapping tissue structures (Fig. 13.10). If tomosynthesis is available at the time of diagnostic mammography, it can simplify the workup of asymmetries identified at 2D mammography. A single tomosynthesis sweep may be obtained in the projection on which an asymmetry was originally seen at 2D mammography to determine whether the 2D finding is a summation artifact or real finding (Fig. 13.11). The location of a finding can be predicted at tomosynthesis, even if it is only seen on one projection, because the location within the image stack can help predict its position.

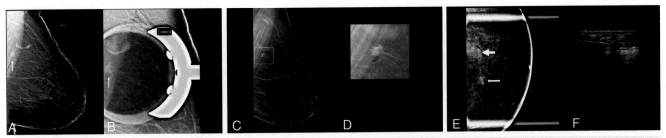

Fig. 13.11 (A) An asymmetry (*solid white arrow*) is identified in the upper left breast overlying the pectoralis muscle, seen on the screening mediolateral oblique (MLO) view only. (B) The asymmetry (*solid white arrow*) persists on the spot compression magnification MLO view but could not be visualized on the exaggerated craniocaudal lateral (XCCL) view (not shown). (C) An MLO tomosynthesis sweep demonstrates a spiculated mass (*white rectangle*), shown enlarged in (D). Because the mass is identified within the medial tomosynthesis slices, it is predicted to be in the upper inner quadrant. Spot compression magnification view of the upper inner breast (E) confirms a spiculated mass (*long white arrow*). The nipple (*short white arrow*) is rolled underneath the breast. (F) Targeted ultrasound of the left breast demonstrates a corresponding irregular hypoechoic mass at the 10 o'clock position, which underwent ultrasound-guided core biopsy revealing invasive ductal carcinoma.

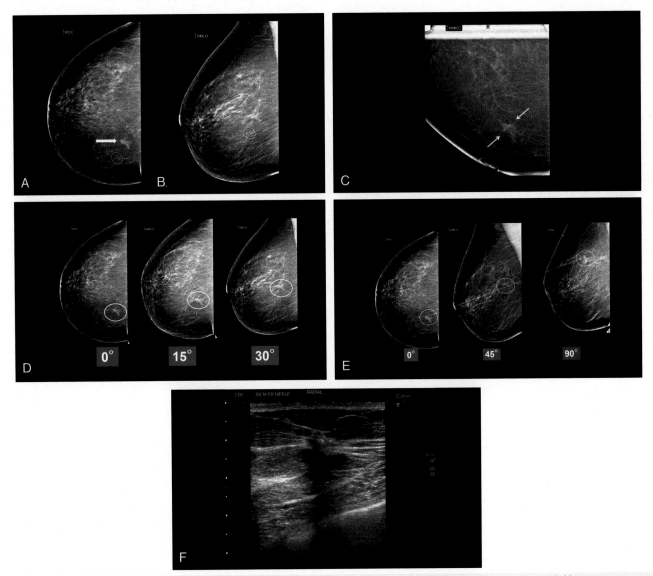

Fig. 13.12 Screening craniocaudal (CC) view of the right breast (A) demonstrates a developing asymmetry (*arrow*) in the medial breast, not present on the prior mammograms. The finding is not well localized on the mediolateral oblique (MLO) view (B). Spot compression CC magnification view (C) demonstrates persistence of the asymmetry (*arrows*), which appears to be spiculated. (D) On step oblique views obtained at 15 and 30 degrees (D), the asymmetry (*circled*) moves superiorly. Lining up the CC, 45-degree MLO, and 90-degree lateral views, the lesion can be more confidently localized on the 45-degree MLO view (*circled*). (E) Based on the step obliques, the asymmetry can be localized on the true lateral view (*circled*). (F) Targeted ultrasound demonstrates a corresponding irregular hypoechoic mass with angular margins and posterior shadowing at the 10 o'clock position, which proved malignant on ultrasound-guided core biopsy.

If an asymmetry persists after the above-described views are obtained, then it is likely to be a true space-occupying lesion. A true lateral projection may be obtained to precisely localize the lesion. For findings that remain visible only on one view, two possible explanations remain: (1) The asymmetry is a true lesion that is obscured by overlapping tissue on the other views or (2) it represents the rare summation artifact that is reproduced on multiple views that were obtained with similar technique. Step oblique views may be obtained to further evaluate these more challenging cases. These should be obtained at 15-degree increments, starting from the view on which the finding was originally seen, progressing toward the view on which the finding was not seen. If the asymmetry resolves on step oblique views, then it represents a summation artifact. If the asymmetry changes significantly in size, shape, and density on step oblique views, then it most likely represents a focal collection of fibroglandular tissue, which may be considered benign unless it is new in comparison to prior mammograms (see section on developing asymmetry). If the asymmetry persists on step oblique views, then it is a true space occupying lesion and can be further characterized with spot compression views. The location of the lesion can be predicted on the orthogonal CC and lateral views based on the step oblique views. Once the lesion has been precisely localized, targeted ultrasound may be performed (Fig. 13.12).

While it might be tempting at times to forego the above-described systematic workup of asymmetries and proceed directly to ultrasound, such a strategy is risky. Asymmetries have a high likelihood of representing summation artifacts. Therefore proceeding directly to ultrasound may result in a lengthy search for a finding that is ultimately not real. Alternatively, if the finding is real, one may miss it at ultrasound or identify an unrelated finding because one does not know precisely where to look. Lastly, it should be emphasized that a suspicious mammographic abnormality without a sonographic correlate still warrants biopsy. For all of these reasons, it is important to fully evaluate asymmetries at mammography prior to ultrasound.

FOCAL ASYMMETRY WORKUP

The workup of a focal asymmetry at 2D mammography includes spot compression views with or without magnification and targeted ultrasound. The purpose of diagnostic evaluation is to exclude an underlying mass, architectural distortion, or suspicious microcalcifications. If tomosynthesis is performed, then spot compression views may not provide additional information and may be omitted at the radiologist's discretion.

In the absence of any associated suspicious findings after full diagnostic evaluation, a focal asymmetry has a less than 2% probability of malignancy and can therefore be given a probably benign, BI-RADS 3 assessment and undergo short interval follow-up. Note that these rules only apply to a focal asymmetry identified on a baseline examination, not any finding that is new or increasing. The latter would be defined as a developing asymmetry, which is discussed in the following section.

DEVELOPING ASYMMETRY WORKUP

As its name implies, a developing asymmetry refers to a focal asymmetry that is new or increased in comparison to prior studies (see Fig. 13.12). The likelihood of malignancy among developing asymmetries approaches 13%, and therefore these lesions warrant biopsy, unless the diagnostic workup reveals a typically benign finding such as a simple cyst or lymph node. The diagnostic imaging algorithm for a developing asymmetry is the same as for a focal asymmetry.

Suggested Reading

Chong A, Weinstein SP, McDonald ES, Conant EF. Digital breast tomosynthesis: concepts and clinical practice. *Radiology*. 2019;292(1):1–14.

Gupta D, Friedewald MD, Sarah M. Lesion localization using digital breast tomosynthesis: where did i go wrong? *J Breast Imaging*. 2019;1(2):143–150.

Leung JW, Sickles EA. The probably benign assessment. *Radiol Clin North Am*. 2007;45(5). 773-vi.

Leung JWT, Sickles EA. Developing asymmetry identified on mammography: correlation with imaging outcome and pathologic findings. *Am J Roentgenol*. 2007;188(3):667–675.

Pearson KL, Sickles EA, Frankel SD, Leung JW. Efficacy of step-oblique mammography for confirmation and localization of densities seen on only one standard mammographic view. *Am J Roentgenol*. 2000;174(3):745–752.

Sickles EA. Practical solutions to common mammographic problems: tailoring the examination. *Am J Roentgenol*. 1988;151(1):31–39.

Sickles EA. The spectrum of breast asymmetries: imaging features, workup, management. *Radiol Clin North Am*. 2007;45(5):765–771.

14 *The Symptomatic Breast*

AMIE Y. LEE

OVERVIEW | *This chapter reviews the imaging evaluation and differential considerations in patients with breast symptoms, including the scenarios of palpable lump, nipple discharge, other nipple changes, breast pain, and breast swelling.*

Despite early detection of asymptomatic cancers from screening mammography, the breast radiologist will still frequently encounter women presenting with signs and symptoms of breast cancer. Symptomatic breast malignancies remain widely prevalent due to several factors. The cancer may be occult or missed on screening mammography, the woman may not be of screening age or is not undergoing routine screening, and interval cancers may arise in between scheduled screenings.

Diagnostic breast imaging is always indicated in women with a new concerning breast symptom, such as a palpable abnormality, suspicious nipple discharge, other nipple changes such as inversion/retraction or rash, or unilateral breast swelling. The breast radiologist plays a central role in the management of these symptomatic women, with the workup and diagnosis often fully completed within the breast imaging facility.

Knowledge of the appropriate imaging workup of breast signs and symptoms can help you, the radiologist, better triage the symptomatic woman and more accurately diagnose malignancy.

Palpable Breast Lump

A palpable breast abnormality is the most common presenting breast symptom. A lump may be found on clinical breast examination or self-identified by the patient. While most palpable lumps are benign in etiology, a palpable finding remains the most common symptom of a breast malignancy. Furthermore, palpable breast cancers are often more advanced and aggressive than asymptomatic cancers detected by screening. Therefore, prompt workup and diagnosis upon symptom recognition are critical.

Diagnostic imaging with mammography and/or ultrasound should be used to appropriately and safely triage women with a palpable lump. These two imaging modalities can determine whether the cause of the palpable lump is benign (Breast Imaging Reporting and Data System [BI-RADS] 1 or 2), probably benign (BI-RADS 3), suspicious (BI-RADS 4), or highly suggestive of malignancy (BI-RADS 5). The specific imaging and management algorithm used is outlined in the American College of Radiology (ACR) Appropriateness Criteria and is largely dictated by the patient's age. Other factors to consider include pregnancy status, lactational status, history of trauma, or suspected infection.

PALPABLE LUMP ≥40 YEARS OLD

For women aged 40 years or older with a palpable breast symptom (Box 14.1), the first step in evaluation is diagnostic mammography with a radiopaque marker placed over the site of palpable concern on full-field views (Fig. 14.1). This consists of craniocaudal and mediolateral oblique views, with additional supplemental views at the discretion of the interpreting radiologist or institutional policy. For conventional two-dimensional mammography, this should be followed by spot compression views at the site of concern with or without magnification. Magnification improves detection and characterization of associated calcifications (Fig. 14.2). Breast tomosynthesis with a tomosynthesis-compatible skin marker may also be utilized. If the patient is due for screening of the contralateral breast or if it is the patient's baseline mammogram, the contralateral breast should also be imaged. Including both breasts can allow for better detection of asymmetries and is also an opportunity to screen for contralateral asymptomatic cancers (Fig. 14.3).

In nearly all cases, diagnostic mammography should be followed with an ultrasound targeted to the site of clinical concern. The rare exception is when there is a definitively benign mammographic lesion clearly corresponding to the palpable lump, such as a lipoma, hamartoma, fat necrosis, morphologically benign intramammary lymph node, or calcified involuting fibroadenoma (Figs. 14.4–14.5). In addition, the ACR appropriateness criteria states that if there is only entirely fatty tissue at the site of the palpable lump, then ultrasound may not be necessary, although data in this particular scenario is sparse.

In all other scenarios, targeted ultrasound is required. If the mammogram is negative, ultrasound can identify

---

Box 14.1 Palpable Lump ≥40 Years Old[a]

- Start with diagnostic mammography.
- Almost always follow with ultrasound.
  - Unless, clearly benign mammographic correlate.
  - If only entirely fatty tissue, ultrasound is not mandatory.
- Screening mammography is not a substitute for diagnostic workup.

[a]For age 30–39: The same algorithm may be followed. The ACR Appropriateness Criteria states ultrasound may also be the initial step for this age group, at the discretion of the radiologist.

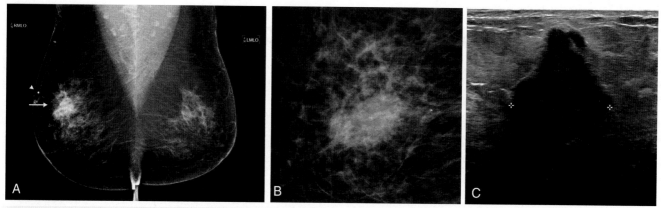

Fig. 14.1 A 62-year-old woman with a palpable lump in the upper outer right breast. (A) Bilateral full-field mediolateral oblique (MLO) views shows a round radiopaque marker (*arrowhead*) placed on the skin over the palpable abnormality in the right breast. There is an underlying irregular mass with spiculated margins. (B) Lateral spot compression magnification image shows the mass and associated subtle amorphous calcifications. (C) Targeted ultrasound of the palpable lump shows a corresponding irregular hypoechoic mass with indistinct margins, nonparallel orientation, and posterior shadowing. This lesion is highly suggestive of malignancy (BI-RADS 5). Ultrasound-guided core biopsy demonstrated invasive ductal carcinoma.

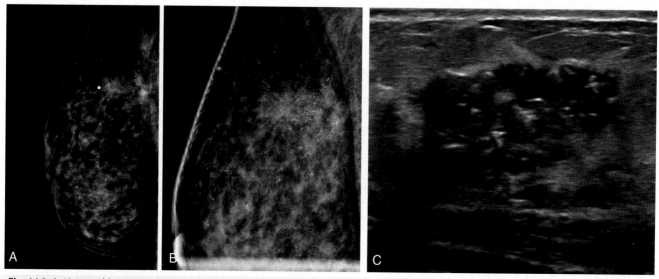

Fig. 14.2 A 43-year-old woman with a palpable lump in the right breast. (A) Full-field mediolateral oblique (MLO) mammogram demonstrates an irregular spiculated mass underlying the round radiopaque marker placed at the site of the palpable lump. There are associated calcifications extending anterior and posterior to the mass. (B) Spot compression magnification view better demonstrates the morphology and extent of the segmental fine pleomorphic calcifications. This lesion is highly suggestive of malignancy (BI-RADS 5). Core biopsy of the corresponding sonographic mass (C) demonstrated invasive ductal carcinoma and ductal carcinoma in situ.

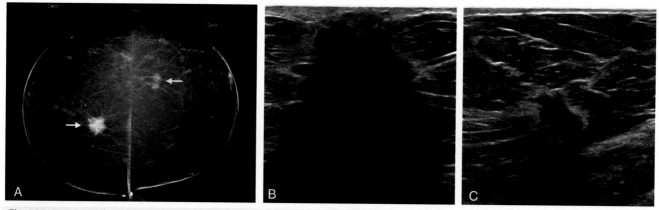

Fig. 14.3 A 73-year-old woman with a palpable right breast lump. (A) Bilateral full-field craniocaudal (CC) views show a dominant irregular spiculated mass (*white arrow*) corresponding to the palpable lump in the right breast. There is a smaller irregular spiculated mass (*yellow arrow*) incidentally found in the asymptomatic left breast. (B) Targeted ultrasound of the right breast palpable lump shows a corresponding irregular hypoechoic mass with spiculated mass and posterior shadowing. (C) Targeted ultrasound of the left breast mass shows a corresponding irregular hypoechoic spiculated mass. Ultrasound-guided core biopsies demonstrated invasive ductal carcinoma in the right breast and invasive lobular carcinoma in the left breast.

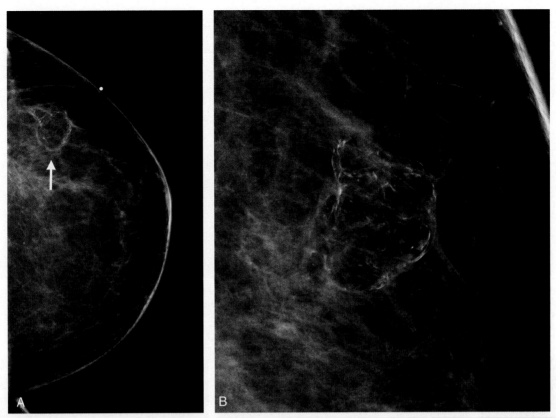

Fig. 14.4 A 60-year-old woman with history of left lumpectomy for invasive ductal carcinoma 1 year ago presents with a new palpable lump in the upper outer left breast. Full-field (A) and spot compression magnification (B) craniocaudal (CC) views demonstrate a rim-calcified fat-containing lesion (*arrow*), consistent with benign fat necrosis. This corresponds to the patient's palpable lump. No further diagnostic workup is needed for this benign finding (BI-RADS 2).

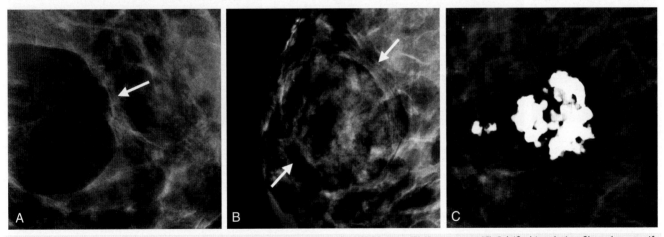

Fig. 14.5 Other characteristically benign palpable masses on mammography. (A) Lipoma. (B) Hamartoma. (C) Calcified involuting fibroadenoma. If these findings on mammography clearly correlate to the palpable lump, no further diagnostic imaging is needed.

mammographically occult lesions (Fig. 14.6). If there is a suspicious mammographic finding, ultrasound can further characterize the lesion and determine whether ultrasound-guided percutaneous biopsy is feasible.

When both diagnostic mammography and targeted ultrasound are negative with no suspicious correlate to the palpable lump, the negative predictive value is very high (97%–100%). The patient may be reassured of the negative examination with recommendation for clinical follow-up.

However, if the clinical breast examination is highly suspicious, palpation-guided percutaneous biopsy should be considered.

PALPABLE LUMP IN WOMEN 30 TO 39 YEARS OLD

The ACR Appropriateness Criteria advises that for women 30 to 39 years old, either diagnostic mammography or targeted ultrasound may be used as the first step in imaging

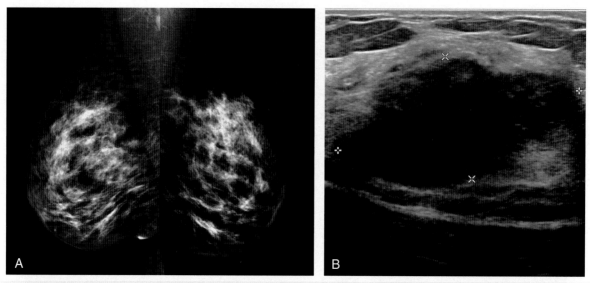

Fig. 14.6 Mammographically occult cancer. (A) A 45-year-old woman with negative screening mammogram. One week later, she returned because her physician palpated a lump in the upper outer left breast. Diagnostic mammography demonstrated no correlate to the lump. (B) Targeted ultrasound demonstrates a 4.6-cm hypoechoic oval mass with indistinct margins (calipers). This lesion is suspicious (BI-RADS 4). Ultrasound-guided core biopsy demonstrated invasive ductal carcinoma.

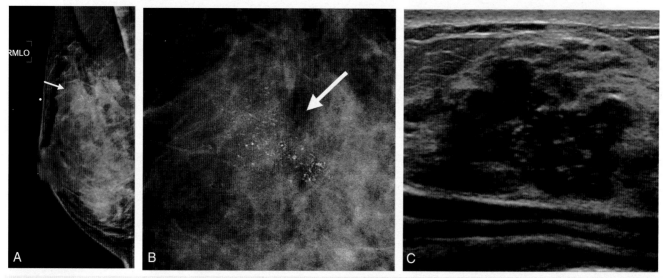

Fig. 14.7 A 31-year-old woman with a palpable right breast lump. (A) Full-field mediolateral oblique (MLO) and (B) spot compression magnification mammogram at the site of the lump demonstrates a group of fine pleomorphic and fine linear calcifications. (B) Targeted ultrasound demonstrates a corresponding hypoechoic irregular mass with indistinct margins. Echogenic foci within this mass correspond to the mammographic calcifications. Ultrasound-guided core biopsy demonstrated invasive ductal carcinoma.

evaluation of a palpable lump (Fig. 14.7). Ultrasound alone has been shown, in a few studies, to have high sensitivity for detection of malignancy in this age group. Whether to begin with mammography or ultrasound is at the discretion of the radiologist or institutional policy.

PALPABLE LUMP IN WOMEN <30 YEARS OLD

For women less than 30 years old with a palpable breast symptom, the first step in evaluation is a breast ultrasound targeted to the site of clinical concern (Box 14.2). Mammography is not routinely performed due to the very low incidence of breast cancer and the low yield of mammography in younger patients with dense breasts. There is

---

Box 14.2   Palpable Lump in Women <30 Years Old

- Targeted ultrasound is the initial and primary modality.
- Mammography is rarely used but not contraindicated.
  - Mammography can be helpful if clinical and ultrasound findings are highly suggestive of malignancy.
  - Mammography may resolve suspected benign fat-containing lesions or benign calcifications.

---

also a desire to avoid unnecessary radiation, albeit a very low dose, in younger more radiosensitive patients.

If a definitively benign correlate to the palpable symptom is identified on targeted ultrasound, no further evaluation

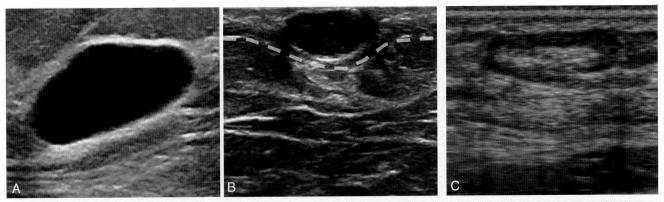

Fig. 14.8 Characteristically benign palpable breast lesions on ultrasound: (A) Simple cyst. (B) Intradermal cysts, such as epidermal inclusion cyst. (C) Intramammary lymph node. These lesions should be assessed as benign (BI-RADS 2).

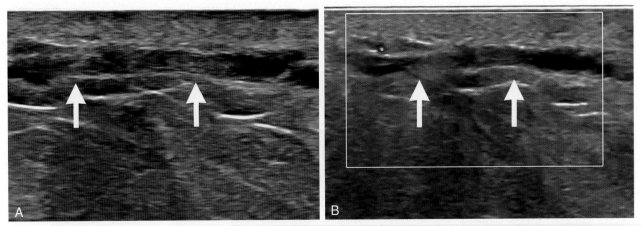

Fig. 14.9 A young woman presents 1 week after sudden-onset superficial breast pain with focal swelling and cord-like palpable lump. Pain has improved, but the lump persists. (A) Targeted ultrasound demonstrates a superficial tubular structure with internal echogenic material (*arrows*). (B) On Doppler, no flow is present within this structure. Findings are consistent with superficial venous thrombophlebitis (Mondor disease), a benign and self-limiting condition (BI-RADS 2).

is needed. Most commonly, this will be a simple cyst. Other characteristically benign lesions on ultrasound include morphologically benign intramammary lymph nodes and intradermal lesions, such as sebaceous cysts and epidermal inclusion cysts (Figs. 14.8–14.9). These lesions should be assessed as BI-RADS 2. The patient can be reassured of the benign etiology of the lump, can undergo clinical follow-up, and may begin screening mammography at age 40.

If targeted ultrasound is negative, showing only normal breast tissue, then typically no further workup is needed. In very rare cases, if the clinical breast examination is highly suspicious for malignancy, diagnostic mammography or palpation-guided percutaneous biopsy could be considered. However, targeted ultrasound alone has been shown to have very high sensitivity and negative predictive value for cancer in women less than 30.

While mammography is rarely used in women less than 30, use of this imaging modality is not contraindicated. Mammography can be helpful if clinical and ultrasound findings are highly suggestive of malignancy to better characterize the suspected malignancy (Fig. 14.10). Mammography may resolve suspected benign fat-containing lesions or benign calcifications, which may be indeterminate with ultrasound alone (Fig. 14.11). Lastly,

bilateral mammography should be performed in any patient with a recent diagnosis of breast cancer regardless of age.

THE PROBABLY BENIGN MASS

In the evaluation of palpable masses, one will commonly encounter a sonographic mass that is oval in shape with circumscribed margins, parallel orientation, uniformly hypoechoic echotexture, and no posterior shadowing (Fig. 14.12). This is defined in BI-RADS as "probably benign" imaging features. Masses with these features most commonly are fibroadenomas. In the prior 2003 edition of BI-RADS, the BI-RADS 3 assessment was reserved only for nonpalpable masses. Due to multiple studies showing the rate of malignancy less than 2% for palpable masses with probably benign features, the current 2013 edition of BI-RADS now supports the application of the BI-RADS 3 assessment for palpable masses with these probably benign sonographic features.

In such cases, the patient should be reassured that the mass is almost certainly benign. The woman should undergo short-interval follow-up ultrasound in 6 months, with imaging confirmation of stability for 2 to 3 years, per standard protocol for BI-RADS 3 lesions. However, the

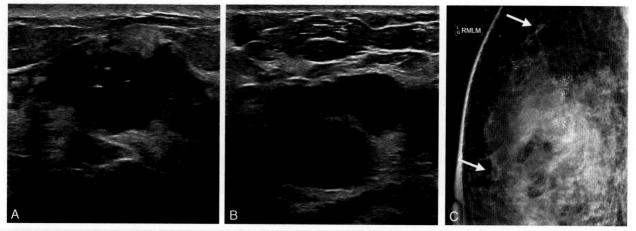

Fig. 14.10 A 27-year-old with a palpable right upper outer breast lump. (A) Targeted ultrasound shows a corresponding 2.5 cm hypoechoic irregular mass with angular margins. Echogenic foci within this mass are suggestive of calcifications. (B) Targeted ultrasound of the right axilla demonstrates a suspicious enlarged lymph node. Given the suspicious sonographic findings, a diagnostic mammogram was performed. (C) Lateral spot compression magnification image demonstrates extensive segmental fine pleomorphic calcifications (*arrows*). Findings are highly suspicious for malignancy (BI-RADS 5), and core biopsies demonstrated invasive ductal carcinoma and ductal carcinoma in situ with axillary metastasis.

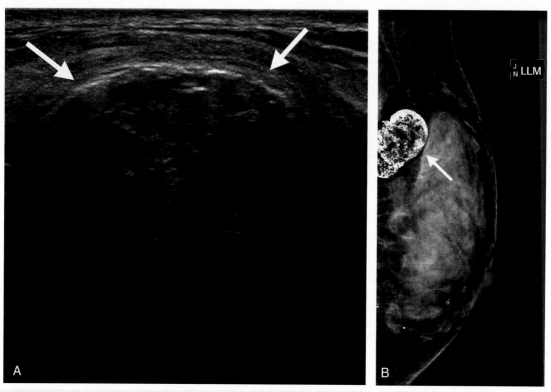

Fig. 14.11 A 26-year-old with a palpable left upper outer breast lump. (A) Targeted ultrasound demonstrates an oval hypoechoic mass with heterogeneous echotexture and marked posterior shadowing. The marked shadowing and suggestion of a superficial echogenic rim (*arrows*) raised the possibility of rim calcifications. Therefore, a mammogram (B) was performed, which confirms fat necrosis with rim calcifications (*arrow*). Due to the mammographic finding, this could be assessed a benign (BI-RADS 2).

literature on palpable masses with probably benign features is strong only for women less than age 40, and caution should be used in older symptomatic women.

PALPABLE LUMP: SPECIAL SCENARIOS

In addition to age, other unique scenarios to consider when evaluating a woman with a palpable lump include whether the patient is pregnant or lactating, has history of recent breast trauma, or has a suspected infection.

Imaging management of the pregnant and lactating patient is covered in greater detail in Chapter 19 (Special Populations in Breast Imaging). Briefly, diagnostic imaging workup of a palpable lump should never be delayed due to the fact that a woman is pregnant or breastfeeding. A palpable lump is the most common symptom of a pregnancy-associated breast cancer, which is defined as malignancy occurring during pregnancy, within 12-months postpartum, or anytime while lactating. The ACR appropriateness criteria recommends breast ultrasound as the first-line imaging modality in pregnant and lactating women, paralleling the management algorithm of women younger than 30 years old. While not routinely performed, mammography is not contraindicated and may be considered if malignancy is suspected. Pathologically benign lesions unique to the pregnant and lactating population include galactoceles (Fig. 14.13) and lactating adenomas.

In the clinical setting of recent breast trauma, a newly palpable lump may arise from hematoma or evolving fat necrosis. While the imaging features of fat necrosis are often characteristically benign on mammography, the features of hematomas are nonspecific and may overlap with the appearance of malignancies. If a lesion is clinically suspected to be posttraumatic in etiology (i.e., overlying ecchymosis after direct breast trauma), close follow-up with repeat imaging in 1 to 2 months is reasonable to assess for resolution of the lesion (Fig. 14.14). If the lesion is unchanged or growing at follow-up, biopsy should be performed.

When a palpable symptom is clinically suspected to be infectious in etiology, close clinical management and treatment of the infection are indicated. However, if an abscess is suspected or if the palpable lump does not resolve with antibiotic therapy, diagnostic imaging is indicated (Fig. 14.15). If an abscess is identified on ultrasound, particularly if larger than 2 to 3 cm, image-guided percutaneous drainage of the fluid may be offered for diagnostic (for cultures

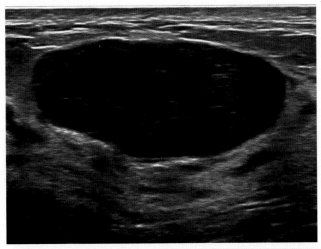

Fig. 14.12 A 28-year-old woman with a palpable right breast mass. Targeted ultrasound demonstrates a corresponding oval, uniformly hypoechoic solid mass with circumscribed margins, parallel orientation, and no posterior shadowing. This mass was assessed as probably benign (BI-RADS 3) with a recommendation for a 6-month follow-up ultrasound.

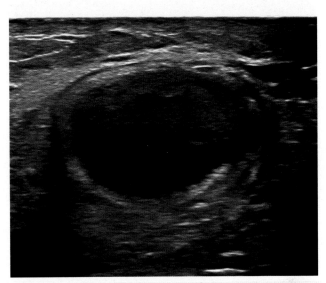

Fig. 14.13 A 33-year-old lactating patient with a painless palpable lump in the right breast. Targeted ultrasound demonstrates a corresponding oval, circumscribed mass with a fat-fluid level. Findings are consistent with a benign galactocele (BI-RADS 2)

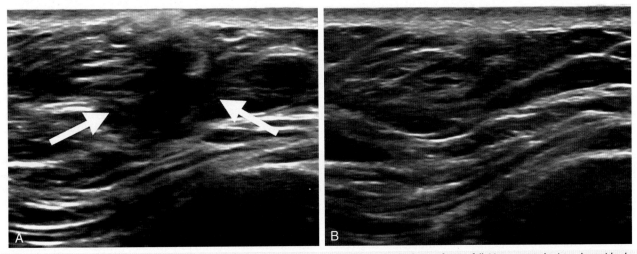

Fig. 14.14 A 62-year-old with a palpable lump in her lower inner left breast after trauma to the breast from a fall. Mammography (not shown) had no correlate to the palpable lump. (A) Targeted ultrasound at the site of the lump shows a hypoechoic, irregular mass with indistinct margins (*arrows*). Given this mass was directly underlying the site ecchymosis, findings were suggestive of a posttraumatic hematoma, and short interval follow-up was recommended. (B) Follow-up ultrasound 6 weeks later shows resolution of the lesion, consistent with a resolved hematoma.

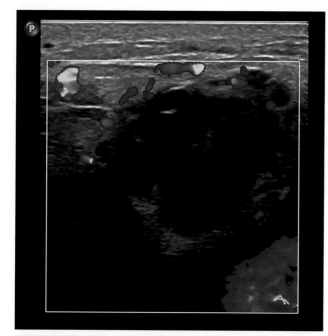

Fig. 14.15 A 34-year-old lactating woman with a palpable lump and associated erythema, warmth, and induration in the upper inner right breast, clinically concerning for abscess. Targeted ultrasound demonstrated a fluid collection with surrounding hyperemia, consistent with abscess. Purulent fluid was aspirated for therapeutic and diagnostic purposes, sent for cultures and sensitivities.

and sensitivities) and therapeutic purposes. Drainage of the infected fluid collection can help facilitate recovery in conjunction with antibiotic treatment.

Nipple Changes

Signs and symptoms involving the nipple that require diagnostic workup include pathologic nipple discharge, new nipple inversion or retraction, and persistent nipple-areolar skin changes. As with the evaluation of palpable breast lumps, the initial diagnostic breast imaging tests should consist of mammography and ultrasound, with the precise algorithm dependent on the patient's age.

NIPPLE DISCHARGE

The first step in evaluation of the patient with nipple discharge is reviewing the clinical history, determining the characteristics of the nipple discharge, and categorizing the discharge as pathologic or physiologic (Box 14.3). Pathologic nipple discharge is bloody or clear in color, spontaneous, unilateral, and usually arises from a single duct orifice.

In contrast, physiologic nipple discharge is neither bloody nor clear and can be a variety of colors, including milky, yellow, green, blue, or black. It is typically nonspontaneous, occurring only with breast manipulation or compression. It is often bilateral and originating from multiple ducts. In the absence of pathologic features, patients with physiologic nipple discharge can undergo routine screening mammography. Diagnostic breast imaging is not indicated, as breast

cancer is not the cause of physiologic nipple discharge. If there is persistent spontaneous milky discharge in a patient who is not pregnant or breastfeeding, medical evaluation for a systemic cause of galactorrhea and testing of prolactin levels may be indicated.

In contrast, pathologic nipple discharge requires diagnostic imaging workup (Box 14.4). Pathologic nipple discharge is most commonly due to a benign intraductal papilloma (Fig. 14.16). However, pathologic nipple discharge may also be symptom of an underlying breast cancer, with risk of malignancy increasing with age. In patients age 40 years or older, diagnostic mammography is the first-line imaging modality, paralleling the imaging algorithm for palpable breast lumps. Similarly, the ACR appropriateness criteria states that in women 30 to 39 years of age with pathologic nipple discharge, either mammography or ultrasound may be used as the initial imaging modality. In addition to standard full-field mammographic views, spot compression magnification images of the subareolar region could be considered. Mammography should be followed by breast ultrasound, which includes targeted evaluation of the subareolar breast. Targeted ultrasound may also better characterize suspicious lesions identified on mammography.

When both mammography and ultrasound are negative in the evaluation of pathologic nipple discharge, either ductography or contrast-enhanced breast magnetic resonance imaging (MRI) may be performed. A ductogram, also known as a galactogram, is a procedure in which the single duct orifice secreting the clear or bloody nipple discharge is cannulated and injected with iodinated contrast (Fig. 14.17). The breast is immediately imaged with mammography to identify and localize intraductal abnormalities. Most commonly, this will be a filling defect or a cut-off sign due to an intraductal mass. While ductography was historically the procedure of choice after negative

mammography and ultrasound, recent studies have shown that contrast-enhanced MRI is a more sensitive tool for detecting papillary lesions and malignancies. For example, deep, peripheral lesions would be difficult to detect with ductography. Furthermore, MRI has been shown to have both a higher positive predictive value and negative predictive value than ductography in the evaluation of patients with pathologic nipple discharge, leading many radiologists to prefer this modality (Fig. 14.18).

OTHER NIPPLE SYMPTOMS

Other nipple symptoms women may present with include nipple inversion or retraction and nipple and areolar skin changes.

Chronic or gradual bilateral nipple retraction or inversion can be benign in etiology, due to processes such as aging and duct ectasia. However, unilateral new or rapidly worsening nipple retraction or inversion requires prompt clinical evaluation. Such symptoms should raise concern for a possible underlying malignancy pulling back the nipple areolar complex. Imaging workup with diagnostic mammography and ultrasound is indicated, with the patient's age dictating the initial modality of choice, paralleling the imaging algorithm of palpable breast lumps and nipple discharge. In addition to standard full-field mammographic views, spot compression magnification images of the subareolar region could be considered. Mammography may be followed by targeted ultrasound to better evaluate the subareolar region or further characterize suspicious lesions identified on mammography (Fig. 14.19).

Persistent rash, redness, scaling, or crusting of the nipple and areola are also suspicious symptoms and could be due to Paget disease of the breast. A classic scenario is a patient initially thought to have eczema or dermatitis of the areola for whom symptoms do not resolve with standard

Fig. 14.16 A 29-year-old with spontaneous clear left nipple discharge. Targeted ultrasound demonstrates an oval intraductal mass (*arrow*) in the subareolar left breast. Ultrasound-guided core biopsy showed benign intraductal papilloma.

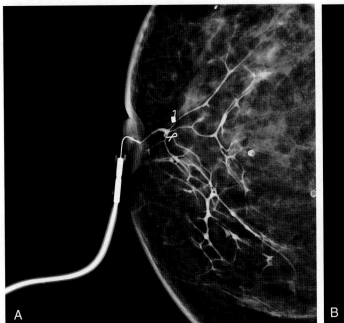
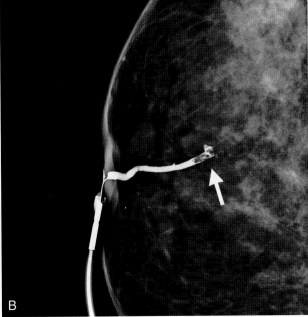

Fig. 14.17 (A) Normal ductogram showing normal caliber ducts with no filling defects or other abnormalities. Two clips are from remote prior benign biopsies. (B) Abnormal ductogram with filling defect (*arrow*) and abrupt cut-off of the iodinated contrast.

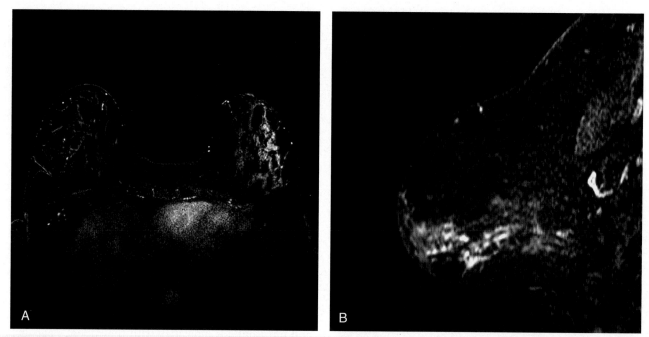

Fig. 14.18 A 34-year-old with spontaneous bloody left nipple discharge. Diagnostic mammography and ultrasound were negative, with no correlate to the left breast symptom. Axial (A) and sagittal (B) subtracted T1 postcontrast magnetic resonance imaging (MRI) demonstrates extensive segmental clumped non-mass enhancement in the outer central left breast. MRI guided core biopsy demonstrated invasive ductal carcinoma and ductal carcinoma in situ.

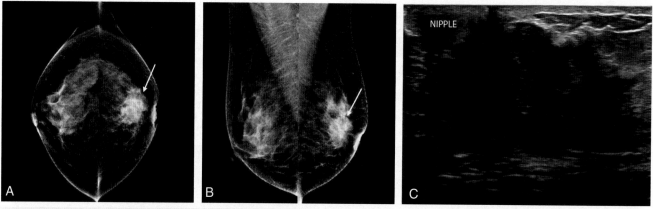

Fig. 14.19 A 46-year-old woman with new left nipple retraction. Bilateral (A) craniocaudal (CC) and (B) mediolateral oblique (MLO) views from the diagnostic mammogram shows left nipple retraction and an underlying irregular spiculated subareolar mass (*arrow*). (C) Targeted ultrasound shows the corresponding hypoechoic irregular spiculated mass extending into the nipple.

topical treatments. Paget disease of the breast, also known as Paget disease of the nipple, is a rare form of breast cancer accounting for 1% to 5% of breast malignancies. It is characterized by malignant cells infiltrating and proliferating in the epidermis of the nipple. In the majority of cases of Paget disease, there is an associated cancer within the breast parenchyma. Therefore, if Paget disease is clinically suspected, diagnostic mammography is indicated to detect an underlying carcinoma. Even when the mammogram is negative, clinical consultation and skin biopsy, typically by a dermatologist or breast surgeon, are usually warranted. In patients with biopsy-proven Paget disease with no suspicious mammographic or sonographic finding, MRI can be useful to identify malignancy within the breast parenchyma.

Diffuse Breast Swelling and Edema

In addition to the focal symptoms covered above, patients may present with diffuse breast swelling and enlargement, with or without associated erythema. On mammography, diffuse edema will appear as skin and trabecular thickening, due to thickening of the fibrous septa of the breast. The differential considerations for unilateral breast swelling are summarized in Box 14.5.

The most common cause of unilateral breast swelling is mastitis, which typically has associated signs and symptoms of infection, such as erythema, fever, and leukocytosis. However, if symptoms of a clinically suspected mastitis

Box 14.5 Unilateral Diffuse Skin and Trabecular Thickening: Top Differential Diagnoses

- Mastitis
- Inflammatory breast cancer
- Axillary lymphatic obstruction
- Venous obstruction
- Post-radiation therapy

Box 14.6 Bilateral Diffuse Skin and Trabecular Thickening: Top Differential Diagnoses

- Systemic fluid overload
- Congestive heart failure
- Renal failure
- Liver failure, hypoalbuminemia

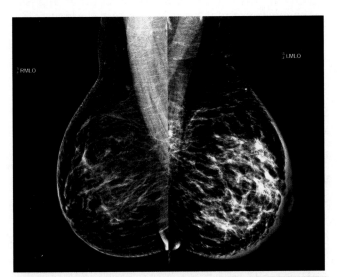

Fig. 14.20 A 31-year-old woman with diffuse left breast swelling and erythema worsening over the past month. Her primary care physician initially treated her for suspected mastitis, but symptoms were unresponsive to antibiotics. Bilateral mediolateral oblique (MLO) views from her diagnostic mammogram shows diffuse skin and trabecular thickening of the left breast. Skin punch biopsy showed extensive tumor emboli in the dermal lymphatics, the pathologic hallmark of inflammatory breast cancer.

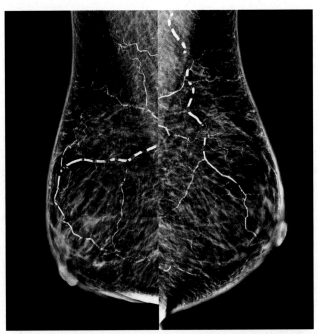

Fig. 14.21 A 49-year-old woman with end-stage renal disease. The mediolateral oblique (MLO) views from a screening mammogram show bilateral and symmetric diffuse skin and trabecular thickening. Findings are consistent with breast edema due to fluid overload.

do not fully resolve with antibiotic treatment, or if the clinical presentation is not consistent with infection, inflammatory breast cancer must be considered. Inflammatory breast cancer is a rare but aggressive form of breast cancer with very poor prognosis (Fig. 14.20). It is categorized as T4d by the American Joint Committee on Cancer (AJCC) TNM classification system. Inflammatory carcinoma is primarily a clinical diagnosis, with a classic presentation of rapid-onset erythema and edema involving greater than one-third of the breast, with a peau d'orange appearance of the skin caused by tumor obstructing the dermal lymphatics. When there is clinical concern for inflammatory breast cancer, skin punch biopsy may be performed, usually by a breast surgeon or dermatologist. However, the sensitivity of skin punch biopsy is limited (i.e., results are positive in less than three-quarters of cases of inflammatory breast cancer), and a positive skin punch biopsy is not a requirement for diagnosis. The characteristic pathologic finding is tumor emboli within the dermal lymphatics.

Lymphedema, due to axillary lymphatic obstruction, can also present as unilateral breast swelling. This can be seen in a patient with active axillary nodal metastasis (i.e., obstruction of axillary lymphatic drainage by bulky tumor involvement in the lymph nodes) or in a patient with a history of surgical dissection of the axillary lymph nodes.

In contrast to unilateral breast swelling, bilateral breast swelling indicates a systemic benign process, such as fluid overload. The differential diagnosis of bilateral breast skin and trabecular thickening is summarized in Box 14.6. Although systemic fluid overload usually presents as symmetric bilateral edema (Fig. 14.21), asymmetric breast swelling is possible if a patient tends to lie decubitus only on one side, resulting in dependent edema.

Pain

Breast pain is a common symptom, but one that is rarely due to cancer in the absence of other associated suspicious clinical findings. In women presenting with breast pain alone, the incidence of malignancy is 0% to 3%. Nonfocal (greater than one quadrant), diffuse, intermittent, or cyclical pain without other suspicious clinical findings is not associated with malignancy, and diagnostic breast imaging usually is not appropriate in these scenarios.

Breast pain that is focal and persistent (noncyclical) is overwhelmingly benign in etiology, but in very rare cases may be associated with cancer. The ACR Appropriateness Criteria currently recommends diagnostic imaging workup of persistent and focal breast pain. The specific imaging

Box 14.7   Imaging for Breast Pain

- Nonfocal, diffuse, or cyclical
  - Diagnostic imaging not indicated for any age group
  - Routine screening mammography per screening guidelines
- Focal and persistent[a]
  - Age <30: Targeted ultrasound
  - Age 30–39: Mammography and ultrasound are equivalent alternatives
  - Age ≥40: Mammography and ultrasound (mammography may be omitted if performed within the last 3–6 months)

[a]Necessity of imaging evaluation for breast pain is controversial. In the absence of other suspicious symptoms, there is little association between pain alone and cancer.

modality recommended is based on age, largely paralleling the imaging algorithm for palpable breast lumps (Box 14.7).

The necessity of diagnostic imaging evaluation for focal breast pain alone remains controversial, given the low to no cancer yield. However, if the breast pain is associated with other suspicious breast symptoms, such as a palpable abnormality, pathologic nipple discharge, other nipple changes such as inversion/retraction or rash, or unilateral breast swelling, diagnostic imaging is always indicated as outlined in the respective sections above.

KEY POINTS

- A palpable breast lump is the most common symptom of breast cancer.
- Imaging algorithm for a palpable lump is largely dictated by the patient's age.
- For women 40 or older, start with mammography, usually followed by ultrasound.
- For women 30 to 39, either mammography or ultrasound may be the initial modality.

- For women <30, start with targeted ultrasound.
- Pathologic nipple discharge is bloody or clear in color, spontaneous, unilateral, and usually arises from a single duct orifice.
- If mammography and ultrasound are negative in the evaluation of pathologic nipple discharge, magnetic resonance imaging (MRI) or ductography are usually indicated.
- Other suspicious nipple symptoms requiring diagnostic evaluation include new inversion or retraction and skin changes concerning for Paget disease of the breast.
- Inflammatory breast cancer is an aggressive form of breast cancer characterized by rapid-onset breast erythema and edema with a peau d'orange appearance of the skin.

Suggested Readings

Moy L, Heller SL, Bailey L, et al. ACR appropriateness criteria palpable breast masses. *J Am Coll Radiol.* 2017;14(5S):S203–S224. Review.

Lehman CD, Lee AY, Lee CI. Imaging management of palpable breast abnormalities. *AJR.* 2014;203:1142–1153.

Lee SJ, Trikha S, Moy L, et al. ACR appropriateness criteria evaluation of nipple discharge. *J Am Coll Radiol.* 2017;14(5S):S138–S153.

Nicholson BT, Harvey JA, Cohen MA. Nipple-areolar complex: normal anatomy and benign and malignant processes. *Radiographics.* 2009;29(2):509–523.

Da Costa D, Taddese A, Cure ML, Gerson D, Poppiti R, Jr Esserman LE. Common and unusual diseases of the nipple-areolar complex. *Radiographics.* 2007;27(Suppl 1): S65–77.

Yeh ED, Jacene HA, Bellon JR, et al. What radiologists need to know about diagnosis and treatment of inflammatory breast cancer: a multidisciplinary approach. *Radiographics.* 2013;33(7):2003–2017.

Holbrook AI, Moy L, Akin EA, et al. ACR appropriateness criteria breast pain. *J Am Coll Radiol.* 2018;15(11S):S276–S282.

Holbrook AI. Breast pain, a common grievance: guidance to radiologists. *Am J Roentgenol.* 2020;214(2):259–264.

15 Breast Cancer Staging: What the Surgeon and Oncologist Want To Know

HAYDEE OJEDA-FOURNIER AND MOHAMMAD EGHTEDARI

OVERVIEW *This chapter reviews the imaging and molecular tumor profiling used in the eighth edition of the TNM staging system developed and maintained by the American Joint Committee on Cancer. The aim of staging is to guide treatment and provide prognosis for patients diagnosed with breast cancer. With significant advances in immunohistochemical and molecular profiling of tumors, staging continues to evolve from simple anatomic information to include molecular information that guides investigational and standard of care information.*

Background

The staging of breast cancer has been developed and is maintained by the American Joint Committee on Cancer (AJCC) since 1977. Initially, the goal of breast cancer staging was to identify those patients who would not benefit from radical mastectomy due to their already advanced disease. Traditionally, patients were grouped according to the anatomic extent of their disease based on the TNM system: tumor size, lymph nodes involved, and distant metastasis.

Since the initial implementation of breast cancer staging, it has been found that the anatomic extent of disease is not the only factor that determines outcomes. For example, a large low-grade tumor may have a better outcome compared with a small high-grade tumor. Molecular staging was first introduced in the sixth edition of AJCC but was not fully implemented in clinical breast cancer practice due to lack of prospective data and lack of worldwide availability. Currently, AJCC committee has not switched completely to molecular staging in the current eighth edition because molecular tests are still not available worldwide. Staging is used to guide breast cancer treatment and provide a prognosis to patients. In addition, staging has facilitated less aggressive surgeries, reduced axillary dissection, and decreased mortality by identifying those patients who may benefit from neoadjuvant therapy (Box 15.1).

Box 15.1 Radiologist's Role in the Clinical Staging of Breast Cancer

- Provide accurate primary tumor size.
- Assess skin or chest wall involvement.
- Assess lymph nodes.
- Assess the presence or absence of distant metastasis.

Eighth Edition of AJCC Cancer Staging Manual

The AJCC staging system provides a strategy for grouping patients for prognosis. The eighth edition of AJCC was implemented on January 1, 2018. The main changes from the prior editions include the implementation of a prognostic staging protocol. In prognostic staging, biological factors such as tumor nuclear grade, hormone receptor status (estrogen receptor [ER]/progesterone receptor [PR]), and human epidermal growth factor 2 (HER2) status are incorporated into the traditional anatomic TNM staging. Commercially available multigene panels (e.g., Oncotype DX, MammaPrint, PAM 50) are also incorporated in limited subgroups. Risk profiles calculated from these biological factors can estimate the 5-year overall survival and disease-specific survival for each anatomic stage of the disease.

Principles and Rules of Staging

At the time of diagnosis, the stage of cancer is a critical factor that defines prognosis and determines the appropriate treatment. Accurate staging is necessary to facilitate the exchange of information among treatment centers and serve as a basis for clinical cancer research. Fig. 15.1 illustrates the AJCC TNM system, which classifies cancers by the size and extent of the primary tumor (T), involvement of lymph nodes (N), and presence or absence of distant metastases (M).

Tumor classification based on the molecular profile is summarized in Table 15.1. The profiles include Luminal A (71% of tumors, ER or PR is highly positive, the tumor is less aggressive), Luminal B (12% of tumors, ER or PR is low positive, more aggressive than Luminal A), HER2 enriched (5% of tumors, most aggressive tumor), and basal-like. ER and PR are nuclear hormone receptors that modulate the activity of certain genes that control breast cell proliferation; staining of 1% of cells or more is considered positive.

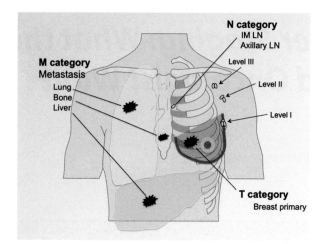

Fig. 15.1 Schematic illustrating the TNM system: *T*, Primary tumor size; *N*, node status; *M*, metastasis.

Table 15.1   Tumor Classification Based on the Molecular Profile

Molecular Subtype	Descriptors[a]	Comments
Luminal A	ER +	Low grade
	PR +	Grows slowly
	HER2 −	Best prognosis
	↓ Ki-67	71% of tumors
Luminal B	ER +	High grade
	PR + or −	Grows slightly faster
	HER2 + or −	Slightly worse prognosis
	↑ Ki-67	12% of tumors
Triple-negative (basal-like)	ER −	Aggressive with poorer prognosis
	PR −	Often responds well to chemotherapy
	HER2 −	Common with *BRCA1* +
		Common with younger individuals
		Common with African ancestry
HER2-enriched	ER −	Aggressive with poorer prognosis
	PR −	HER2-targeted therapies have improved outcomes
	HER2 +	
		5% of tumors

ER, Estrogen receptor; *HER2*, human epidermal growth factor receptor; PR, progesterone; +, positive; −, negative
[a]Note: The most common descriptors are listed; rare variations may exist.

HER2 is a member of epidermal growth factor receptors. HER2 is first evaluated by immunohistochemistry: score 0 and 1+ equals HER2 negative, score 2+ equals needs fluorescent in situ hybridization assays (FISH), and score 3+ equals HER2 positive. Additional tumor markers include Ki67, a proliferation marker (graded as <10%, 10%–20%, >20% positivity). Finally, the tumor grade is determined by microscopic evaluation of tubule formation, mitotic count, and nuclear pleomorphism. The tumor grade is classified as low, intermediate, or high grade with an increasing number of scores.

Table 15.2   Types of Staging

Staging	Definition	Comments
Clinical	Physical examination Imaging tests Percutaneous biopsies	Will not change based on response to chemotherapy
Pathology	Pathology from excision of the primary tumor, lymph nodes, and metastatic sites	Only on patients who have had surgery
Restaging	Determine the extent of the disease after recurrence	Directs treatment options

Clinical Versus Pathologic Staging

(Table 15.2)

CLINICAL STAGING

Prefix *c* is added in front of staging, for example, cT1N1. Clinical staging determines how much cancer is present based on physical examination, imaging tests, and percutaneous biopsies of the affected areas before surgery. The clinical stage is not changed after the administration of neoadjuvant chemotherapy; however, prefix *yc* is used to clarify that the patient received neoadjuvant therapy (e.g., ycT1N1).

PATHOLOGY STAGING

Prefix *p* is added in front of the staging, for example, pT2N1. Pathology stage (also called the surgical stage) includes pathology from the primary tumor, lymph nodes, and metastatic sites. Pathologic staging is only performed on patients who have undergone surgery to remove or explore the extent of cancer. If the patient received neoadjuvant therapy, the prefix *yp* is used to clarify that patient received neoadjuvant therapy (e.g., ypT2N1).

RESTAGING

Restaging is used to determine the extent of the disease if cancer comes back after treatment. Other important terms include synchronous and metachronous cancers. Synchronous cancers are those found in the same organ (or paired organs) within 4 months, while metachronous cancers are those found greater than 4 months apart and consequently will need a separate staging. The prefix *r* indicates recurrence; for example, rcT1N1. The prefix *a* indicates cancer found on autopsy. Table 15.2 summarizes the types of staging.

Imaging Modalities Used to Stage Breast Cancer

Mammography, with or without digital breast tomosynthesis (DBT), is the primary imaging modality for breast cancer screening and diagnosis. Ultrasound (US) is the most commonly used adjunct imaging modality to mammography and complements physical examination. Mammography,

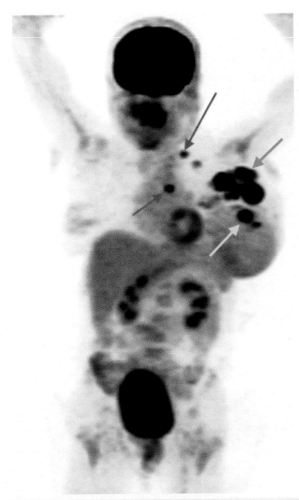

Fig. 15.2 PET-CT image for the detection of systemic disease. PET-CT in a 54-year-old with invasive ductal carcinoma demonstrates increased FDG uptake in the known left breast mass (*yellow arrow*), ipsilateral axillary lymph nodes (*green arrow*), infraclavicular nodes, and mediastinal nodes (*orange arrows*), consistent with stage IV disease.

tumors, or breast lymphoma. The T classification measures the size of the tumor to the nearest millimeter. When multiple tumors are in a breast, the largest individual tumor mass is used to provide the T classification. Satellite masses are not added up for the T parameter. Box 15.2 summarizes the T category.

For the T parameter, *chest wall* invasion (T4a) includes involvement of ribs, intercostal muscles, and serratus anterior muscle. Involvement of the pectoralis muscles does not constitute chest wall invasion. In addition, the term *inflammatory carcinoma* should not be used for locally advanced

---

Box 15.2   T Parameter Definitions

- Tx Primary tumor cannot be assessed.
- T0 No evidence of primary tumor.
- Tis carcinoma in situ or Tis (DCIS) ductal carcinoma in situ (Fig. 15.3).
- Tis (Paget) Paget disease of the nipple not associated with invasive carcinoma and/or carcinoma in situ in the underlying breast parenchyma (Fig. 15.4).
- T1 Tumors are less than 2 cm.
  - T1mi Less than 0.1 cm
  - T1a Greater than 0.1 cm up to 0.5 cm (Fig. 15.5)
  - T1b Greater than 0.5 cm up to 1.0 cm (Fig. 15.6)
  - T1c Greater than 1.0 cm up to 2.0 cm (Fig. 15.7)
- T2 Tumors are greater than 2 cm but up to 5 cm (Fig. 15.8).
- T3 Tumors are greater than 5 cm (Fig. 15.9).
- T4 Tumor of any size with direct extension to the chest wall and/or to the skin.
  - T4a Extension to the chest wall (ribs, intercostal muscles, serratus anterior muscle), not including only pectoralis muscle adherence/invasion (Fig. 15.10)
  - T4b Non-inflammatory skin involvement; Ulceration and/or ipsilateral satellite nodules and/or edema of the skin, which do not meet the criteria for inflammatory carcinoma (Fig. 15.11)
  - T4c Both T4a and T4b (Fig. 15.12)
  - T4d Inflammatory breast cancer (Fig. 15.13)

DBT, and US are covered in detail in earlier chapters. With regard to breast cancer staging, US, in conjunction with mammography, can help assess tumor size and extent, stage the axilla, and guide interventions. Magnetic resonance imaging (MRI) is often used to evaluate the extent of disease in a patient with a new diagnosis of breast cancer, assess for multifocal or multicentric disease, screen for contralateral disease, and guide biopsy or localization. Computed tomography (CT) and positron emission tomography (PET)/CT are reserved for patients with locally advanced breast cancer to evaluate for metastatic disease. PET has been shown to be 89% sensitive and 84% specificity in staging systemic disease (Fig. 15.2).

TNM

ASSESSMENT OF THE T (TUMOR) PARAMETER

Note that the breast TNM staging applies only to invasive (infiltrating) breast carcinoma and ductal carcinoma in situ. It is not used to stage breast sarcomas, phyllodes

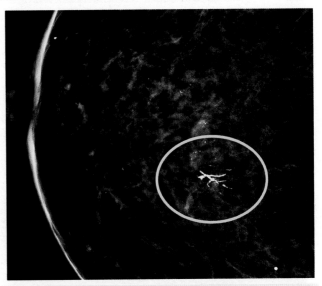

Fig. 15.3 Tis ductal carcinoma in situ (DCIS) Stage 0. A 74-year-old with mammographically detected fine linear branching grouped calcifications (*circle*). Pathology from stereotactic biopsy demonstrated high-grade DCIS with no upgrade at lumpectomy.

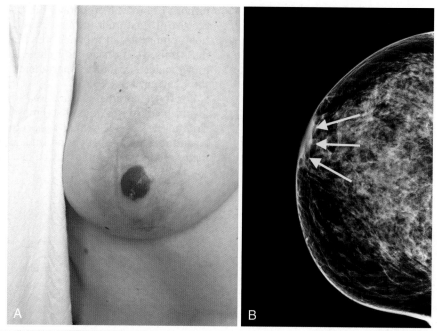

Fig. 15.4 Tis (Paget) Stage 0. A 62-year-old presenting with a persistent right nipple wound (A). Pathology from punch biopsy showed Paget disease of the nipple. Mammographic evaluation (B) shows subtle thickening of the areolar region (*arrows*). The patient opted for mastectomy rather than central lumpectomy and was shown at final pathology to have 1.5 cm of mammographically occult high-grade ductal carcinoma in situ (DCIS).

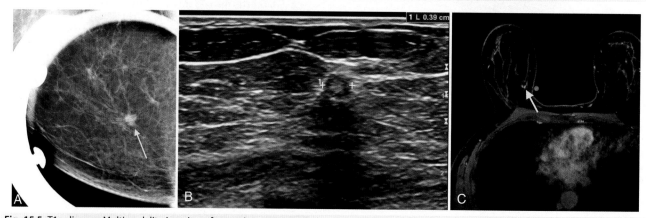

Fig. 15.5 T1a disease. Multimodality imaging of screening mammography detected right breast 0.4-cm invasive mixed ductal and lobular invasive carcinoma in a 69-year-old patient. (A) Spot compression view at the time of diagnostic evaluation demonstrates an irregular mass with spiculated margins (*arrow*). (B) Ultrasound demonstrates a corresponding irregular mass with angular margins measuring a maximum of 0.4 cm. (C) Preoperative breast magnetic resonance imaging (MRI) dynamic postcontrast sequence demonstrates the mass to be partially obscured by the signal void from the marker clip placed at the time of biopsy. No other sites of disease were present.

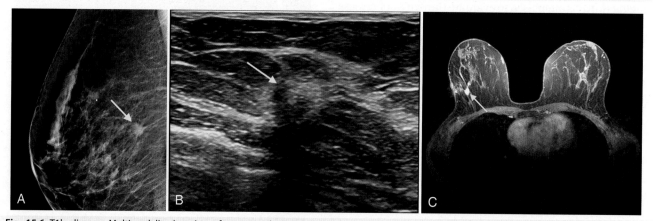

Fig. 15.6 T1b disease. Multimodality imaging of a screen-detected right breast 0.7-cm invasive ductal carcinoma in a 56-year-old patient. (A) Mammography demonstrates an irregular mass with spiculated margins (*arrow*). (B) Ultrasound demonstrates a corresponding nonparallel hypoechoic irregular mass with indistinct margins and posterior shadowing measuring 0.7 cm (*arrow*). (C) Preoperative breast magnetic resonance imaging (MRI) dynamic postcontrast image demonstrates unifocal irregular mass with irregular margins (*arrow*).

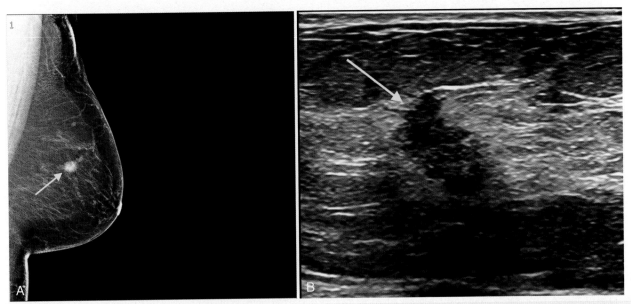

Fig. 15.7 T1c disease. A 66-year-old with a screen-detected 1.2- cm invasive ductal carcinoma in the left breast. (A) Mediolateral oblique (MLO) mammographic view demonstrates the irregular mass (*arrow*). (B) Ultrasound demonstrates a corresponding nonparallel irregular mass with angular margins and posterior shadowing, measuring a maximum dimension of 1.2 cm (*arrow*).

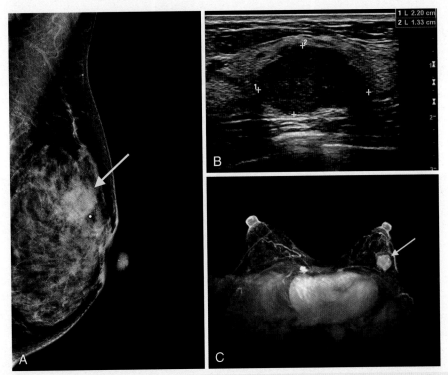

Fig. 15.8 T2 disease. A 45-year-old with a palpable 2.2- cm invasive ductal carcinoma in the left breast. (A) Mediolateral oblique (MLO) mammographic view demonstrates an obscured oval mass (*arrow*). (B) Ultrasound evaluation of the palpable finding demonstrates a corresponding oval mass with angular margins and posterior enhancement. (d) Subtracted maximum intensity projection (MIP) image from preoperative contrast enhance breast MR demonstrates a corresponding irregular mass with heterogeneous internal enhancement measuring 2.6 cm (*arrow*).

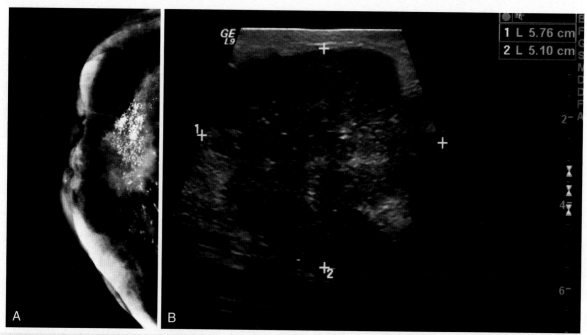

Fig. 15.9 T3 disease. A 65-year-old with a 5.8-cm locally advanced invasive ductal carcinoma in the right breast. (A) Craniocaudal (CC) mammographic view demonstrates an irregular mass with associated fine pleomorphic calcifications, skin thickening, and nipple retraction. (B) Ultrasound demonstrates a corresponding large irregular mass exceeding the width of the transducer.

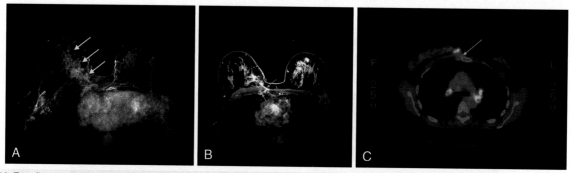

Fig. 15.10 T4a disease. A 61-year-old with a palpable estrogen receptor/progesterone receptor (ER/PR)-negative, human epidermal growth factor receptor (HER2)-positive invasive breast cancer. (A) Subtracted maximum intensity projection (MIP) image from contrast-enhanced breast magnetic resonance imaging (MRI) shows clumped segmental nonmass enhancement (*arrows*). (B) Delayed postcontrast sequence demonstrates tumor enhancement extending into the medial insertion of the pectoralis muscle and into the chest wall (*arrows*), including the intercostal muscle, surrounding the sternum. (C) Positron emission tomography–computed tomography (PET-CT) fusion image demonstrates uptake in the chest wall with a distribution similar to disease seen on breast MRI (*arrow*).

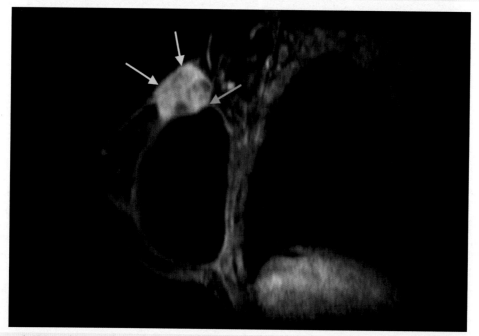

Fig. 15.11 T4b disease. A 47-year-old with estrogen receptor/progesterone receptor (ER/PR)-positive, human epidermal growth factor receptor (HER2)-negative invasive ductal carcinoma (IDC) that grew over a 2-year period with the patient presenting with clinical skin invasion. Sagittal T1 fat-saturated dynamic postcontrast magnetic resonance imaging (MRI) shows the mass invading the skin (*yellow arrows*) and mass effect on subglandular implant (*green arrow*).

cancers that directly invade the adjacent skin. Inflammatory carcinoma, T4d, is primarily a clinical diagnosis in a patient with a rapid onset of skin inflammation characterized by redness and peau d'orange and diffuse breast swelling involving greater than one-third of the breast.

ASSESSMENT OF THE N (LYMPH NODE) PARAMETER

Combination of axillary, supraclavicular, and internal mammary nodal involvement determines N. Imaging assessment

of the lymph nodes is covered in detail in Chapter 17. Ultrasound is highly sensitive when used in conjunction with fine-needle aspiration (FNA) or core biopsy to determine axillary lymph node involvement. Compared with surgery, imaging assessment of axillary status is relatively inexpensive. Evaluation of regional axillary lymph nodes is based on morphology and not size. Normal lymph nodes are oval in shape with a homogenously thin cortex. Suspicious features include round shape, thickened cortex, and complete or partial effacement of the fatty hilum. Box 15.3 summarizes lymph node imaging assessment criteria. The goal of axillary ultrasound was to identify nodal involvement before surgery to direct patients to a single-step axillary dissection or before neoadjuvant therapy to provide accurate pretreatment clinical nodal staging.

Fig. 15.16 is an illustration of regional axillary lymph nodes stations pertinent to breast cancer. The pectoralis minor is the landmark to determine the axillary node station. Level I is lateral/inferior to, level II is deep to, and level III is medial/superior to the pectoralis minor. Note that interpectoral, also known as Rotter, nodes are equivalent to level II in staging.

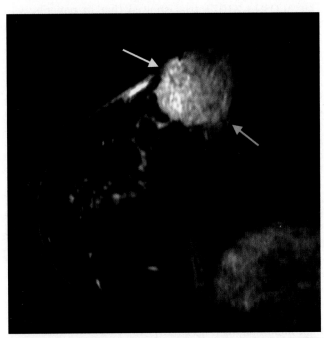

Fig. 15.12 T4c disease. A 56-year-old with biopsy-proven triple-negative invasive breast cancer. Sagittal T1 fat-saturated dynamic postcontrast magnetic resonance imaging (MRI) shows an irregular mass with heterogeneous internal enhancement invading both the skin (*yellow arrow*) and the chest wall (*green arrow*), including the intercostal muscles.

Box 15.3 Characterizing Lymph Node Morphology

- Normal morphology (Fig. 15.14)
  - Fatty hilum
  - Thin symmetric cortex
  - Reniform or oval shape
  - Circumscribed
  - Variable size (not as important as morphology)
  - T2 hyperintense on MRI
- Abnormal morphology (Fig. 15.15)
  - Compressed or obliterated fatty hilum
  - Thickened cortex >3 mm, asymmetric
  - Focal cortical bulge
  - Round or irregular shape
  - Indistinct margins

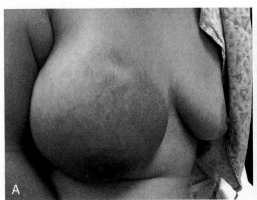
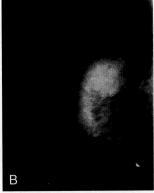
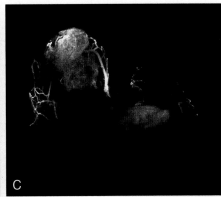

Fig. 15.13 T4d disease, inflammatory breast cancer. A 27-year-old with biopsy-proven triple-negative invasive ductal carcinoma with axillary nodal metastasis, subsequently found to have a *BRCA1* mutation. (A) Clinical image with diffuse enlargement, redness, and peau d'orange appearance throughout the entire right breast. (B) Mammographic mediolateral oblique (MLO) view demonstrates an irregular mass with indistinct margins and associated fine pleomorphic calcifications in the upper central right breast measuring 8 cm. There is associated skin thickening and trabecular thickening. (C) Subtracted maximum intensity projection (MIP) image from contrast-enhanced breast magnetic resonance imaging (MRI) demonstrates a heterogeneously enhancing irregular mass occupying the near entirety of the right breast measuring 12.1 cm in maximum extent. Tumor enhancement extends into the nipple-areolar complex anteriorly. The diagnosis of inflammatory breast cancer is based on clinical presentation. However, imaging features of skin and trabecular thickening, as in this case, can suggest inflammatory breast cancer.

Sentinel lymph node biopsy involves identifying and excising the sentinel lymph node(s) after intratumoral or periareolar injection of a traceable substance. This is the gold standard in evaluating axillary nodes. Traditionally, this involves preoperative lymphoscintigraphic mapping with the use of dual radiocolloid tracers (Fig. 15.17). This may be supplemented with intraoperative blue dye detection and intraoperative gamma probe. Newer methods include the detection of injected superparamagnetic iron oxide particles. Sentinel node biopsy may be therapeutic and is also essential for pathologic staging.

Clinical node-negative patients with invasive breast malignancy require a sentinel node biopsy. If the sentinel node(s) are positive, historically, a complete axillary lymph node dissection (ALND) would have been indicated. However, the ACOSOG Z0011 trial results demonstrated that in the absence of neoadjuvant therapy and for T1/T2 disease, patients with one or two positive sentinel lymph nodes (without extranodal extension) can be treated in the same manner as node-negative patients, without completion ALND. Further, in patients with axillary nodal metastasis who have undergone neoadjuvant therapy, breast surgeons increasingly perform targeted axillary dissection. The ACOSOG Z1071 trial showed that in patients with initially clinically positive axilla treated with neoadjuvant therapy, sentinel node biopsy alone had a false-negative rate of greater than 12% for detecting residual metastatic nodes. Thus the latest recommendations for patients with initially cN1 or cN2 disease with good response to neoadjuvant therapy are for targeted axillary dissection with excision of both the previously biopsied clipped positive node in addition to the sentinel node, which was found to reduce the false-negative rate to 2%. This emphasizes the importance of placing marker clips in lymph nodes that have undergone FNA or core biopsy.

The staging of lymph nodes can be performed based on clinical and imaging information (cN) or after surgical intervention (pN). Box 15.4 highlights the N categories. The full details can be found in AJCC Cancer Staging Manual eighth edition.

Involvement of the cervical lymph nodes or the contralateral axillary or internal mammary chain lymph nodes is considered M1 (Fig. 15.23). Ipsilateral intramammary lymph nodes are considered N1, while interpectoral lymph nodes (i.e., Rotter nodes) are considered equivalent to level II for nodal staging (Fig. 15.24).

ASSESSMENT OF THE M (METASTASES) PARAMETER

The National Comprehensive Cancer Network (NCCN) guidelines state that workup for metastasis (e.g., with PET,

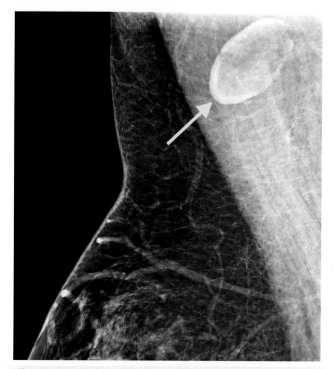

Fig. 15.14 Normal morphology node. Mammographic example of a normal morphology level I axillary lymph node demonstrating oval shape with circumscribed margins and thin cortex surrounding a fatty hilum.

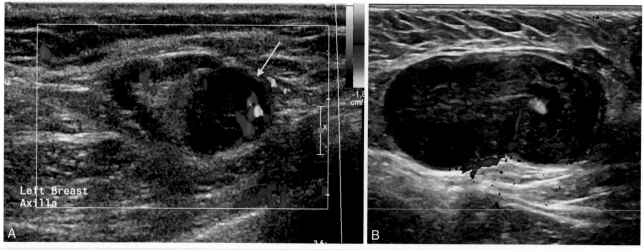

Fig. 15.15 Abnormal morphology lymph node. (A) A 56-year-old with a new diagnosis of invasive ductal carcinoma. Targeted ultrasound of the axilla demonstrates eccentric cortical thickening (*arrow*) in a level I axillary lymph node with associated compression of the fatty hilum. (B) A second example of abnormal morphology lymph node in a 60-year-old patient with invasive ductal carcinoma demonstrating complete obliteration of the fatty hilum.

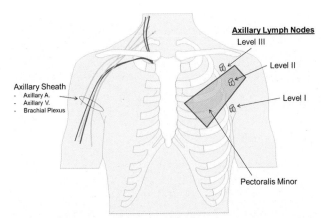

Fig. 15.16 Regional lymph node schematics. The axillary lymph nodes are evaluated based on the surgical levels determined by location relative to the pectoralis minor muscle. Level I: lateral/inferior to pectoralis minor. Level II: deep/posterior to pectoralis minor; interpectoral (Rotter) nodes are equivalent to level II in staging. Level III: medial and superior to pectoralis minor.

bone scintigraphy, or CT scan of chest/abdomen/pelvis) should be considered for patients with clinical stage IIIA or higher disease (i.e., primary tumor larger than 5 cm and/or skin or chest wall tumor involvement) or for patients with symptoms of metastasis. Systemic staging is also appropriate in patients with fixed axillary nodes, positive supraclavicular/infraclavicular and/or internal mammary chain lymph nodes, and inflammatory cancer. No clinical or radiographic evidence of distant metastases is classified as M0. M1 is used for distant detectable metastases as determined by classic clinical and radiographic means (cM1) and/or histologically proven metastasis in

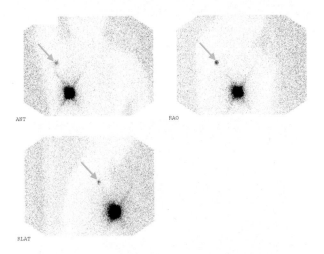

Fig. 15.17 Lymphoscintigraphy. A 57-year-old with invasive ductal carcinoma scheduled to undergo lumpectomy with sentinel lymph node biopsy. Preoperative lymphoscintigraphy demonstrates radiotracer uptake in a single sentinel lymph node in the right axilla (*arrow*).

Box 15.4   N Parameter Definitions

- NX Lymph node cannot be assessed
- N0 No regional metastatic disease
- N1 Metastases to movable ipsilateral level I and II axillary lymph nodes (Fig. 15.18)
- N2 Metastases in ipsilateral level I, II axillary lymph nodes that are clinically fixed or matted or in clinically detected ipsilateral internal mammary nodes in the absence of clinically evident axillary lymph node metastases
  N2a Metastases in ipsilateral level I, II axillary lymph nodes fixed to one another (matted) or to other structures (Fig. 15.19)
  N2b Metastases only in clinically detected ipsilateral internal mammary nodes and in the absence of clinically evident level I, II axillary lymph node metastases (Fig. 15.20)
- N3 Metastases in ipsilateral infraclavicular (level III axillary) lymph node(s) with or without level I, II axillary lymph node involvement or in clinically detected ipsilateral internal mammary lymph node(s) with clinically evident level I, II axillary lymph node metastases or metastases in ipsilateral supraclavicular lymph node(s) with or without axillary or internal mammary lymph node involvement
  N3a Metastases in ipsilateral infraclavicular lymph node(s) (Fig. 15.21)
  N3b Metastases in ipsilateral internal mammary lymph node(s) and axillary lymph node(s)
  N3c Metastases in ipsilateral supraclavicular lymph node(s) (Fig. 15.22)

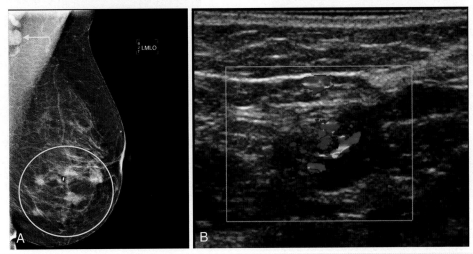

Fig. 15.18 N1 disease. A 58-year-old with a new diagnosis of left breast invasive ductal carcinoma and high-grade ductal carcinoma in situ (DCIS) presents with a palpable lump in the left axilla. (A) Mammographic mediolateral oblique (MLO) view demonstrates multicentric irregular breast masses (*circle*) with one associated biopsy clip. Within the axilla, there is a morphologically abnormal lymph node with loss of fatty hilum and round shape (*arrow*). (B) Ultrasound (US) evaluation with Doppler interrogation demonstrates a morphologically abnormal level I lymph node with obliteration of the fatty hilum.

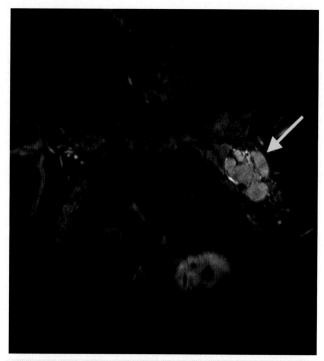

Fig. 15.19 N2a disease. Coronal T2 sequence from breast magnetic resonance imaging (MRI) demonstrates matted appearance of bulky left level I and II axillary lymph nodes (*arrow*).

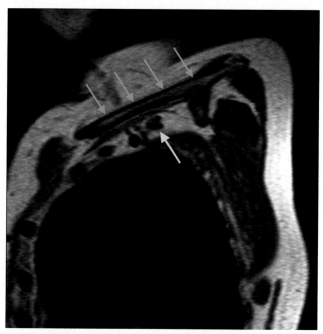

Fig. 15.21 N3a disease. T1 sagittal oblique view of the axilla in a 54-year-old with infraclavicular lymph node metastasis (*yellow arrow*). Green arrows outline the clavicle.

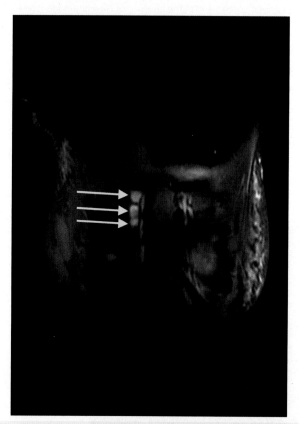

Fig. 15.20 N2b disease. A 35-year-old with right breast invasive mucinous carcinoma that is estrogen receptor/progesterone receptor (ER/PR) positive and human epidermal growth factor receptor (HER2) negative. Coronal T2 sequence from preoperative breast magnetic resonance imaging (MRI) shows ipsilateral internal mammary nodal metastasis (*arrows*). Level I and II axillary nodes were normal (not shown).

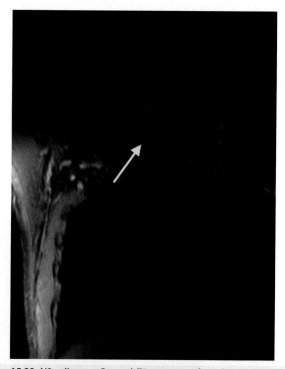

Fig. 15.22 N3c disease. Coronal T2 sequence from breast magnetic resonance imaging (MRI) demonstrates right supraclavicular lymphadenopathy. The patient initially presented with a right neck lump for which biopsy demonstrated metastatic invasive ductal carcinoma.

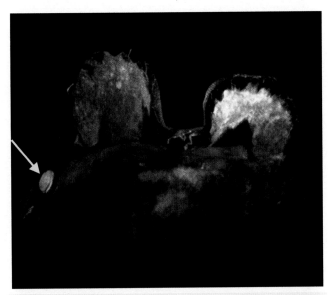

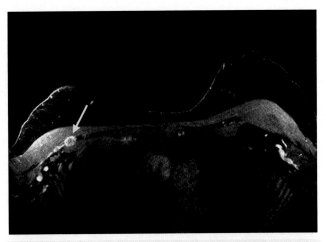

Fig. 15.24 Interpectoral lymph node, also known as Rotter lymph node (*arrow*) metastasis, is demonstrated in this axial T1 postcontrast breast magnetic resonance imaging (MRI). Interpectoral lymph nodes are equivalent to level II lymph nodes for the purposes of breast cancer staging.

Fig. 15.23 M1 disease. Axial thick maximum intensity projection (MIP) image from contrast-enhanced breast magnetic resonance imaging (MRI) of a patient clinically presenting with "vanishing" left breast (biopsy-proven invasive mammary carcinoma) and contralateral lymphadenopathy. Contralateral nodal metastasis is staged as M1 disease.

distant organs or larger than 0.2 mm deposits in nonregional lymph nodes (pM1). Examples of metastatic imaging findings are shown in Fig. 15.25. The four common sites for breast cancer metastasis include bone, lung, brain, and liver.

Multifocal and Multicentric Disease

Multifocal breast cancer is defined by the presence of two more tumor masses within a single quadrant of the breast (Fig. 15.26). Multicentric breast cancer is defined by the presence of two more tumor masses within different

quadrants of the same breast (Fig. 15.27). For TNM staging, tumor size is assessed by the largest individual tumor mass. Satellite masses are not added up for the T stage. Total disease extent is used to determine resectability. Multifocal/multicentric breast cancer is an independent breast cancer prognostic factor.

Putting It All Together

Anatomic stage is summarized in Table 15.3. The stage is a major prognostic factor for breast cancer. As the stage at the time of diagnosis increases, the survival rate dramatically decreases. The goal of screening mammography, and supplemental screening MRI and US, is to find breast cancers when they are small (less than 1.5 cm) in size and early-stage to reduce patient morbidity and mortality.

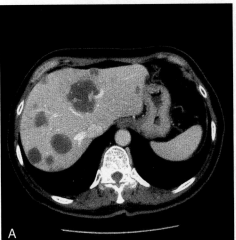

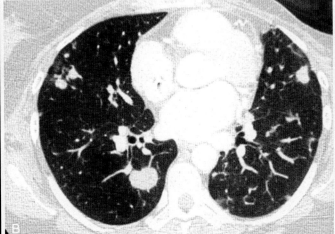

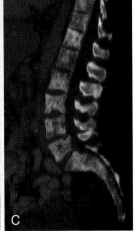

Fig. 15.25 Metastasis. Examples of metastatic disease in different patients. (A) Abdominal computed tomography (CT) demonstrating liver metastases in a 57-year-old with inflammatory breast cancer. (B) Chest CT demonstrating bilateral pulmonary metastases in a 54-year-old with breast cancer that invades the chest wall. (C) Sagittal reformatted CT with bone window in a 69-year-old with invasive ductal carcinoma demonstrating diffuse sclerotic and lytic lesions throughout the spine consistent with osseous metastases.

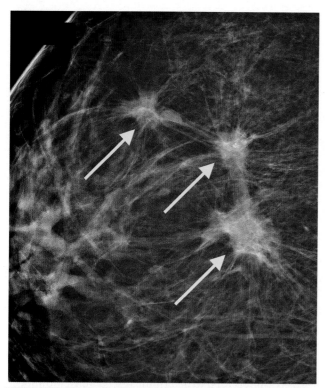

Fig. 15.26 Multifocal disease. Spot compression magnification mammogram shows three irregular masses with spiculated margins (*arrows*). Masses on mammography and magnetic resonance imaging (MRI) (not shown) were found to be confined to a single quadrant of the breast.

Table 15.3   Anatomic StageAnatomic Stage/Prognostic Groups

Stage	Tumor	Node	Metastasis
Stage 0	Tis	N0	M0
Stage IA	T1*	N0	M0
Stage IB	T0	N1mi	M0
Stage IIA	T0	N1**	M0
	T1*	N1**	M0
	T2	N0	M0
Stage IIB	T2	N1	M0
	T3	N0	M0
Stage IIIA	T0	N2	M0
	T1*	N2	M0
	T2	N2	M0
	T3	N1	M0
	T3	N2	M0
Stage IIIB	T4	N0	M0
	T4	N1	M0
	T4	N2	M0
Stage IIIC	Any T	N3	M0
Stage IV	Any T	Any N	M1

Used with permission of the American College of Surgeons, Chicago, Illinois. The original source for this information is the AJCC Cancer Staging System (2020).

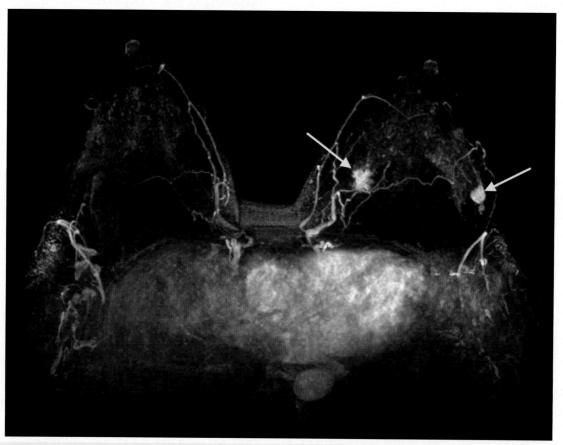

Fig. 15.27 Multicentric disease. A 54-year-old woman with estrogen receptor/progesterone receptor (ER/PR) positive, human epidermal growth factor receptor (HER2) positive, multicentric invasive ductal breast cancer. Subtracted maximum intensity projection (MIP) image from contrast-enhanced breast magnetic resonance imaging (MRI) demonstrates two masses in the medial and lateral left breast (*arrows*).

- The anatomic stage of breast cancer, along with its biological type, determines treatment options and prognosis.
- Traditional anatomic staging is based only on the anatomic extent of the tumor as defined by the T, N, and M categories.
- The eighth edition of the American Joint Committee on Cancer (AJCC) staging guidelines implemented the prognostic stage, which incorporates tumor biomarkers (tumor grade, estrogen receptor [ER], progesterone receptor [PR], human epidermal growth factor receptor [HER2]) to calculate 5-year survival.
- Luminal A cancers have the best prognosis, while triple-negative cancers and HER2-enriched cancers are more aggressive and have a poorer prognosis.
- The goal of screening is to diagnose breast cancers at an earlier stage when treatments are more effective and survival is improved.

Suggested Reading

AJCC . In: Amin MB, ed. *Cancer Staging Manual.* 8th ed. New York: Springer-Verlag; 2017.

American Cancer Society. *Breast Cancer Facts and Figures 2019-2020.* Atlanta, Ga: American Cancer Society; 2019.

Adrada BE, Candelaria R, Rauch GM. MRI for the staging and evaluation of response to therapy in breast cancer. *Top Magn Reson Imaging.* 2017;26(5):211–218. https://doi.org/10.1097/RMR.0000000000000147.

D'Orsi CJ, Sickles EA, Mendelson EB, Morris EA, et al. ACR BI-RADS® Atlas, Breast Imaging Reporting and Data System. Reston, VA, American College of Radiology; 2013.

Cools-Lartigue, et al. Pre-operative axillary ultrasound and fine-needle aspiration biopsy in the diagnosis of axillary metastases in patients with breast cancer; predictors of accuracy and future implications. *Ann Surg Oncol.* 2013;20(3):819–827.

Giuliano AE, Edge SB, Hortobagyi GN. Eighth Edition of the AJCC Cancer Staging Manual: Breast Cancer. *Ann Surg Oncol.* 2018;25(7):1783–1785. https://doi.org/10.1245/s10434-018-6486-6.

Günhan-Bilgen I, Ustün EE, Memiş A. Inflammatory breast carcinoma: mammographic, ultrasonographic, clinical, and pathologic findings in 142 cases. *Radiology.* 2002;223(3):829–838.

Hortobagyi GN, Connolly JL, D'Orsi CJ, et al. Breast. In: Amin MB, Edge S, Greene F, eds. *American Joint Committee on Cancer. AJCC cancer staging manual.* 8th ed. New York, NY: Springer; 2017:589–636.

Hortobagyi GN, Edge SB, Giuliano A. New and Important Changes in the TNM Staging System for Breast Cancer. *Am Soc Clin Oncol Educ Book.* 2018;38:457–467. https://doi.org/10.1200/EDBK_201313.

Houssami N, Ciatto S, Macaskill P, et al. Accuracy and surgical impact of magnetic resonance imaging in breast cancer staging: systematic review and meta-analysis in detection of multifocal and multicentric cancer. *J Clin Oncol.* 2008;26(19):3248–3258.

Kriege M, Brekelmans CTM, Boetes C, et al. Efficacy of MRI and mammography for breast-cancer screening in women with a familial or genetic predisposition. *N Engl J Med.* 2004;351(5):427–437.

Kuhl CK, Schrading S, Leutner CC, et al. Mammography, breast ultrasound, and magnetic resonance imaging for surveillance of women at high familial risk for breast cancer. *J Clin Oncol.* 2005;23(33):8469–8476.

Key Statistics for Breast Cancer. How common is breast cancer? American Cancer Society. https://www.cancer.org/cancer/breast-cancer/about/how-common-is-breast-cancer.html. Last revised January 12, 2022. Accessed January 28, 2022.

Lowes S, Leaver A, Cox K, Satchithananda K, Cosgrove D, Lim A. Evolving imaging techniques for staging axillary lymph nodes in breast cancer. *Clin Radiol.* 2018;73(4):396–409. https://doi.org/10.1016/j.crad.2018.01.003.

Lynch SP, Lei X, Chavez-MacGregor M, et al. Multifocality and multicentricity in breast cancer and survival outcomes. *Ann Oncol.* 2012;23(12):3063–3069.

Macia F, et al. Factors affecting 5- and 10-year survival of women with breast cancer: an analysis based on a public general hospital in Barcelona. *Cancer Epidemiology.* 2012 Dec;36(6):544–549.

Mittendorf EA, Bartlett JMS, Lichtensztajn DL, Chandarlapaty S. Incorporating biology into breast cancer staging: American Joint Committee on Cancer, Eighth Edition, revisions and beyond. *Am Soc Clin Oncol Educ Book.* 2018;38:38–46. https://doi.org/10.1200/EDBK_200981.

Morrow M, Waters J, Morris E. MRI for breast cancer screening, diagnosis, and treatment. *Lancet.* 2011;378(9805):1804–1811.

Plichta JK, Campbell BM, Mittendorf EA, Hwang ES. Anatomy and breast cancer staging: is it still relevant? *Surg Oncol Clin N Am.* 2018;27(1):51–67. https://doi.org/10.1016/j.soc.2017.07.010.

Ravaioli A, Pasini G, Polselli A, et al. Staging of breast cancer: new recommended standard procedure. *Breast Cancer Res Treat.* 2002;72(1):53–60.

Rosen et al. FDG PET, PET/CT, and breast cancer imaging. *Radiographics.* 2007 Oct;27:S215–S229.

Rosenberg RD, Yankaskasb C, Abrahaml A, et al. Performance benchmarks for screening mammography. *Radiology.* 2006;241(1):55–66.

Saslow D, Boetes C, Burke W, et al. for the American Cancer Society Breast Cancer Advisory Group. American Cancer Society guidelines for breast screening with MRI as an adjunct to mammography. *CA Cancer J Clin.* 2007;57:75–89. Available at: http://caonline.amcancersoc.org/cgi/content/full/57/2/75. Accessed July 17, 2008.

Selleck M, Senthil M. Implications of abnormal pre-operative axillary imaging in the post Z011 era. *Gland Surg.* 2016;5(3):372–374. https://doi.org/10.21037/gs.2016.04.03.

Sicklese A, Miglioretti Dl, Ballard-Barbash R, et al. Performance benchmarks for diagnostic mammography. *Radiology.* 2005;235(3):775–790.

The California Breast Density Information Group: A Collaborative Response to the Issues of Breast Density, Breast Cancer Risk, and Breast Density Notification Legislation. *Radiology.* 2013:131–217.

Voduc KD, Cheang MC, Tyldesley S, Gelmon K, Nielsen TO, Kennecke H. Breast cancer subtypes and the risk of local and regional relapse. *J Clin Oncol.* 2010;28(10):1684–1691.

Weiss A, King TA, Hunt KK, Mittendorf EA. Incorporating Biologic Factors into the American Joint Committee on Cancer Breast Cancer Staging System: Review of the Supporting Evidence. *Surg Clin North Am.* 2018;98(4):687–702. https://doi.org/10.1016/j.suc.2018.03.005.

Whitman GJ, Sheppard DG, Phelps MJ, Gonzales BN. Breast cancer staging. *Semin Roentgenol.* 2006;41(2):91–104.

Yamashita M, Hovanessian-Larsen L, Sener SF. The role of axillary ultrasound in the detection of metastases from primary breast cancers. *Am J Surg.* 2013;205(3):242–244. discussion 244–245.

Yang WT. Staging of breast cancer with ultrasound. *Semin Ultrasound CT MR.* 2011;32(4):331–341. https://doi.org/10.1053/j.sult.2011.02.008.

Yen TW, Hunt KK, Ross MI, et al. Predictors of invasive breast cancer in patients with an initial diagnosis of ductal carcinoma in situ: a guide to selective use of sentinel lymph node biopsy in management of ductal carcinoma in situ. *J Am Coll Surg.* 2005;200(4):516–526.

16 After Breast Conservation Therapy

GAIANE M. RAUCH, MARY S. GUIRGUIS, AND BEATRIZ E. ADRADA

OVERVIEW *This chapter will review the definition of breast conservation therapy, indications for this therapy, principles of preoperative tumor localization and surgical specimen radiography, surveillance after breast conservation therapy, expected changes after breast conservation therapy, and typical imaging findings of residual disease or recurrent cancer.*

The optimal therapy for breast cancer is based on a multidisciplinary approach and collaborative effort of breast radiologists, surgeons, oncologists, pathologists, breast reconstructive surgeons, and radiation oncologists who together develop the best treatment plan for each patient. The aims of treatment are to completely excise the tumor using the appropriate surgical option (i.e., the option that optimizes locoregional control and overall survival while ensuring an acceptable cosmetic outcome) and to eradicate any possible microscopic tumor deposits with radiation therapy and/or systemic therapy. The choice of treatment plan depends on multiple factors, including cancer stage, hormonal subtype, local disease extent, tumor multicentricity and multifocality, contraindications to radiation therapy, and the patient's own preference. Tumor excision is achieved with either mastectomy, which is surgical removal of the whole tumor-harboring breast, or lumpectomy, also referred to as breast conservation surgery (BCS), which is excision of the tumor with a safe margin. BCS is usually followed by whole-breast radiation therapy.

Radiologists play an important role in the care of patients who undergo breast conservation therapy (BCT) and thus must be familiar with the principles of this treatment approach. Specifically, radiologists play an important role in patient selection, presurgical planning, and intraoperative imaging guidance in patients undergoing BCT. Furthermore, radiologists must have knowledge of the imaging appearance and evolution of benign posttreatment changes in the breast after BCT to ensure appropriate posttreatment surveillance and timely detection of residual or recurrent disease.

This chapter will review the definition of BCT, indications for BCT, principles of preoperative tumor localization and surgical specimen radiography, post-BCT surveillance, expected post-BCT changes, and typical imaging findings of residual or recurrent cancer.

Breast Conservation Therapy

DEFINITION AND HISTORY

BCT includes tumor excision followed by adjuvant whole-breast radiation therapy (Box 16.1). Surgical staging of the axilla usually is also performed. Additionally, systemic hormonal therapy or cytotoxic therapy may be administered after surgery to eradicate microscopic residual disease ("adjuvant systemic therapy") or before surgery to downstage the primary malignancy ("neoadjuvant systemic therapy").

BCS was first described by Sir Geoffrey Keynes, an English surgeon at St. Bartholomew's Hospital in London in 1924. BCS is defined as the removal of a breast cancer with clear surgical margins. It has also been referred to as "lumpectomy," "wide local excision," "segmental resection," "partial mastectomy," "quadrantectomy," and "tylectomy."

Studies showed that whole-breast radiation therapy after BCS significantly improved outcomes of breast cancer patients. Multiple randomized trials have been conducted showing similar overall survival after mastectomy and BCT. In 1990, a National Institutes of Health consensus panel advised that BCT is an appropriate primary therapy for the majority of women with early (stage I or II) breast cancer. More recently, neoadjuvant systemic therapy has increasingly been used for preoperative treatment of patients with more advanced breast cancer, rendering some patients eligible for BCT rather than total mastectomy, depending on the response to the treatment.

ONCOPLASTIC BCS

The term "oncoplastic surgery" was introduced by a German surgeon, Dr. Werner Audretsch, in 1993, when he first described the technique of repairing defects from BCS

Box 16.1 Breast Conservation Therapy: Definition and Requirements

Definition

- Surgical excision of the primary tumor (breast conservation surgery) followed by whole-breast radiation therapy

Requirements for Successful BCT

- Surgical excision of the primary tumor with negative margins
- Acceptable postsurgical cosmetic appearance of the breast
- Patient's ability to receive radiation therapy
- Ability to perform follow-up breast imaging

using plastic surgery. Oncoplastic BCS gained popularity, since it provided patients with better cosmetic results than simple BCS. Oncoplastic BCS encompasses a variety of techniques that allow resection of a breast cancer with wide surgical margins while preserving the shape and appearance of the breast. Oncoplastic BCS usually includes excision of the primary tumor with clear margins, immediate soft tissue rearrangement, and if needed, contralateral breast procedures to achieve symmetry. The two most commonly used oncoplastic techniques are (1) repair of the defect by transposition of tissue from elsewhere in the breast and (2) filling of the defect with local tissue or with autologous fat grafting. Collaboration between breast surgery and plastic surgery teams is necessary to achieve the best oncological and cosmetic outcomes.

SURGICAL MANAGEMENT OF THE AXILLA

The initial site of metastatic disease for breast cancer patients is usually axillary lymph nodes. Therefore correct assessment of axillary nodal status is of outmost importance for breast cancer patients. For patients undergoing BCT who have a clinically negative axillary nodes (i.e., by physical examination and/or imaging), sentinel lymph node biopsy during BCT is generally the standard initial approach. Intraoperative injection of blue dye, radioactive tracer, or both is traditionally used to identify the sentinel lymph node. At some institutions, presurgical lymphoscintigraphy following radioactive tracer injection, usually in the peritumoral or periareolar region, is used to localize the sentinel lymph node before surgery (Fig. 16.1). Axillary lymph node management, including sentinel lymph node biopsy, targeted axillary dissection, and indications for complete axillary dissection are covered in detail in Chapters 15 and 17.

Patient Selection for BCT

Careful patient selection for BCT is very important to minimize risk of recurrence. In order to achieve successful BCT, it must be possible to excise the primary tumor with negative margins and acceptable cosmetic results, the patient typically must be able to receive radiation therapy, and the patient must be amenable to performing follow-up imaging of the breast to detect local recurrence (see Box 16.1).

Patients who are generally not candidates for BCT include those with a high probability of recurrence, those with contraindications to radiation therapy, those at risk for a poor cosmetic outcome, and those who prefer mastectomy.

CONTRAINDICATIONS TO BCT

Patients with extensive malignant microcalcifications occupying the majority of the breast are not suitable candidates for BCT (Box 16.2). This mammographic presentation suggests diffuse ductal carcinoma in situ (DCIS), which precludes achievement of negative margins. In addition, patients in whom negative surgical margins are not achievable without compromising the cosmetic appearance of the breast are not candidates for BCT. A history of prior therapeutic radiation therapy delivered to the breast region or mediastinum/lung also often excludes BCT as a treatment option. This category includes patients with Hodgkin disease who received chest wall radiation during adolescence or early adulthood. Pregnancy is a major contraindication to radiation therapy, which cannot be administered during any gestational period because of scatter exposure to the fetus. However, BCS may be performed during the third trimester of pregnancy, with radiation therapy deferred to after delivery.

Multifocal and multicentric breast cancers are no longer absolute contraindications to BCT. However, the number of lesions, their size, location, and relationship to each other determine whether it is possible to resect all tumors with negative margins and an acceptable cosmetic outcome and thus influence whether BCT is feasible (Fig. 16.2). Specific types of collagen vascular disease, including active scleroderma and, to a lesser degree, active systemic lupus erythematosus, are relative contraindications because of the risk of radiation toxicity (see Box 16.2). Tumor size relative to breast size is another important consideration in selecting patients for BCT. A large tumor in a small breast is a relative contraindication, since an adequate resection would result in poor cosmetic outcome. Neoadjuvant chemotherapy or hormonal therapy can reduce tumor size significantly and allow for BCT with acceptable rates of local recurrence. Eligibility for BCT depends on the extent of tumor after, not before, neoadjuvant systemic therapy.

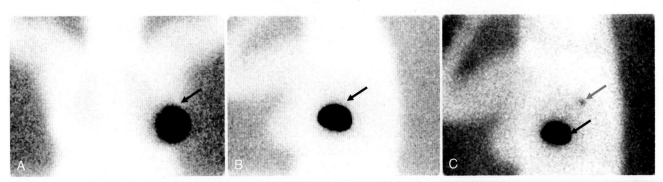

Fig. 16.1 Lymphoscintigraphy for sentinel lymph node localization. (A, B) Anterior (A) and lateral (B) views obtained 1 hour after peritumoral injection of radiotracer show intense radiotracer activity in the injection site in the left breast (*arrows*). (C) Lateral view obtained 3 hours after radiotracer injection shows focal uptake in the axillary sentinel lymph node (*blue arrow*).

Box 16.2   Contraindications to Breast Conservation Therapy

Absolute

- Diffuse, malignant microcalcifications on the preoperative mammogram
- Inability to achieve negative surgical margins with satisfactory cosmetic result
- Pregnancy (possible if radiation performed after delivery)

Relative

- Multicentric disease
- Collagen vascular disease (e.g., active scleroderma and active systemic lupus erythematosus)
- Prior radiation therapy delivered to breast or chest wall
- Large primary tumor size relative to breast size

Preoperative Tumor Localization for BCT and Specimen Radiography

Preoperative tumor localization and adequate postoperative assessment of the radiograph of the excised surgical specimen are crucial components of successful BCT. These techniques help achieve negative margins, the most important factor influencing locoregional recurrence. Surgical margin is defined as the closest distance between the free inked edge of the excised surgical specimen and cancer cells. As mentioned above, a negative margin after BCS is a prerequisite for successful BCT.

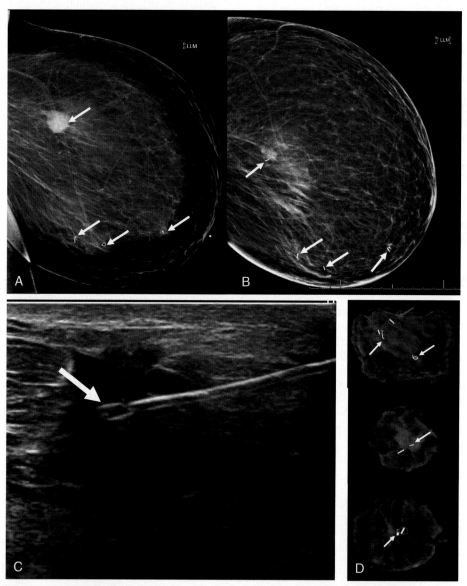

Fig. 16.2 Breast conservation therapy (BCT) in multicentric breast cancer. (A) Lateromedial mammogram in a woman with multicentric invasive ductal carcinoma denoted by four clips in the breast (*arrows*). She received neoadjuvant chemotherapy, with a good response. Given the large size of the breast, she underwent BCT. (B) Lateromedial mammogram after preoperative localization shows four areas of residual malignancy with ^{125}I radioactive seeds (*arrows*) placed next to the clips for intraoperative guidance. (C) A representative ultrasound image shows deployment of a ^{125}I radioactive seed (*arrow*) within the index mass under ultrasound guidance. (D) Intraoperative specimen radiographs demonstrate removal of all four lesions with associated clips (*arrows*) and ^{125}I radioactive seeds (*red circles*) with clear margins. One of the seeds (*blue arrow*) migrated during specimen handling.

Box 16.3 Preoperative Tumor Localization and Intraoperative Specimen Radiography

Preoperative Tumor Localization Methods

- Wire localization
  - Performed same day as surgery
  - External wire
  - Inexpensive
- Nonwire localization
  - Radioactive seed
  - Magnetic seed (Magseed)
  - Radar reflector (SAVI SCOUT)
  - Radiofrequency identification tag
  - Scheduling flexibility
  - No external component
  - Higher cost than wire

Intraoperative Specimen Radiography

- Confirm complete removal of target lesion
- Evaluate status of surgical margins
- Document removal of all targeted biopsy clip(s) and localization device(s) placed before surgery

---

Preoperative localization procedures and intraoperative specimen radiography are reviewed in detail in Chapter 7, but we provide a brief overview here.

PREOPERATIVE TUMOR LOCALIZATION

BCT usually requires preoperative image-guided placement of a device in or adjacent to the tumor to help the surgeon identify and successfully excise the target lesion (Box 16.3). Careful review of preoperative imaging and histopathologic findings is necessary for adequate planning of preoperative localization procedures. In carefully selected patients with multifocal or multicentric breast cancer, accurate presurgical tumor localization makes BCT possible (see Fig. 16.2).

For decades, the standard technique for preoperative tumor localization was wire-guided localization, in which a wire is percutaneously introduced into the tumor under ultrasound, mammographic, or magnetic resonance imaging (MRI) guidance. With this technique, surgery must be performed on the same day as wire placement, and care must be taken to assure stability of wire position before surgery. More recently, nonwire-guided localization devices have emerged as a safe alternative. These include use of radioactive and magnetic seeds (Magseed), radar reflectors (SAVI SCOUT), and radiofrequency identification tags. These devices can be placed percutaneously in the tumor many days before surgery, with some even placed at the time of biopsy, allowing scheduling flexibility and convenience for patients. A special probe is usually needed for intraoperative detection of these nonwire devices.

INTRAOPERATIVE SPECIMEN RADIOGRAPHY

Intraoperative specimen radiography is an essential part of BCT. Final pathologic evaluation of the breast surgical specimen is time consuming, and results usually are not available until days after surgery. Intraoperative specimen radiography is used to confirm complete removal of the target lesion and evaluate the status of the surgical margins during surgery. Intraoperative specimen radiography is also used to document removal of the clip placed in the target lesion during biopsy, as well as removal of the localization device if presurgical tumor localization was performed (see Box 16.3).

Collaboration between the breast surgeon, pathologist, and radiologist is needed for timely and accurate evaluation of the specimen radiograph. The excised surgical specimen is marked by the surgeon in the operating room to indicate orientation of the tumor margins. A radiograph of the en bloc specimen then is acquired, and the edges of the specimen are marked with ink to indicate margins. Some institutions also slice the specimen in thin sections and acquire a radiograph of the tissue slices as an additional tool for margin evaluation. If intraoperative specimen radiography review by radiologist reveals positive margins, the surgeon is immediately notified, and the surgeon reexcises the edges of the surgical cavity where the specimen radiograph indicates that the target lesion abuts the inked edge of the specimen (Fig. 16.3). It has been shown that intraoperative specimen radiography impacts intraoperative decision making in patients undergoing BCT and substantially decreases the rate of reexcision due to positive margins found at final surgical pathology.

Posttreatment Surveillance

According to the National Comprehensive Cancer Network (NCCN) and the American Society of Clinical Oncology (ASCO) guidelines, surveillance in patients with history of breast cancer should include physical examination and mammography. Approximately 50% of recurrences are detected by mammography, while the rest are detected by clinical examination or reported by the patient. Imaging surveillance in patients who have undergone BCT includes postoperative mammography and correlation of findings with pertinent elements of the patient's clinical history, such as the date and type of surgical treatment, the presence of surgical complications, palpable masses, and comparison with previous mammograms (Box 16.4).

The American College of Radiology (ACR) has not put forth a universal post-BCT imaging protocol but rather allows surveillance to vary per local institutional protocols. Mammography is a critical element of post-BCT imaging, while breast ultrasound and breast MRI are used in certain subsets of patients.

MAMMOGRAPHY

After BCT, mammography remains the modality of choice for surveillance, both to evaluate for tumor recurrence in the treated breast and to screen for contralateral breast cancer. Both the NCCN and ASCO recommend that patients undergo bilateral mammography no sooner than 6 months after the completion of radiation therapy and annually thereafter (Box 16.5). Ipsilateral tumor recurrence more commonly occurs within the first 5 years after BCT and is more likely to occur at the site of the original tumor. Therefore the NCCN and ASCO recommend that patients who have undergone BCT be closely

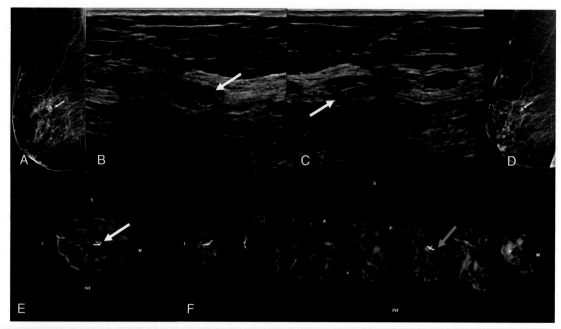

Fig. 16.3 Preoperative tumor localization and intraoperative specimen radiography. (A) Mediolateral oblique mammogram shows a 1.2-cm obscured mass with a clip (*arrow*) in the right breast representing biopsy-proven invasive ductal carcinoma. (B) Ultrasound image shows a corresponding hypoechoic mass with a clip (*arrow*). (C) A magnetic seed (*arrow*) was placed in the lesion adjacent to the clip under sonographic guidance. (D) Mediolateral oblique mammogram after ultrasound-guided preoperative localization confirms magnetic seed placement next to the clip (*arrow*). (E) Intraoperative whole-specimen radiograph demonstrates removal of the target lesion with clip and magnetic seed (*arrow*) without suspicious margins. (F) Intraoperative radiographic evaluation of the sliced specimen shows the target lesion at the posterior margin (*blue arrow*), suggestive of a positive margin. The surgeon was immediately notified and the posterior edge of the surgical cavity was reexcised by surgeon while patient was still in the operating room. Pathologic evaluation confirmed a positive initial posterior margin and a negative posterior margin after reexcision. *S*, Superior; *L*, lateral; *M*, medial; *I*, inferior; *P*, posterior; *A*, anterior.

Box 16.4   Mammographic Surveillance After Breast Conservation Therapy

- Correlation of findings with patient's clinical history
  - Type of cancer (e.g., invasive lobular carcinoma, invasive ductal carcinoma, ductal carcinoma in situ)
  - Date and type of surgical treatment and date of radiation therapy
  - History of early and late surgical complications
- Mammogram with additional views as needed
- Comparison of postoperative mammogram with preoperative mammogram
- Placement of radiopaque markers to indicate the surgical scar, dermal lesions, and palpable abnormalities

Box 16.5   Protocol for Surveillance After Breast Conservation Therapy

Mammography

- Baseline postoperative mammogram performed 6 months after the completion of radiation therapy
- The American College of Radiology allows institutions to vary their imaging protocol to best serve their patient population
- Many institutions perform diagnostic mammography annually or every 6 months for the first 3–5 years after completion of radiation therapy, after which patients are returned to routine screening mammography

Breast Ultrasound

- Usually reserved for evaluation of suspicious or indeterminate mammographic findings and for evaluation of focal breast signs/symptoms

Breast Magnetic Resonance Imaging

- May be considered for problem solving when mammographic or sonographic findings are indeterminate
- The ACR recommends annual supplemental surveillance in women with a personal history of breast cancer and dense breast parenchyma and women with a history of breast cancer diagnosed by age 50 years

followed clinically during that period. Correspondingly, during the first 3 to 5 years after BCT, most institutions perform diagnostic mammography annually or every 6 months, with specific protocols varying by institution. Afterward, patients are returned to routine screening mammography.

The mammographic workup should include standard views (craniocaudal, mediolateral oblique, and lateromedial views) and any additional views as deemed necessary by the radiologist (e.g., spot compression, tomosynthesis, tangential, and magnification views). Placement of radiopaque markers on the breast to indicate scars, dermal lesions, and palpable masses is critical to ensure an adequate mammographic evaluation. The interpretation of mammographic findings after BCT can be challenging because of

postsurgical and postradiation changes. Stability of mammographic findings after BCT can be established when there is no interval change in serial mammographic examinations and often occurs within 2 to 3 years after completion of radiation therapy.

BREAST ULTRASOUND AND BREAST MRI

Breast ultrasound is not routinely performed for surveillance after BCT. Instead, breast ultrasound is usually reserved for further workup of suspicious or indeterminate mammographic findings or for concerning clinical signs or symptoms, such as a palpable lump, nipple retraction, or signs of infection.

There is no consensus regarding the role of breast MRI as an adjunct to mammography in patients with a history of breast cancer. Several studies have advocated the addition of breast MRI in patients with history of breast cancer given the low sensitivity of mammography secondary to BCT changes and reported two-fold increase in incremental cancer yield with breast MRI. Therefore in addition to the established indications for high-risk screening, the ACR now also recommends annual breast MRI for two groups: (1) women with a personal history of breast cancer and dense breast parenchyma and (2) women with a history of breast cancer diagnosed by age 50 (see Box 16.5). In some scenarios, breast MRI may also be used as a problem-solving tool to further characterize indeterminate mammographic or sonographic findings, though this should be done sparingly and with discretion.

Imaging Features of Benign Posttreatment Findings

The most common benign posttreatment breast findings are fluid collection (e.g., seroma/hematoma), skin and trabecular thickening, postsurgical scar with architectural distortion, fat necrosis and rim calcifications, and other benign calcifications (e.g., dystrophic and suture) (Box 16.6).

SEROMA

After BCS, fluid and blood products often accumulate in the surgical cavity, resulting in a seroma. Mammographically, a seroma presents as an oval or round mass with circumscribed or obscured margins. Because of the associated scarring, the margins can also appear indistinct or spiculated. The collection may become more evident as the surrounding postoperative inflammatory changes subside. Sonographically, postsurgical fluid collections can have varying complexity, presenting as a circumscribed simple or complex cystic mass with debris and septations. On MRI, postoperative collections demonstrate high T2 signal and circumscribed margins. A thin rim of enhancement is sometimes seen and is considered benign. High T1 signal can be seen if imaging is performed shortly after surgery (Fig. 16.4). Seromas are seen in up to 50% of patients at 4

Box 16.6   Benign Posttreatment Imaging Findings After Breast Conservation Therapy

- Seroma or hematoma
- Postradiation skin and trabecular thickening
- Postsurgical scar
- Architectural distortion
- Fat necrosis and associated rim or dystrophic calcifications
- Suture calcifications

---

weeks and 25% of patients at 6 months after surgery. The collection gradually resorbs over the subsequent months, usually resolving completely by 12 to 18 months, as scarring and fibrosis develop within the postsurgical cavity (Fig. 16.5). In some instances, however, a chronic seroma can persist for years.

POSTRADIATION SKIN AND TRABECULAR THICKENING

Unlike postsurgical changes, which tend to be confined to the postsurgical cavity, postradiation changes typically involve the breast diffusely. On mammography, findings include diffuse skin and trabecular thickening, overall increased breast density, and subcutaneous edema (Fig. 16.6). Periareolar edema is frequently observed because of disruption of the lymphatic channels. These findings are most pronounced in the months after completion of radiation therapy, often apparent at the time of the first posttreatment mammogram at approximately 6 months after the completion of radiation therapy. The findings typically subside or remain stable over the following 2 to 3 years. Sonographically, patients present with diffuse edema, skin thickening, increased trabecular echogenicity, and shadowing. On MRI, diffuse skin thickening and edema is seen without skin enhancement (Fig. 16.7). The degree of skin thickening should improve or remain stable over time. Worsening skin thickening warrants further workup and correlation with physical examination findings, as in some instances this could represent tumor recurrence or inflammatory breast cancer. The differential considerations for unilateral skin thickening include infection, lymphedema, and obstructed venous drainage.

POSTSURGICAL SCAR AND ARCHITECTURAL DISTORTION

The postsurgical scar at the lumpectomy site is usually easily identified by mammography. Often, surgical clips or a BioZorb device are implanted by the surgeon within the postsurgical cavity to mark the site of the malignancy to guide radiation therapy (see Fig. 16.6). Mammographically, the scar presents as a focal asymmetry or an obscured or spiculated mass. The prominence of the postsurgical scar will decrease with time, especially over the first 2 years after BCT, after which the scar usually remains stable.

Sonographically, the postsurgical scar is seen as a disruption of the normal breast parenchymal planes, or a hypoechoic irregular mass with associated posterior shadowing. The surgical clips or BioZorb device can sometimes be seen as echogenic foci with shadowing or "comet-tail" artifact. The scar can sometime be traced extending vertically to the skin surface when scanning in real time. The appearance of the scar on ultrasound and the associated shadowing will become less prominent over time and then remain stable.

Architectural distortion is frequently associated with the postsurgical scar or fat necrosis on all imaging modalities. Mammographically, architectural distortion associated with the postsurgical scar at the lumpectomy cavity should become less prominent and then remain stable over time. Sonographically, disruption of the parenchymal planes is evident, corresponding to the mammographic architectural distortion, which should also remain stable.

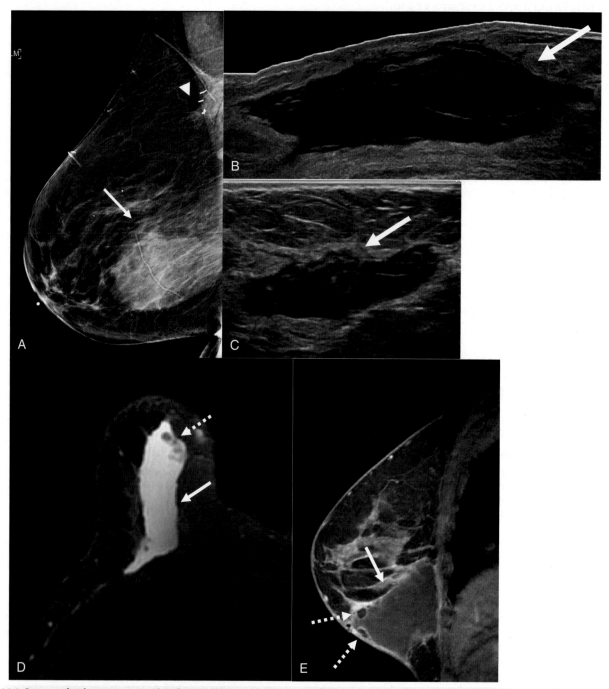

Fig. 16.4 Seroma after breast conservation therapy (BCT). (A) Mediolateral oblique mammogram in a woman treated with BCT shows a large oval mass (*arrow*) with indistinct margins at the site of the lumpectomy. There is a focal asymmetry with surgical clips (*arrowhead*) representing the axillary scar at the site of sentinel lymph node biopsy. (B, C) Ultrasound shows (B) a corresponding fluid collection (*arrow*) with internal septations consistent with a seroma in the breast and (C) a smaller similar-appearing collection (*arrow*) in the axilla. (D) Axial T2-weighted magnetic resonance imaging (MRI) in a different patient shows a T2-hyperintense collection (*arrow*) with areas of debris (*dashed arrow*). (E) Postcontrast sagittal MRI in the same patient as in panel D shows a fluid collection with a thin peripheral rim of enhancement (*arrow*) and nonenhancing internal contents and debris (*dashed arrows*), consistent with a seroma.

On MRI, architectural distortion is seen at the site of the postsurgical cavity, sometimes with an associated signal void artifact related to surgical clips or a BioZorb device (see Fig. 16.7). Associated areas of enhancement at the lumpectomy site can sometimes be seen. If present, this enhancement will decrease over time, often showing slow and persistent enhancement kinetics.

If the patient has undergone a sentinel lymph node biopsy or axillary lymph node dissection, a postsurgical scar and susceptibility artifacts from clips may also be seen within the axilla.

FAT NECROSIS

Fat necrosis has a wide spectrum of appearances, reflecting its various stages of evolution, and this largely depends on the time after surgery. Some of the imaging features of fat necrosis are pathognomonically benign, while others

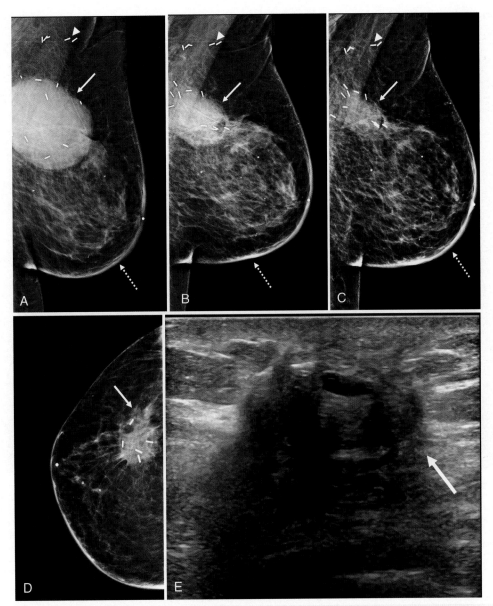

Fig. 16.5 Evolution of seroma after breast conservation therapy (BCT). (A) Mediolateral oblique mammogram in a woman treated with BCT shows a high-density oval mass with circumscribed margins and surgical clips consistent with a postsurgical seroma or hematoma (*arrow*). Associated skin thickening is seen (*dashed arrow*). A postsurgical scar with surgical clips is seen in the axilla at the site of sentinel lymph node biopsy (*arrowhead*). (B, C) Subsequent mammograms performed (B) 1 year and (C) 2 years after treatment show gradual decrease in the size and density of the postoperative collection (*arrows*). Improving diffuse trabecular thickening is seen, representing evolving postradiation changes. There is a stable axillary scar (*arrowhead*). Persistent skin thickening is seen (*dashed arrows*), which in some women can persist for years. (D) Craniocaudal mammogram in a different patient shows an oval mass with spiculated margins (*arrow*) along the postsurgical scar with surgical clips that had been stable over several years. (E) Ultrasound of the same patient as in panel D shows a corresponding circumscribed mass with layering echogenic debris (*arrow*), consistent with a chronic seroma.

are difficult to distinguish from new or recurrent breast cancer.

On mammography, characteristically benign features of fat necrosis include oil cysts, which are circumscribed fat density masses. When they calcify, they exhibit characteristic rim calcifications (Fig. 16.8) or lucent centered calcifications. As fat necrosis evolves over time, these calcifications may become coarser and develop into dystrophic calcifications, also a characteristically benign morphology of fat necrosis (Fig. 16.9). Extensive inflammatory changes sometimes associated with fat necrosis may lead to development of diffuse changes in the breast with skin thickening

and breast deformity (Fig. 16.10). Mammographically indeterminate features of fat necrosis include an irregular mass, focal asymmetry, architectural distortion, and morphologically suspicious calcifications, including coarse heterogeneous, amorphous, pleomorphic, and fine linear calcifications.

Sonographically, fat necrosis can present as a simple circumscribed anechoic oil cyst with characteristic posterior enhancement, or as a benign appearing circumscribed hyperechoic mass. More commonly, however, fat necrosis is associated with indeterminate or suspicious features on ultrasound, such as a hypoechoic mass with

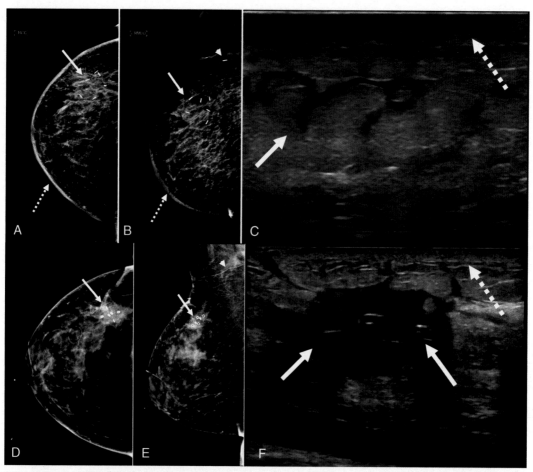

Fig. 16.6 Mammographic and sonographic findings after breast conservation therapy (BCT). (A, B) Craniocaudal (A) and mediolateral oblique (B) mammograms in a woman treated with BCT show architectural distortion with surgical clips corresponding to the lumpectomy site (*arrows*). There is expected trabecular thickening diffusely involving the breast parenchyma. Skin thickening is seen diffusely involving the breast and is most pronounced in the periareolar region because of disruption of the lymphatics (*dashed arrows*). A scar with a surgical clip (*arrowhead*) is seen in the axilla at the site of sentinel lymph node biopsy. (C) Ultrasound shows corresponding skin thickening (*dashed arrow*) and diffuse subcutaneous edema (*arrow*) diffusely involving the breast. (D, E) Craniocaudal (D) and mediolateral oblique (E) mammograms in a different patient show focal asymmetry with a BioZorb device (*arrows*) at the site of the lumpectomy. A scar marker (*arrowhead*) in the axilla denotes the site of sentinel lymph node biopsy. (F) Ultrasound shows the BioZorb device as linear echogenic structures (*arrows*) within the postsurgical scar. Skin thickening (*dashed arrow*) is also seen.

circumscribed, indistinct, or spiculated margins. These features can make it difficult to confidently distinguish fat necrosis from malignant masses, sometimes necessitating biopsy for definitive diagnosis (Fig. 16.11). Posterior shadowing due to associated calcifications is sometimes seen. Correlation with mammographic findings is key.

On MRI, fat necrosis can be associated with areas of macroscopic internal fat with signal following fat on all sequences, supporting the benign diagnosis. However, fat necrosis on MRI can also be associated with suspicious imaging features making it indistinguishable from malignancy. Fat necrosis can present as an irregular mass, can present as clumped or heterogeneous non-mass enhancement, and can have associated washout enhancement kinetics.

SUTURE AND OTHER BENIGN CALCIFICATIONS

In addition to the calcifications associated with fat necrosis described above, linear or knot-shaped calcifications can sometimes be seen after BCT. These are related to

calcifications of suture material that was placed at the time of the surgery and are benign (Fig. 16.12). Other characteristically benign calcifications that can occur at or near the surgical site include large rod-like calcifications and postsurgical/postradiation dystrophic calcifications not necessarily associated with fat necrosis.

Imaging Assessment of Residual Disease

Prospective randomized trials have demonstrated equivalent survival rates for BCS and mastectomy when BCS achieves negative margins. However, the reported incidence of positive margins after BCS ranges from 25% to 70%. Positive margins in patients with invasive tumors are defined as "ink on tumor." What is considered positive margins in patients with DCIS is more controversial, but most guidelines including NCCN recommend that margins

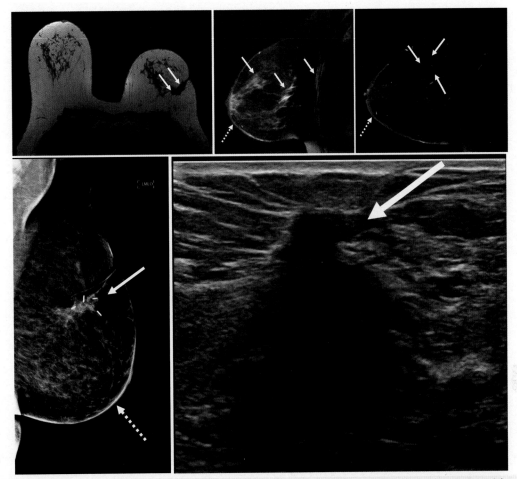

Fig. 16.7 Magnetic resonance imaging (MRI) findings after breast conservation therapy (BCT). (A) Posttreatment axial non-fat-saturated T1-weighted MRI shows a postsurgical scar in the upper outer left breast with signal void artifact (*arrows*) corresponding to the surgical clips placed within the surgical cavity. The treated breast is smaller than the opposite breast. (B) Sagittal T2-weighted MRI shows diffuse increased T2 signal within the breast parenchyma and the pectoralis muscle related to edematous posttreatment changes (*arrows*), as well as skin thickening (*dashed arrow*). (C) Sagittal postcontrast subtraction MRI shows the signal void artifact (*arrows*) corresponding to the surgical clips within the scar as well as skin thickening (*dashed arrow*). No suspicious enhancement is noted within the breast or within the skin, consistent with benign posttreatment change. (D) Corresponding mediolateral oblique mammogram shows the postsurgical scar with associated surgical clips in the upper breast (*arrow*) and skin thickening (*dashed arrow*). (E) Ultrasound image shows corresponding ill-defined irregular hypoechoic mass with architectural distortion with posterior shadowing (*arrow*), corresponding to the surgical scar.

for DCIS treated with lumpectomy and radiation should be greater than 2 mm (Box 16.7). Positive margins for invasive cancer and margins less than 2 mm for DCIS are associated with increased risk of local recurrence and generally warrant reexcision.

The workup of patients with positive margins after BCS includes an early postoperative diagnostic mammogram and review of preoperative imaging, clinical history, type of surgical procedure performed, and pathologic findings. Scar markers may be helpful to document the surgical site. An important step in the evaluation for possible residual disease is comparison with presurgical mammograms. If the initial cancer contained microcalcifications, magnification views (craniocaudal and lateromedial projections) are essential to establish whether residual calcifications remain (Fig. 16.13). If calcifications are present, they can be localized under mammographic guidance at the time of reexcision. Conversely, if the initial cancer did not contain calcifications, the mammographic evaluation for residual disease is limited, as the postsurgical hematoma/seroma can easily obscure a residual mass. In all patients, regardless of whether calcifications were present initially, mammographic evaluation of the postoperative breast is limited due to decreased breast compressibility, architectural distortion, and increased density related to postsurgical inflammatory changes.

Ultrasound is not helpful for evaluation for residual calcifications but is the imaging modality of choice for characterization of masses detected on mammography. Ultrasound in the early postoperative period can be useful to distinguish between hematoma/seroma and solid masses related to residual disease.

Breast MRI has been considered the most accurate imaging modality to evaluate patients with positive margins, with reported sensitivity ranging from 61% to 95%. The sensitivity of MRI increases with increasing burden of residual disease. Residual microscopic disease at the surgical margin cannot be reliably detected with MRI. Nonetheless, microscopic residual disease is usually successfully excised at reexcision regardless of the imaging results. MRI is most

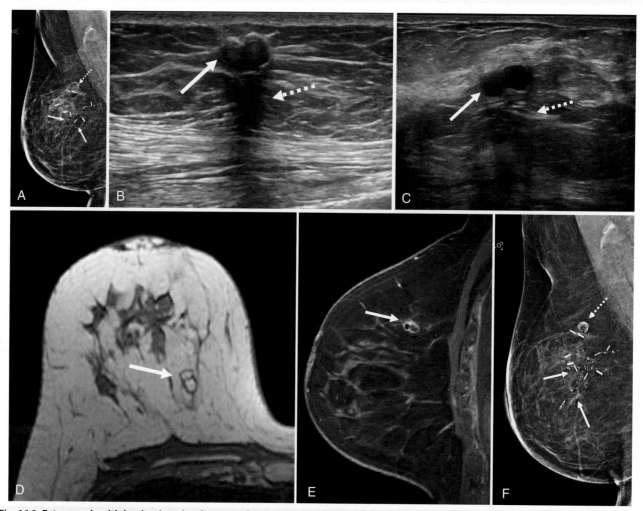

Fig. 16.8 Fat necrosis with benign imaging features after breast conservation therapy (BCT). (A) Mediolateral oblique mammogram after BCT shows fat necrosis at the site of the postsurgical scar (*arrows*). A partially calcified oil cyst is seen (*dashed arrow*) with characteristic rim calcification. (B) Corresponding ultrasound shows the characteristic appearance of a calcified oil cyst (*arrow*) as a hypoechoic circumscribed oval mass with a thin hyperechoic rim and associated posterior shadowing (*dashed arrow*). (C) This patient also had a noncalcified oil cyst (*arrow*) in another region of the scar seen as an anechoic oval mass with associated posterior enhancement (dashed arrow); the noncalcified oil cyst was not identified on mammography. (D) Corresponding T1-weighted non-fat-saturated axial magnetic resonance imaging (MRI) shows an oval circumscribed mass with fat signal (*arrow*) consistent with macroscopic fat. (E) Sagittal postcontrast fat-saturated MRI demonstrates corresponding fat saturation of the oval fat-containing mass with a thin rim of enhancement (*arrow*). These are benign MRI features characteristic of fat necrosis. (F) Mediolateral oblique mammogram performed the following year shows interval increase of the dystrophic and large rod-like calcifications along the postsurgical scar (*arrows*) with increasing rim calcification of the previously noted partially calcified oil cyst (*dashed arrow*).

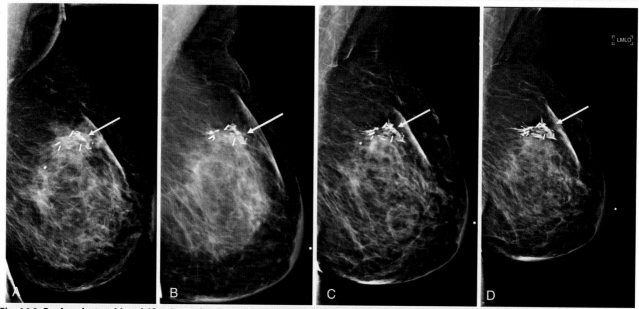

Fig. 16.9 Benign dystrophic calcifications after breast conservation therapy (BCT). (A–D) Mediolateral mammograms at 1 year (A), 2 years (B), 3 years (C), and 4 years (D) after BCT show increasing benign dystrophic calcifications (*arrows*) associated with the postsurgical scar.

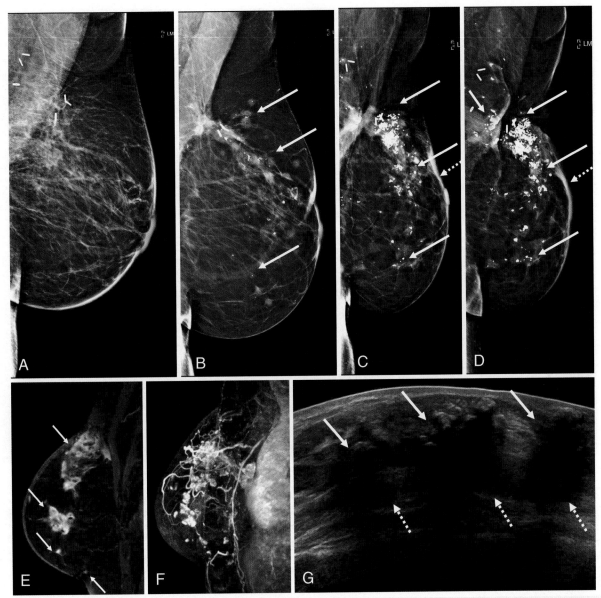

Fig. 16.10 Diffuse fat necrosis after breast conservation therapy (BCT). (A–D) Mediolateral mammograms at 1 year (A), 2 years (B), 3 years (C), and 4 years (D) after BCT show development and increase in number of circumscribed masses and diffuse dystrophic calcifications (*arrows*) secondary to progressive diffuse fat necrosis. There is increasing deformity and shrinkage of the breast, as well as development of skin thickening (*dashed arrows*) secondary to inflammatory changes associated with diffuse fat necrosis. (E, F) Sagittal postcontrast fat-saturated magnetic resonance imaging (MRI) (E) and maximum intensity projection reconstruction image (F) demonstrate multiple areas of mass and non-mass enhancement (*arrows*) corresponding to fat necrosis seen on mammogram. (G) Ultrasound image shows multiple hypoechoic ill-defined masses (*arrows*) with intense shadowing (*dashed arrows*) due to dense calcifications. Knowledge of the patient's history of BCT and the typical mammographic appearance are essential for the correct diagnosis of diffuse fat necrosis in this patient who has suspicious features on MRI and ultrasound.

useful for assessment of bulky residual disease at the resection margin so that the surgeon can be directed to the specific area of surgical cavity for reexcision (Fig. 16.14). Imaging features of residual disease on MRI vary and may include residual mass or clumped non-mass enhancement with suspicious enhancement kinetics at the border of surgical cavity. Advantages of breast MRI in assessment for residual disease are the lack of need for breast compression and the lack of impact of breast density on the findings. There is no consensus regarding the optimal time interval between lumpectomy and performance of breast MRI to assess margins.

Imaging Features of Recurrent Disease

The risk of tumor recurrence after BCT is approximately 1% to 2% per year for 10 years. The recurrence risk is highest within the first 5 years and then gradually decreases over time. Factors associated with increased risk of recurrence in the ipsilateral breast include lymphovascular invasion, higher nodal stage, multifocality, positive margins at surgical pathology, age less than 50 years, and certain biological markers including triple-negative status and HER-2

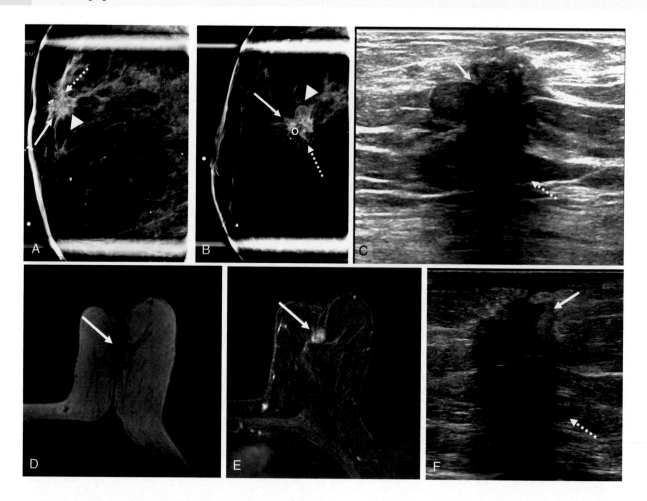

Fig. 16.11 Fat necrosis with suspicious imaging features after breast conservation therapy (BCT). (A, B) Spot lateral (A) and craniocaudal (B) mammographic views after BCT show an irregular mass with spiculated margins (*arrows*) in the retroareolar region adjacent to the postsurgical scar. There are associated coarse heterogeneous calcifications (*dashed arrows*) and an oil cyst (*arrowheads*). (C) Ultrasound shows a corresponding irregular hypoechoic mass with spiculated margins (*arrow*) and posterior shadowing (*dashed arrow*). Biopsy was recommended and demonstrated fat necrosis. (D) Axial T1-weighted noncontrast breast magnetic resonance imaging (MRI) in a different patient who was previously treated with BCT shows a T1 hypointense irregular mass (*arrow*). (E) Postcontrast fat-saturated axial MRI in the same patient as in panel D shows a corresponding heterogeneously enhancing irregular mass (*arrow*). (F) Ultrasound in the same patient as in panel D shows a hypoechoic irregular mass (*arrow*) with indistinct margins and posterior shadowing (*dashed arrow*). Biopsy was recommended and demonstrated fat necrosis.

enrichment. New cancers after BCT in the ipsilateral breast are categorized as either true recurrences or new breast primary tumors. True recurrence is defined as a regrowth of residual malignant disease remaining after surgery. True recurrences are usually located in the vicinity of the surgical site and have a shorter time to detection (Box 16.8). New primary breast tumors are suspected when the cancer occurs in a location remote from the original surgical site. New primary breast tumors often present more than 10 years after BCT (Fig. 16.15).

Recurrent breast tumors can be invasive or in situ regardless of the pathology of the original tumor. Early detection of local recurrence provides a significant survival advantage. Studies show that about 61% of recurrences exhibit mammographic findings similar to those of primary tumors. About 94% of DCIS recurrences have calcifications similar in morphology to the original DCIS. The standard approach for an ipsilateral breast cancer recurrence after BCT is usually mastectomy, provided there is no evidence of distant metastatic disease.

MAMMOGRAPHY

Because the usual site of breast cancer recurrence after BCT is near the postsurgical scar, careful inspection of the lumpectomy bed is recommended (Box 16.9). Masses related to the seroma/hematoma or scar should decrease in size and density or stabilize after 1 year. Therefore any increase in size or density or interval development of new convex margins of the surgical scar should raise a suspicion of recurrence (Fig. 16.16). Architectural distortions related to the scar should decrease or stabilize over time. An architectural distortion that exhibits an increase in size, density, or nodularity should raise suspicion of recurrence. Comparison to prior examinations is critical to differentiate a postsurgical scar from a new architectural distortion. Scar markers can also be helpful to localize the incision site. Digital breast tomosynthesis might help address the limitations of two-dimensional mammographic evaluation of the posttreatment breast because it resolves overlapping normal tissue and improves lesion characterization.

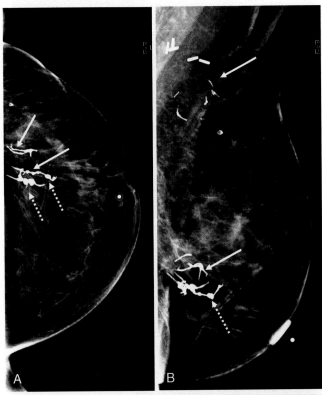

Fig. 16.12 Suture calcifications after breast conservation therapy (BCT). (A, B) Craniocaudal (A) and mediolateral (B) mammograms show linear (*arrows*) and knot-shaped (*dashed arrows*) calcifications along the lumpectomy scar and along the axillary scar related to sentinel lymph node biopsy after BCT.

Box 16.7   Recommended Margins After Breast Conservation Surgery

- Invasive cancer: no ink on tumor
- Ductal carcinoma in situ: DCIS >2 mm from the margin

As described above, skin and trabecular thickening is a common mammographic finding after radiation therapy. This finding is most pronounced within 6 months after radiation therapy and then usually decreases or stabilizes over the subsequent 2 to 3 years. New or increased skin and trabecular thickening should raise concern for recurrence, warranting further workup and correlation of clinical examination findings. The differential diagnosis of unilateral increased skin and trabecular thickening includes infection, lymphedema, or inflammatory breast cancer. Congestive heart and renal failure can also present with skin and trabecular thickening, but this would usually be a bilateral presentation.

New microcalcifications in the posttreatment breast is a common mammographic finding, seen in about 25% of patients, and often poses a challenge for the radiologist. Although most microcalcifications are benign, especially within the first 2 years after BCT, they can also represent a new or recurrent malignancy. Therefore in the case of new microcalcifications in the treated breast, the appropriate workup should include magnification views and comparison with prior mammograms (Fig. 16.17). Evaluation of the morphology and distribution of microcalcifications follows the criteria of the ACR Breast Imaging Reporting and Data System (BI-RADS) lexicon, fifth edition. If microcalcifications demonstrate suspicious morphology and distribution, vacuum-assisted stereotactic-guided biopsy is recommended.

One of the areas often overlooked on mammography is the axillary region. In the posttreatment breast, careful evaluation of the axillary region is needed because early recurrences can manifest as axillary lymphadenopathy.

A thorough workup is needed for any new or growing mass, new calcifications, developing asymmetry, new or worsening architectural distortion, or lymphadenopathy. Biopsy should be considered for any indeterminate or suspicious findings.

BREAST ULTRASOUND

Ultrasound is a valuable adjunct to mammography and helps overcome the limitations of mammography in the

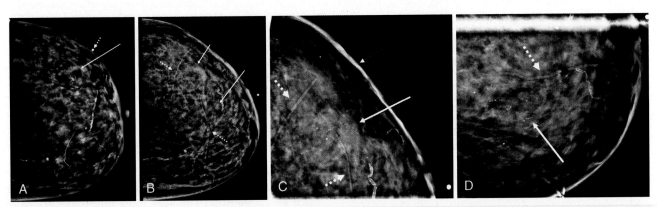

Fig. 16.13 Residual disease after breast conservation surgery (BCS): calcifications. (A–D) Mammograms of a woman who had BCS for invasive ductal carcinoma and ductal carcinoma in situ (DCIS) in the left breast. Surgical pathology showed invasive carcinoma at multiple inked margins. (A) Presurgical craniocaudal mammogram shows initial mammographic appearance of known carcinoma as pleomorphic calcifications in regional distribution (*arrow*) correlating with the palpable marker in the lateral breast (*dashed arrow*). (B) Postsurgical craniocaudal mammogram shows residual pleomorphic calcifications (*arrows*) in the lateral left breast. Scar markers (*dashed arrows*) are seen denoting incision scar. Comparison with presurgical mammograms and additional magnification views helped determine the extent of residual calcifications. (C, D) Craniocaudal (C) and lateromedial (D) magnification views show the residual pleomorphic calcifications (*arrows*) anterior and inferior to the postsurgical scar markers (*dashed arrows*). Skin thickening (*dashed and dotted arrow*) related to postsurgical changes is seen. Surgical reexcision with negative final margins was performed based on the mammographic findings.

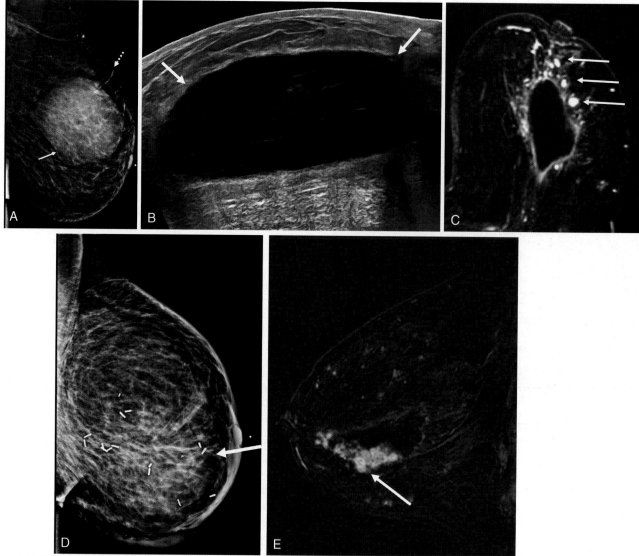

Fig. 16.14 Residual disease after breast conservation surgery (BCS): mass. (A–C) Postoperative imaging of a woman with invasive mammary carcinoma in the left breast who underwent BCS with multiple positive margins. (A) Mediolateral oblique mammogram shows a large seroma (*arrow*) involving the entire superior region of the breast. A scar marker is seen denoting incision scar (*dashed arrow*). Mammography has limited value for evaluation of residual disease in this patient because of decreased compressibility, large seroma, and increased breast density related to the edema and inflammatory changes after surgery. The initial presentation of malignancy was obscured mass without calcifications on the presurgical mammogram (not shown). (B) Ultrasound shows a fluid collection with septations and debris in the area of the surgical scar consistent with a seroma (*arrows*) without suspicious sonographic findings. (C) Axial T1 weighted contrast-enhanced breast magnetic resonance imaging (MRI) shows multiple small masses (*arrows*) at the anterolateral margin of the surgical cavity consistent with residual disease. (D) In a different patient who underwent BCS for invasive ductal carcinoma and DCIS with positive margins, mediolateral oblique mammogram shows the postsurgical scar in the inferior region of the breast (*arrow*). There are marked postsurgical changes with increased trabecular and skin thickening without mammographic evidence of residual disease. (E) Sagittal T1 weighted contrast-enhanced breast MRI in the same patient as in panel D shows a focal area of confluent clumped non-mass enhancement at the inferior margin of the surgical cavity (*arrow*) consistent with residual disease. MRI findings were used to guide surgical reexcision in both patients. Negative margins were documented at final pathology.

Box 16.8   True Local Recurrence Versus New Primary Breast Tumor After Breast Conservation Therapy

True Recurrence

- Defined as proliferation of residual malignant cells after surgical removal of the primary tumor
- Usually located at or near the surgical site
- Shorter time to occurrence, usually within first 5 years after BCT

New Primary Breast Tumor

- Often occurs in a different quadrant, remote from the surgical site
- Often occurs more than 10 years after BCT

posttreatment breast. Ultrasound is used to evaluate any suspicious findings detected on mammography as well as new palpable masses even if no mammographic abnormality is identified.

The postsurgical scar often stabilizes to its final appearance at 12 months. The scar most often appears as an irregular hypoechoic mass with posterior shadowing. The posterior shadowing becomes more prominent as the fibrosis progresses. Often, it is difficult to distinguish between postsurgical scarring and tumor recurrence (Fig. 16.18). Obtaining imaging in two orthogonal views can sometimes help distinguish the two, as the scar can be seen as a more discrete round or irregular mass in one

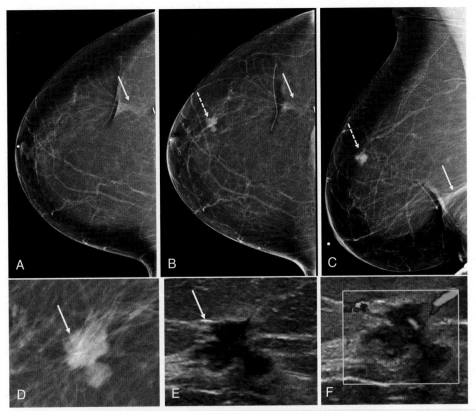

Fig. 16.15 New primary breast cancer after breast conservation therapy (BCT). (A) Right craniocaudal mammogram performed after BCT for invasive ductal carcinoma shows a postsurgical scar with a surgical clip in the lower outer quadrant (*arrow*). (B, C) Right craniocaudal (B) and mediolateral (C) mammograms performed 9 years later show a new high-density mass (*dashed arrows*) anterior to the surgical scar (*arrows*) in the upper outer quadrant. (D) Craniocaudal spot compression view shows the noncalcified mass, irregular in shape with spiculated margins (*arrow*). (E) Ultrasound demonstrates corresponding irregular, spiculated hypoechoic mass (*arrow*), suggestive of malignancy. (F) Power Doppler ultrasound shows that the mass has internal vascularity. Ultrasound-guided core needle biopsy showed invasive ductal carcinoma.

Box 16.9 Imaging Findings Suggestive of Recurrence After Breast Conservation Therapy

- Increase in density, size, or interval development of convex margins of the surgical scar
- New architectural distortion
- New or worsening of skin or trabecular thickening
- New suspicious calcifications
- New masses or developing asymmetries
- Enlarged lymph nodes in the axilla

view but a more subtle linear structure in the orthogonal view. Comparison with previous ultrasound images also aids in the detection of subtle changes of the surgical scar. New solid masses with internal vascularity on Doppler evaluation should be considered suspicious and warrant image-guided biopsy.

An additional advantage of ultrasound is its suitability for the evaluation of regional nodal basins. Early detection of locoregional recurrence increases survival. Mammography has limited utility in evaluation of the axilla as mammography permits evaluation of only the low axillary region. Ultrasound of the regional nodal basins is an inexpensive imaging method to detect recurrence. Features suggestive of lymph node recurrence include round or irregular shape

of the lymph nodes, eccentric cortical thickening, and replaced fatty hilum.

BREAST MRI

There is no consensus about use of breast MRI in patients with history of BCT. ACR recommends annual breast MRI surveillance for women with a personal history of breast cancer with dense breast parenchyma and women who had breast cancer diagnosed by age 50 years (Fig. 16.19). Breast MRI may also be helpful when mammography or sonography is indeterminate in the assessment of the surgical scar. MRI can be used to distinguish posttreatment scar tissue from recurrence when performed at least 12 to 18 months after completion of BCT, yielding a sensitivity of 90% to 100% and specificity of 83% to 93%. Posttreatment scar is distinguished from recurrence on the basis of the dynamic enhancement pattern combined with morphology on contrast-enhanced MRI. The presence of a thin smooth rim around the surgical seroma or the absence of enhancement in the lumpectomy bed suggests fibrosis. Conversely, irregular enhancing masses or areas of clumped or heterogeneous non-mass enhancement with fast or washout enhancement kinetics are concerning for recurrence (Fig. 16.20). The differential diagnosis includes fat necrosis, which sometimes is indistinguishable from malignancy. Therefore needle biopsy is often needed to confirm the diagnosis of recurrence.

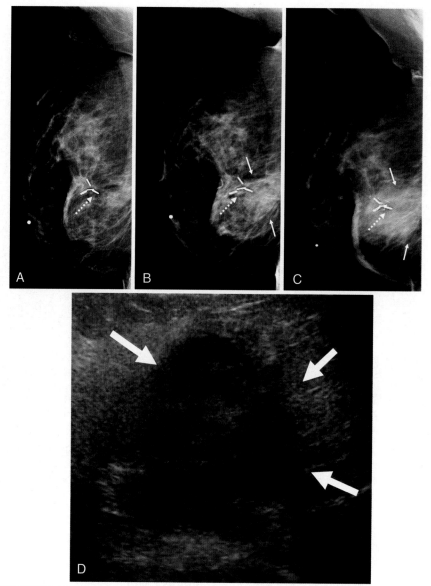

Fig. 16.16 Mammographic and ultrasound features of recurrence after breast conservation therapy (BCT): mass. Posttreatment imaging of a woman who had BCT for invasive ductal carcinoma in the right breast. Mediolateral oblique views at 1 year (A), 2 years (B), and 3 years (C) after treatment show gradual increase in density and interval development of convex margins (*arrows*) at the area of the breast conservation surgery (BCS) scar (*dashed arrows*). (D) Ultrasound shows a round hypoechoic mass with indistinct margins (*arrows*) deep to the surgical scar. Ultrasound-guided core biopsy showed invasive ductal carcinoma.

KEY POINTS

- Breast conservation therapy (BCT) includes surgical excision of the primary tumor followed by whole-breast radiation therapy.
- For successful BCT, the primary tumor must be excised with negative margins and acceptable cosmetic results. The patient should be able to receive radiation therapy, and must be amenable for follow-up breast imaging to detect local recurrence.
- Successful BCT requires careful presurgical planning with appropriate tumor localization and adequate intraoperative assessment of the radiograph of the excised surgical specimen.
- After BCT, mammography is the imaging modality of choice for surveillance and usually performed 6 months after completion of radiation therapy and yearly thereafter.
- Breast ultrasound is typically reserved for evaluation of suspicious/indeterminate mammographic findings or for evaluation of focal breast signs and symptoms.
- The American College of Radiology (ACR) recommends supplemental yearly breast magnetic resonance imaging (MRI) surveillance in women with a personal history of breast cancer and dense breast parenchyma and in women with a history of breast cancer diagnosed by the age 50 years. Breast MRI may also be used in problem solving of indeterminate mammographic or sonographic findings, though this should be done sparingly and with discretion.

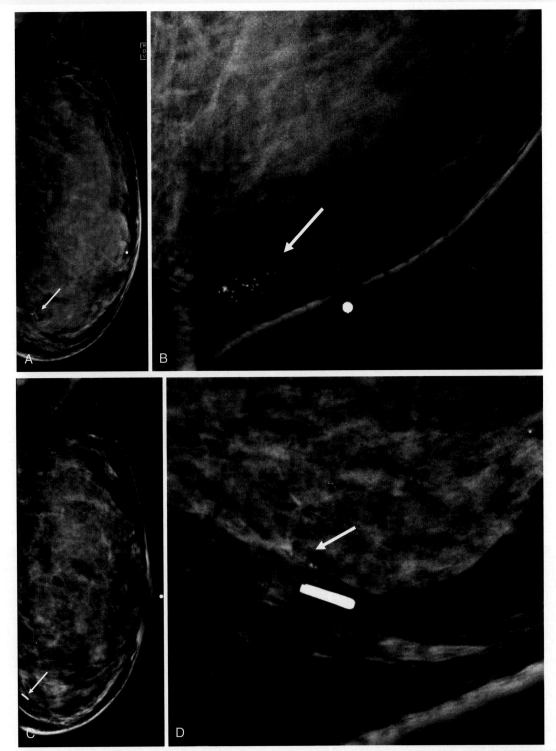

Fig. 16.17 Mammographic features of recurrence: calcifications. (A, B) Presurgical mediolateral oblique mammogram (A) and lateromedial magnification view (B) show pleomorphic calcifications in grouped distribution (*arrows*). Stereotactic biopsy showed ductal carcinoma in situ (DCIS), and the patient underwent breast conservation therapy (BCT) with negative surgical margins. There was no evidence of residual disease on 1-year follow-up imaging (not shown). (C, D) Mediolateral oblique mammogram (C) and lateromedial magnification view (D) 2 years after treatment show new pleomorphic calcifications (*arrows*) adjacent to the surgical clip at the inferior region of the left breast. Stereotactic-guided biopsy confirmed recurrent DCIS.

- Common benign findings after BCT include fluid collection, skin and trabecular thickening, postsurgical scar, architectural distortion, fat necrosis with rim or dystrophic calcifications, and suture calcifications.
- The initial workup of a patient with positive surgical margins after lumpectomy is diagnostic mammography. Knowledge of the patient's clinical history, type of surgical procedure, and comparison with presurgical mammograms are critical to accurately assess for residual disease.
- Breast MRI is the most accurate imaging modality to evaluate positive surgical margins and can help direct the surgeon to the areas of bulky residual disease for reexcision.

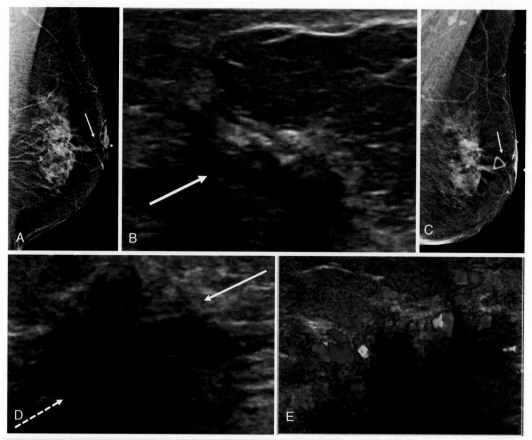

Fig. 16.18 Ultrasound features of recurrence after breast conservation therapy (BCT): mass. (A) Mediolateral oblique mammogram shows the postsurgical scar (*arrow*) in the periareolar region from BCT for invasive ductal carcinoma. (B) Ultrasound shows postsurgical scar (*arrow*) in the retroareolar region as a linear hypoechoic lesion. Two years later, the patient felt a palpable abnormality in the periareolar region and skin dimpling was seen in the area of palpable abnormality on physical examination. (C) Left mediolateral oblique view shows no mammographic abnormality correlating with the palpable abnormality. The postsurgical scar was mammographically stable (*arrow*). (D) Ultrasound demonstrates interval thickening and irregularity at the postsurgical scar (*arrow*), which now appears as an indistinct hypoechoic mass with posterior shadowing (*dashed arrow*). (E) Color Doppler ultrasound shows increased vascularity at this site. Ultrasound-guided core biopsy showed invasive ductal carcinoma.

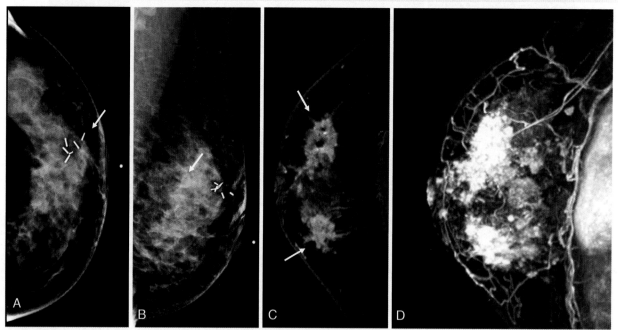

Fig. 16.19 Magnetic resonance imaging (MRI) features of recurrence after breast carcinoma therapy (BCT): multicentric disease. First posttreatment imaging in a 40-year-old woman who underwent BCT for invasive lobular carcinoma 3 years earlier, who declined hormonal therapy, and was then lost to follow-up. (A, B) Craniocaudal (A) and mediolateral oblique (B) mammograms show a postsurgical scar with surgical clips in the upper outer quadrant of the left breast (*arrows*). No mammographic abnormality is seen. (C) Sagittal T1 weighted contrast-enhanced breast MRI shows multiple irregular enhancing masses (*arrows*) involving the entire breast highly suggestive of recurrence. (D) Maximum intensity projection reconstruction shows the multicentric diffuse involvement of the left breast by the recurrent disease. Ultrasound-guided core biopsy confirmed recurrent multicentric invasive lobular carcinoma.

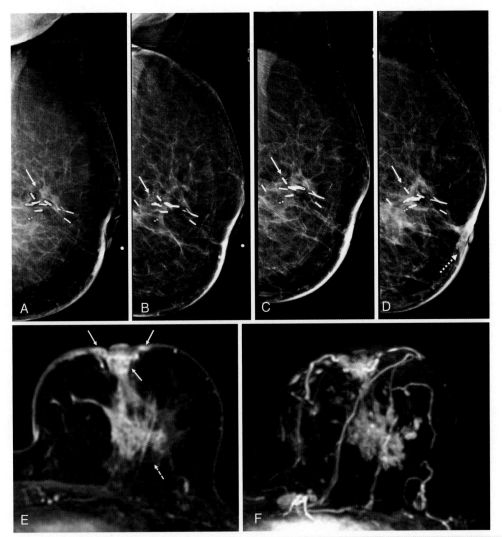

Fig. 16.20 Magnetic resonance imaging (MRI) features of recurrence after breast conservation therapy (BCT). (A–D) Serial mediolateral oblique mammograms after BCT for invasive ductal carcinoma show a gradual developing asymmetry with increase in density (*arrows*) in the area of the surgical scar. The skin thickening is increasingly prominent (*dashed arrow*) predominantly in the periareolar region. (E) Axial T1 weighted contrast-enhanced breast MRI shows regional clumped non-mass enhancement involving the surgical scar (*dashed arrow*) extending to and involving the base of the nipple and the periareolar skin (*arrows*). (F) Maximum intensity projection reconstruction image of the left breast shows the extent of the recurrence in the breast. Ultrasound-guided core biopsy showed recurrent invasive ductal carcinoma.

- Any increase in size, density, or the development of new convex margins of the surgical scar should raise suspicion for local recurrence. Suspicious lesions remote from the surgical site could also represent a new primary breast cancer.
- Any new or growing mass, new microcalcifications, new or worsening areas of architectural distortion, and developing asymmetries should raise suspicion for malignancy. Biopsy should be recommended for any new lesions that are not characteristically benign.
- Breast MRI performed 12 to 18 months after BCT can help distinguish between a postsurgical scar and tumor recurrence when the mammographic and ultrasound findings are equivocal.

Suggested Readings

Chae EY, Cha JH, Kim HH, et al. Evaluation of residual disease using breast MRI after excisional biopsy for breast cancer. *AJR Am J Roentgenol.* 2013;200(5):1167–1173.

Chansakul T, Lai KC, Slanetz PJ. The postconservation breast: part 1, Expected imaging findings. *AJR Am J Roentgenol.* 2012;198(2):321–330.

Chansakul T, Lai KC, Slanetz PJ. The postconservation breast: part 2, Imaging findings of tumor recurrence and other long-term sequelae. *AJR Am J Roentgenol.* 2012;198(2):331–343.

Cho N, Han W, Han BK, et al. Breast Cancer Screening With Mammography Plus Ultrasonography or Magnetic Resonance Imaging in Women 50 Years or Younger at Diagnosis and Treated With Breast Conservation Therapy. *JAMA Oncol.* 2017;3(11):1495–1502.

Drukteinis JS, Gombos EC, Raza S, Chikarmane SA, Swami A, Birdwell RL. MR imaging assessment of the breast after breast conservation therapy: distinguishing benign from malignant lesions. *Radiographics.* 2012;32(1):219–234.

Kapoor MM, Patel MM, Scoggins ME. The wire and beyond: recent advances in breast imaging preoperative needle localization. *Radiographics.* 2019;39(7):1886–1906.

Monticciolo DL, Newell MS, Moy L, Niell B, Monsees B, Sickles EA. Breast Cancer Screening in Women at Higher-Than-Average Risk: Recommendations From the ACR. *J Am Coll Radiol.* 2018;15(3 Pt A):408–414.

Morrow M, Khan AJ. Locoregional management after neoadjuvant chemotherapy. *J Clin Onc.* 2020 May 22:JCO1902576. doi: 10.1200/JCO.19.02576. Online ahead of print.

Neal CH, Yilmaz ZN, Noroozian M, et al. Imaging of breast cancer-related changes after surgical therapy. *AJR Am J Roentgenol.* 2014;202(2):262–272.

Tayyab SJ, Adrada BE, Rauch GM, Yang WT. A pictorial review: multimodality imaging of benign and suspicious features of fat necrosis in the breast. *Br J Radiol.* 2018;91(1092). 20180213.

Teshome M, Kuerer HM. Breast conserving surgery and locoregional control after neoadjuvant chemotherapy. *Eur J Surg Oncol.* 2017;43(5):865–874.

17 | Lymph Node Evaluation in Breast Imaging

AMY M. FOWLER AND MOLLY PETERSON

OVERVIEW | *This chapter provides a framework for the diagnostic approach to axillary lymphadenopathy and its differential considerations including unilateral axillary lymphadenopathy, bilateral axillary lymphadenopathy, and axillary nodal calcifications. A brief overview of the evaluation and management of axillary lymph nodes in newly diagnosed breast cancer patients concludes the chapter.*

Axillary lymphadenopathy can be encountered during the evaluation of a palpable lump in the axilla, as part of locoregional staging for a highly suspicious finding or known biopsy-proven malignancy in the breast, as an incidental finding from other imaging (e.g., computed tomography [CT], magnetic resonance imaging [MRI], positron emission tomography [PET]/CT), or infrequently as an isolated finding from breast cancer screening (<0.5% screening mammography examinations). Though axillary lymph nodes may be visualized on mammography, ultrasound is the preferred imaging modality for specific evaluation of the axilla. Imaging evaluation of a palpable axillary lump starts with diagnostic mammography to evaluate for potential associated findings in the breast (sometimes with specialized views including exaggerated craniocaudal lateral and axillary tail views) followed by targeted ultrasound of the clinical area of concern. For locoregional staging in a patient with newly diagnosed breast cancer, sonographic evaluation of the entire ipsilateral axilla is performed. Suspicious findings on ultrasound can be biopsied by ultrasound-guided fine-needle aspiration (FNA) or ultrasound-guided core biopsy with marker clip placement.

Basic Anatomy

The axilla is composed of nerves, blood vessels, adipose tissue, muscles, lymph nodes, and fibroglandular tissue. It is bounded superiorly by the clavicle, scapula, and first rib; anteriorly by the pectoralis major and minor muscles; medially by the serratus anterior muscle and thoracic wall; and posteriorly by the scapularis, teres major, and latissimus dorsi muscles.

Axillary lymph nodes receive lymphatic drainage from the arm, breast, walls of the thorax, and upper walls of the abdomen. The lymphatic vessels then course through the pectoralis major muscle and enter the internal mammary lymph nodes.

Surgical levels of axillary lymph nodes are defined by their relationship to the pectoralis minor muscle. Level I nodes are located lateral to the pectoralis minor muscle. Level II nodes are located posterior to the pectoralis minor muscle and also include interpectoral nodes located between the pectoralis major and minor muscles (Rotter nodes). Level III nodes are located medial to the pectoralis minor muscle. Fig. 17.1 demonstrates examples of level I, level II, and level III axillary lymph nodes.

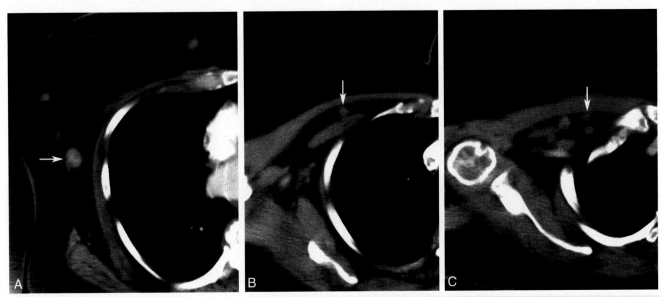

Fig. 17.1 Axillary lymph nodes levels. Computed tomography (CT) of the right axilla demonstrates examples of level I through III lymph nodes. (A) Level I lymph node (*arrow*) lateral to the pectoralis minor muscle. (B) Level II lymph node (*arrow*) between the pectoralis minor and major muscles (Rotter node). (C) Level III lymph nodes (*arrow*) medial to the pectoralis minor muscle.

Normal Versus Abnormal Appearance

Normal axillary lymph nodes can vary in size from a few millimeters to several centimeters in longest dimension. The most important criterion for distinguishing between normal and abnormal lymph nodes is thus based on morphology. The following characteristics should be evaluated: size, shape (oval, round, irregular), cortical thickening (uniform/concentric, focal), margin (circumscribed, not circumscribed), and hilar compression or replacement.

Normal lymph nodes are oval in shape and have a fatty hilum, which is seen as a lucent center or notch on mammography, and an echogenic center on ultrasound. They have a thin uniform cortex (<3 mm), and Doppler evaluation shows vascularization only within the hilum. Fig. 17.2 demonstrates the normal appearance of axillary lymph nodes on mammography, ultrasound, CT, and MRI.

Suspicious features include rounded shape, focal cortical bulge, eccentric cortical thickening, diffuse cortical thickening greater than 3 mm, complete or partial effacement of the fatty hilum, and nonhilar blood flow. An irregular shape and/or indistinct margin may indicate extranodal

extension, a poor prognostic sign. Fig. 17.3 demonstrates the various abnormal appearance of axillary lymph nodes on ultrasound (Box 17.1).

Diagnostic Approach

A variety of benign and malignant processes can result in axillary lymphadenopathy and the loss of normal nodal morphology. Fig. 17.4 provides a framework for the diagnostic approach to breast imaging evaluation of axillary lymph nodes. Reviewing the electronic medical record and prior available imaging are important for identifying potential known causes of axillary lymphadenopathy and for assessing stability.

Box 17.1

Real-time ultrasound scanning is recommended for evaluating lymph node cortical thickness, since projection/positional artifacts such as an oblique angle of insonation can simulate cortical thickening.

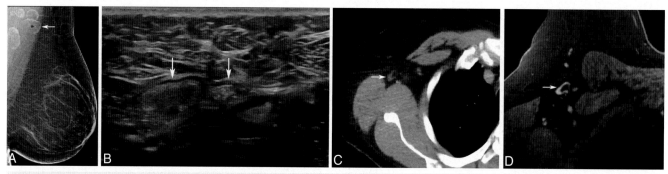

Fig. 17.2 Normal appearance of axillary lymph nodes. (A) On mammogram (mediolateral oblique [MLO] view), normal lymph nodes demonstrate a thin white cortex (*arrow*) and radiolucent fatty hilum (*). (B) On ultrasound, the cortex is thin and hypoechoic (*arrows*) and the fatty hilum is isoechoic. (C) Computed tomography (CT) and (D) magnetic resonance imaging (MRI) show the normal reniform shape with smooth enhancing cortex and central fatty hilum (lymph nodes annotated by arrows).

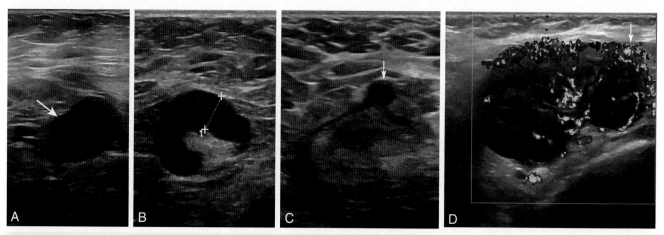

Fig. 17.3 Abnormal appearance of axillary lymph nodes. There are several sonographic presentations of abnormal axillary lymph nodes including: (A) complete or partial effacement of the fatty hilum (*arrow*), (B) diffuse cortical thickening > 3 mm (calipers), (C) focal cortical bulge or eccentric thickening (*arrow*), and (D) nonhilar blood flow (*arrow*).

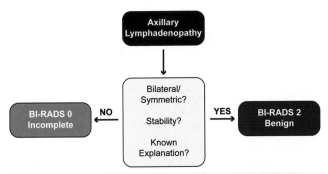

Fig. 17.4 Diagnostic algorithm for axillary lymphadenopathy encountered on screening mammogram. In addition, bilateral axillary lymphadenopathy with no known explanation should be assessed as BI-RADS 0, particularly if new and there is concern for lymphoma/leukemia.

Bilateral Axillary Lymphadenopathy

Bilateral axillary lymphadenopathy usually implies a systemic cause. Box 17.2 summarizes the top differential considerations for both benign and malignant causes of bilateral axillary lymphadenopathy.

Bilateral adenopathy can be seen with infection (Fig. 17.5), granulomatous diseases, and autoimmune diseases. Autoimmune diseases, such as rheumatoid arthritis, scleroderma, and systemic lupus erythematosus, could also present with unilateral axillary lymphadenopathy early in the disease process. Malignant causes are most commonly lymphoma/leukemia (Fig. 17.6) and metastases.

If there is a known reactive or infectious origin or in the setting of known lymphoma/leukemia, Breast Imaging Reporting and Data System (BI-RADS) category 2 (benign) may be assigned and the patient can return to normal screening guidelines based on age and risk factors. It is recommended to include a statement in the impression acknowledging the observed lymphadenopathy and presumed etiology.

If there is no known explanation, particularly if new and there is concern for lymphoma/leukemia, BI-RADS

Box 17.2   Bilateral Axillary Lymphadenopathy: Top Differential Diagnoses

Benign

- Infection
  - Human immunodeficiency virus (HIV)
  - Epstein-Barr virus (EBV) mononucleosis
- Granulomatous disease
  - Sarcoidosis
  - Tuberculosis
- Autoimmune disease
  - Rheumatoid arthritis
  - Scleroderma
  - Systemic lupus erythematosus
  - Psoriasis

Malignant

- Lymphoma/leukemia
- Metastases
  - Nonbreast
  - Breast (typically unilateral)

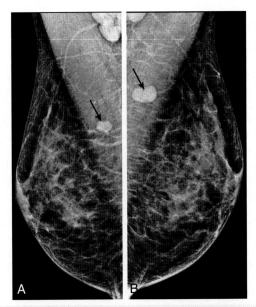

Fig. 17.5 HIV infection. Screening mammogram (mediolateral oblique [MLO] views) of the (A) right and (B) left breasts in a patient with known HIV demonstrate multiple enlarged lymph nodes in both axillae (*arrows*). This was stable compared with prior exams (not shown). This examination was assessed as BI-RADS 2 (benign).

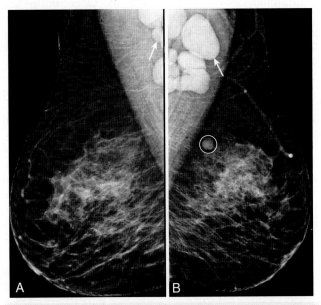

Fig. 17.6 Chronic lymphocytic leukemia. Baseline screening mammogram (mediolateral oblique [MLO] views) of the (A) right and (B) left breasts in a patient with known chronic lymphocytic leukemia demonstrate multiple enlarged lymph nodes in both axillae (*arrows*). There is also an enlarged oval intramammary lymph node (*circle*) in the left breast at 2 o'clock posterior depth. No other significant masses or calcifications are seen in either breast. The examination was assessed as BI-RADS 2 (benign).

category 0 (incomplete) assessment is indicated on a screening mammogram and BI-RADS category 4 (suspicious) assessment is indicated and ultrasound-guided FNA or core biopsy is recommended. If lymphoma is suspected, it is recommended to check with your pathology department for any specific requirements for specimen processing (e.g., cores in saline or media instead of formalin for flow cytometry).

Unilateral Axillary Lymphadenopathy

Unilateral axillary lymphadenopathy can arise from a variety of benign causes but is typically more concerning than bilateral axillary lymphadenopathy. The finding of unilateral axillary lymphadenopathy on mammography should therefore prompt careful search of the ipsilateral breast since metastatic lymphadenopathy from primary breast malignancy is a common cause. To confirm that the lymphadenopathy is indeed unilateral, comparison with the contralateral axilla by ultrasound can be performed.

Box 17.3 summarizes the top differential diagnoses for both benign and malignant causes of unilateral axillary lymphadenopathy. Definitive infectious or inflammatory causes can be designated BI-RADS category 2. If there is no known infectious or inflammatory explanation, BI-RADS category 4 is indicated and ultrasound-guided FNA or core biopsy is recommended.

The most common causes of reactive benign lymphadenopathy are mastitis/breast abscess and ipsilateral arm cellulitis. Reactive lymph nodes typically are enlarged with uniform cortical thickening. Physical examination for signs of infection or inflammation in the ipsilateral breast, axilla, arm, and hand can be performed at the time of ultrasound.

Granulomatous diseases, such as tuberculosis and sarcoidosis, may also cause unilateral axillary lymphadenopathy and frequently demonstrate coarse internal calcifications. If granulomatous disease is suspected, prior chest imaging can confirm pulmonary granulomas and/or calcified mediastinal/hilar lymph nodes.

Recent vaccination in the ipsilateral arm can also be a cause for transient reactive unilateral axillary lymphadenopathy. This finding is a well-documented reaction to COVID-19 vaccination and can also occur less frequently with other vaccines such as human papilloma virus, influenza, and Bacille Calmette-Guérin (BCG) for tuberculosis. Correlation should be made with patient history and information in the electronic medical record regarding the timing and laterality of recently administered vaccines. Persistent unilateral axillary lymphadenopathy (>6 weeks

after vaccine administration) is an indication for further diagnostic evaluation.

A common malignant cause for unilateral lymphadenopathy is metastasis from an ipsilateral breast primary malignancy (Fig. 17.7). For patients with biopsy-proven metastatic axillary lymphadenopathy consistent with breast origin and no suspicious findings on clinical examination and mammography, breast MRI is indicated (Fig. 17.8).

Metastases from melanoma involving the ipsilateral upper extremity (Fig. 17.9) is also included in the differential diagnoses for unilateral lymphadenopathy. Dark pigmentation of the core biopsy tissue can be grossly visualized due to the presence of melanin. Physical examination of the ipsilateral breast, axilla, arm, and hand can be performed at the time of ultrasound to evaluate for suspicious skin lesions. Nonbreast metastases and lymphoma/leukemia may be unilateral but more often cause bilateral axillary lymphadenopathy.

Box 17.3 Unilateral Axillary Lymphadenopathy: Top Differential Diagnoses

Benign

- Infection
  - Mastitis/breast abscess
  - Ipsilateral arm cellulitis
  - Cat scratch disease (*Bartonella henselae*)
  - Tuberculosis
- Granulomatous disease
  - Tuberculosis
  - Sarcoidosis
- Recent ipsilateral upper extremity vaccination
- Silicone implant rupture

Malignant

- Metastases from breast primary malignancy
- Metastases from nonbreast primary malignancy
  - Lung
  - Melanoma (upper extremity)
- Lymphoma/leukemia (typically bilateral)

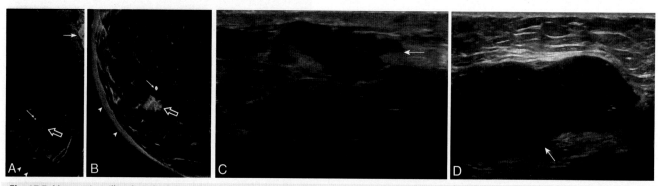

Fig. 17.7 Metastatic axillary lymphadenopathy from ipsilateral primary breast cancer. (A) Mediolateral oblique (MLO) and (B) craniocaudal (CC) mammographic views of the right breast show an irregular mass (*open arrow*) with spiculated margins at the 3 o'clock position with skin thickening (*arrowheads*), which corresponds with the palpable area of concern (radiopaque skin BB marker). Enlarged axillary lymph nodes are partially visualized (*arrow*). (C) Ultrasound of the palpable mass confirms an irregular hypoechoic mass with angular margins (*arrow*) abutting the skin. Case was assessed as BI-RADS 5 (highly suggestive of malignancy). Ultrasound-guided biopsy yielded invasive ductal carcinoma (grade 3, triple negative) with lymphovascular invasion. (D) Ultrasound of the axilla shows a large level I axillary lymph node with complete replacement of the fatty hilum (*arrow*). Ultrasound-guided biopsy confirmed the presence of invasive ductal carcinoma completely replacing the axillary lymph node.

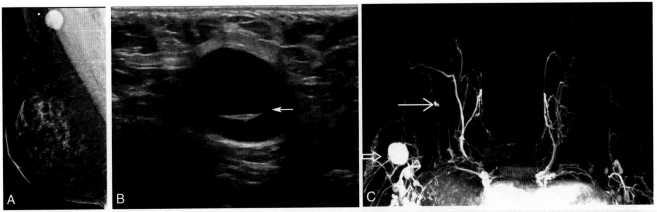

Fig. 17.8 Metastatic axillary lymphadenopathy from mammographically occult ipsilateral primary breast cancer. (A) Mediolateral oblique (MLO) mammographic view of the right breast demonstrates an enlarged round high-density lymph node in the axilla, which corresponds with the palpable area of concern (radiopaque skin BB marker). No suspicious findings are seen in the breast. (B) Ultrasound of the axillary lymph node shows compression of the fatty hilum (*arrow*) by the enlarged cortex. Examination assessed as BI-RADS 4 (suspicious). Ultrasound-guided biopsy yielded metastatic carcinoma consistent with breast primary. (C) Magnetic resonance imaging (MRI) (maximum intensity projection [MIP] view) identifies a small circumscribed mass in the right breast at the 9 o'clock position (*arrow*) and the enlarged biopsy-proven malignant level I axillary lymph node (*open arrow*). MRI-guided biopsy revealed invasive ductal carcinoma.

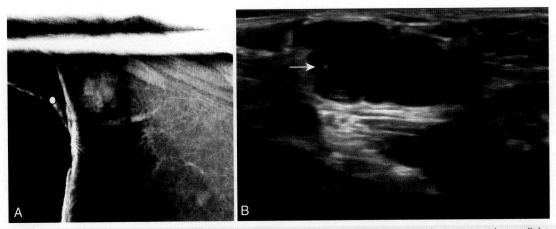

Fig. 17.9 Metastatic axillary lymphadenopathy from ipsilateral upper extremity melanoma. (A) Mammogram (spot compression mediolateral oblique [MLO] view) of a palpable axillary lump (radiopaque skin BB marker) shows an enlarged irregular shaped lymph node. No suspicious mammographic findings were seen within either breast (not shown). (B) Ultrasound shows an irregular heterogeneous mass (*arrow*) with microlobulated margins and posterior acoustic enhancement. The examination was assessed as BI-RADS 4 (suspicious). Tissue from ultrasound-guided core biopsy of the mass appeared black and pathology was consistent with metastatic melanoma. A suspicious appearing skin lesion was subsequently identified on the patient's upper arm, which was confirmed to be the site of primary malignancy.

Axillary Nodal Calcifications

Axillary nodal calcifications may occur in both benign and malignant causes but are more concerning than axillary lymphadenopathy alone. Box 17.4 summarizes the top differential considerations for axillary nodal calcifications.

Benign causes include gold deposits (intramuscular gold injections for treatment of rheumatoid arthritis or juvenile idiopathic arthritis), dye pigments from large upper extremity tattoos, and granulomatous diseases such as tuberculosis, sarcoidosis, and histoplasmosis. Calcifications associated with benign granulomatous diseases have a typical coarse morphology (Fig. 17.10).

Microcalcifications are a particularly concerning feature for malignancy. Malignant causes include metastases from breast cancer most frequently (Fig. 17.11). The morphology

---

Box 17.4   Axillary Nodal Calcifications: Top Differential Diagnoses

Benign

- Gold deposits
- Dye pigments from skin tattoo
- Granulomatous disease
  - Tuberculosis
  - Sarcoidosis
  - Histoplasmosis

Malignant

- Metastases
  - Breast
  - Ovarian
  - Thyroid

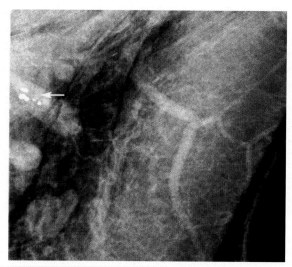

Fig. 17.10 Benign axillary nodal calcifications, granulomatous disease. Mediolateral oblique (MLO) screening mammogram view of the left breast shows coarse calcifications (*arrow*) within a nonenlarged axillary lymph node. The examination was assessed as BI-RADS 2 (benign).

of axillary nodal microcalcifications from metastatic breast cancer are typically similar in appearance to the primary breast malignancy. Axillary nodal microcalcifications can also be seen with metastatic papillary serous ovarian cancer (Fig. 17.12) and metastatic papillary thyroid cancer (e.g., psammoma bodies).

Axillary Lymph Node Management in Breast Cancer Patients

The presence or absence of axillary lymph node involvement in patients with breast cancer is one of the most important prognostic indicators and is used for determining American Joint Committee on Cancer (AJCC) staging and treatment decisions. For patients with clinically palpable or suspicious axillary lymph nodes, ultrasound evaluation and tissue sampling (ultrasound-guided FNA or core biopsy) is recommended generally followed by completion axillary lymph node dissection (ALND) for patients with positive sentinel lymph nodes (SLNs). For patients without clinically

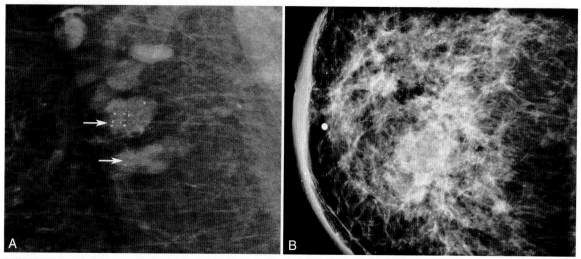

Fig. 17.11 Metastatic axillary nodal calcifications from ipsilateral primary breast cancer. (A) Mediolateral oblique (MLO) mammographic view of the right breast shows pleomorphic calcifications (*arrows*) within several mildly enlarged axillary lymph nodes. (B) Spot compression craniocaudal (CC) view demonstrates fine pleomorphic calcifications associated with a palpable irregular mass with indistinct margins (invasive ductal carcinoma), marked by a radiopaque skin BB marker. Associated skin thickening and erythema is consistent with the patient's clinical diagnosis of inflammatory breast cancer.

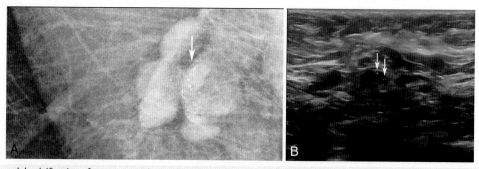

Fig. 17.12 Axillary nodal calcifications from metastatic ovarian cancer. (A) Screening mammogram (mediolateral oblique [MLO] view) shows axillary nodal microcalcifications (*arrow*). No suspicious findings were seen in either breast (not shown). (B) Ultrasound of the axilla demonstrates punctate echogenic foci (*arrows*) within a lymph node corresponding to microcalcifications. The examination was assessed as BI-RADS 4 (suspicious). Ultrasound-guided biopsy yielded metastatic carcinoma with psammomatous calcifications consistent with Mullerian primary origin. Subsequent computed tomography (CT) imaging demonstrated a left adnexal mass (not shown) with surgical pathology confirming ovarian seromucinous carcinoma.

palpable or mammographically suspicious axillary lymph nodes, the indication for performing axillary ultrasound varies among institutions. Currently at our institution, axillary ultrasound is performed at the time of diagnostic imaging evaluation for suspicious (BI-RADS 4 C or 5) breast masses that measure 2 cm in size or greater.

For patients without clinically suspicious lymph nodes, SLN biopsy (SLNB) is the preferred initial approach as it provides reliable staging information with less morbidity than ALND. If the SLNB is negative, no further axillary surgery is required and ALND may be omitted. Completion ALND was previously the standard for all patients with positive SLNs in this setting; however, the American College of Surgeons Oncology Group (ACOSOG) Z0011 trial showed that its utility among patients with limited metastatic SLNs may not be necessary. This trial showed equivalent rates of locoregional failure and survival among patients who underwent SLNB alone compared with SLNB and completion ALND. The patients included in this study had T1-T2 tumors, no palpable adenopathy, and one to two SLNs containing metastasis, and they were treated with breast conservation and systemic therapy. The ACOSOG Z0011 data do not apply to patients with T3 tumors, three or more involved nodes, those undergoing mastectomy, those receiving neoadjuvant chemotherapy, or those receiving partial-breast radiation therapy or radiation therapy in the prone position in which the low axilla is not treated. Completion ALND is still recommended in patients with three or more positive SLNs.

Preoperative/neoadjuvant chemotherapy is frequently used for patients with large primary tumors and/or biopsy-proven metastatic axillary lymph nodes. Accurate determination of residual axillary disease following chemotherapy provides important staging information. SLNB is preferable to ALND as it results in less morbidity; however the role of SLNB in this setting has been widely debated due to relatively high false-negative rates. This was investigated by the ACOSOG Z1071 trial, which showed that the false-negative rate for SLNB following chemotherapy in women presenting with biopsy-proven cN1 breast cancer was 12.6%, exceeding the acceptable threshold of 10%. While their data do not support the use of SLNB as an alternative to ALND following chemotherapy, they identified factors associated with a lower likelihood of false-negative SLNB findings, in particular dual-agent mapping and recovery of more than two SLNs. Reduced false-negative rates of SLNB have also been observed if there is a normal axillary ultrasound after neoadjuvant chemotherapy and if the biopsy-proven malignant lymph node containing the marker clip is retrieved in the specimen.

KEY POINTS

- Axillary lymphadenopathy is common and may be caused by a variety of both benign and malignant processes including infection/inflammation, granulomatous diseases, autoimmune diseases, metastases, and lymphoproliferative diseases.
- Unilateral axillary lymphadenopathy is typically more concerning than bilateral axillary lymphadenopathy and should prompt careful search of the ipsilateral breast and sonographic evaluation of the axilla.
- Bilateral axillary lymphadenopathy usually implies a systemic cause, such as inflammatory/infectious etiology or hematologic malignancy.
- Axillary nodal calcifications are more concerning than axillary lymphadenopathy alone, and microcalcifications are a particularly worrisome feature for malignancy.
- Axillary lymph node involvement in patients with breast cancer is an important factor for staging, treatment, and prognosis.

Suggested Readings

Boughey JC, Suman VJ, Mittendorf EA, et al. Sentinel lymph node surgery after neoadjuvant chemotherapy in patients with node-positive breast cancer. *JAMA.* 2013;310(14):1455–1461.

Chang JM, Leung JWT, Moy L, et al. Axillary nodal evaluation in breast cancer: state of the art. *Radiology.* 2020;295(3):500–515. https://doi.org/10.1148/radiol.2020192534.

Dialani V, James DF, Slanetz PJ. A practical approach to imaging the axilla. *Insights Imaging.* 2015;6(2):217–229.

Ecanow JS, Abe H, Newstead GM, et al. Axillary staging of breast cancer: what the radiologist should know. *Radiographics.* 2013;33:1589–1612.

Giuliano AE, Hunt KK, Ballman KV, et al. Axillary dissection vs no axillary dissection in women with invasive breast cancer and sentinel node metastasis. *JAMA.* 2011;305(6):569–575.

Lehman CD, Lamb LR, D'Alessandro HA. Mitigating the Impact of Coronavirus Disease (COVID-19) Vaccinations on Patients Undergoing Breast Imaging Examinations: A Pragmatic Approach. *AJR.* 2021;217(3):584–586. https://doi.org/10.2214/AJR.21.25688.

Lernevall A. Imaging of axillary lymph nodes. *Acta Oncologica.* 2000;39(3):277–281.

Mittendorf EA, Caudle AS, Yang W, et al. Implementation of the American College of Surgeons Oncology Group Z1071 trial data in clinical practice: is there a way forward for sentinel lymph node dissection in clinically node-positive breast cancer patients treated with neoadjuvant chemotherapy? *Ann Surg Oncol.* 2014;21:2468–2473.

Monaco SE, Khalbuss WE, Pantanowitz L. Benign non-infectious causes of lymphadenopathy: a review of cytomorphology and differential diagnosis. *Diagn Cytopathol.* 2012;40(10):925–938.

Net JM, Mirpuri TM, Plaza MJ, et al. Resident and fellow education feature: US evaluation of axillary lymph nodes. *Radiographics.* 2014;34(7):1817–1818.

Shah-Khan M, Boughey JC. Evolution of axillary nodal staging in breast cancer: clinical implications of the ACOSOG Z0011 trial. *Cancer Control.* 2012;19(4):267–276.

18 The Augmented and Reconstructed Breast

SUJATA V. GHATE

OVERVIEW This chapter reviews the normal and abnormal imaging appearances of the augmented and reconstructed breast. This includes implants and autologous flap reconstructions, as well as associated early, delayed, and rare complications.

Breast surgeries, whether for cosmetic intent or for reconstruction, have evolved considerably over the last several decades. Advances in microsurgical techniques, increased use of autologous flaps, and availability of higher quality of implants have provided more options for both augmentation and reconstruction and have resulted in improved aesthetic outcomes with fewer complications.

Both the cosmetically augmented and reconstructed breast are frequently encountered on imaging; thus, knowledge of the normal appearances, and familiarity with the imaging features of benign changes versus those suspicious for tumor recurrence, is essential for the radiologist to arrive at the correct diagnosis. This chapter will review the normal and abnormal imaging appearances after various breast surgical techniques, including implant augmentation, autologous flap reconstruction, reduction mammoplasty, and explantation, along with their associated risks and complications.

Breast Implants

Breast implants are medical prostheses placed within the breast tissue or under the pectoralis muscle to either augment the breast for cosmesis or reconstruct the breast after cancer surgery, trauma, or for correction of a congenital malformation. Implants were first introduced in the 1960s and have undergone considerable changes and improvements over the last several decades. The U.S. Food and Drug Administration (FDA) has approved two types of implants: saline and silicone.

Both saline and silicone implants consist of a textured or smooth elastomer silicone outer shell filled with either a saline solution or silicone gel. Normal implants have an oval shape and smooth contour on mammography. Saline prostheses will appear radiolucent with a prominent valve, usually seen in a periareolar location. This valve allows for volume adjustment during and after implant placement (Fig. 18.1A). Silicone implants with either viscous or cohesive gel filler are radiopaque on mammography (Fig. 18.1B) and lack the valve seen with saline implants. Double lumen or expandable implants with various combinations of saline and silicone inner and outer lumens are less commonly encountered, as their complicated construction has been

linked to higher rates of implant failure. These dual lumen implants allow gradual expansion and volume adjustment of the saline lumen through a subcutaneous valve after placement—a useful advantage for breast reconstruction (Box 18.1).

The placement of any type of implant will trigger an inflammatory response, which is a normal part of the healing process. The body recognizes the prosthesis as a foreign object and attempts to isolate it by surrounding the implant with a thin, collagenous fibrous capsule. This barrier is a normal finding around all implants, is harmless in most women, and helps stabilize the implant position. The capsule usually is not discernible on conventional imaging unless it calcifies, which may occur in up to 16% of women with implants.[1] Capsular calcifications on mammography vary in morphology from coarse, plaque-like calcifications to amorphous or pleomorphic calcifications along the implant margin.

Implant location or position is defined by its anatomic relationship to the pectoralis muscle. Prepectoral (also known as subglandular) implants are in front of the pectoralis muscle, while retropectoral (also known as subpectoral) implant are behind the pectoralis muscle (see Fig. 18.1A–B). Because the presence of implants may obscure up to 25% of breast tissue on mammography, four implant-displaced (ID) or Eklund views in addition to the four standard craniocaudal (CC) and mediolateral oblique (MLO) views are recommended to visualize as much tissue as possible. The ID technique requires displacing the implant posteriorly and compressing the anterior tissue, allowing for improved visualization of the native breast tissue (Fig. 18.2A–B). ID views are easier to acquire in women with retropectoral implants but are not as successful if marked capsular calcifications or capsular contracture are present (Box 18.2).

Box 18.1   Normal Implants: Imaging Findings

- Thin elastomer outer shell
- Smooth contour, oval shape
- Saline: radiolucent, presence of fill valve
- Silicone: radiopaque

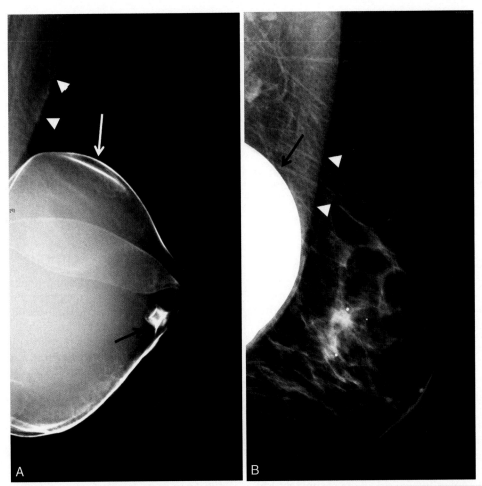

Fig. 18.1 Mediolateral oblique (MLO) implant views in two different women demonstrate (A) a radiolucent, saline implant (*white arrow*) with a characteristic "fill valve" (*black arrow*) in a periareolar location. Note the prepectoral/subglandular placement, with the pectoralis muscle (*arrowheads*) located posterior to the implant. (B) A radiopaque, silicone implant in a retropectoral location (*black arrow*). Note the pectoralis muscle drapes anterior to the implant (*arrowheads*).

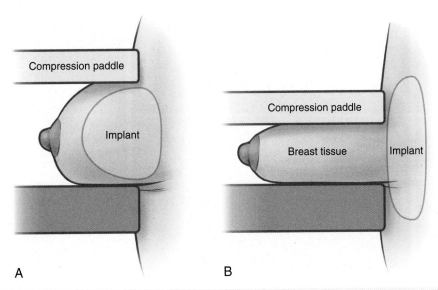

Fig. 18.2 Optimal imaging technique for women with implants should include (A) the implant view, where implant and breast tissue are minimally compressed and (B) the implant displaced view, where the implant is pushed posteriorly and the anterior, native breast tissue is compressed for optimal visualization.

Implant Risks and Complications

Silicone implants are considered safe, but as with any medical device, there are associated risks and complications that are important to recognize. In the 1980s, there was growing concern over silicone implant rupture and its potential association with immunologic disorders. In response, the FDA issued a moratorium on use of silicone breast implants in 1992, which was subsequently lifted in 2006, after a number of published studies revealed no connection to systemic disease.[2–4]

More recently, breast implant–associated anaplastic large cell lymphoma (BIA-ALCL) has emerged as a potential risk of the newer-generation silicone cohesive gel implants, particularly the textured variety. BIA-ALCL is a rare, T-cell lymphoma, with a current estimated risk of approximately 1 in 35,000 women with implants by age 50, with risk increasing with age.[5] The pathogenesis is unknown, but theories suggest that it may be associated chronic peri-implant inflammation in a genetically susceptible host. The most common presentation is a large fluid collection surrounding the implant greater than 1 year after implant placement.

Less commonly, it can present as a capsular mass with or without associated fluid collection (Fig. 18.3). Clinical signs and symptoms include rapid swelling of the affected breast, palpable mass, skin erythema, or ulceration. The presence of a delayed moderate or large fluid collection surrounding the implant greater than 1 year after placement should be further investigated with fluid aspiration to evaluate for infection or BIA-ALCL. BIA-ALCL is uniformly and strongly positive for the CD30 tumor marker and negative for anaplastic lymphoma kinase (ALK). On imaging, ultrasound is more sensitive than mammography for detecting fluid collections and associated capsular masses. Prognosis is dependent on stage at diagnosis; thus, magnetic resonance imaging (MRI) or positron emission tomography–computed tomography (PET-CT) may be helpful for staging (Box 18.3).

EARLY IMPLANT COMPLICATIONS

Potential complications following implant surgery can be broadly divided into two categories: early and late. Early complications are rare and include peri-implant fluid collections, hematomas, and infection. Small, peri-implant fluid collections or seromas are common and can be a normal finding in the immediate postoperative period. Larger collections, however, are problematic and may be associated with pain, disfigurement, and increased risk of infection; thus, therapeutic aspiration or drainage is often advised.

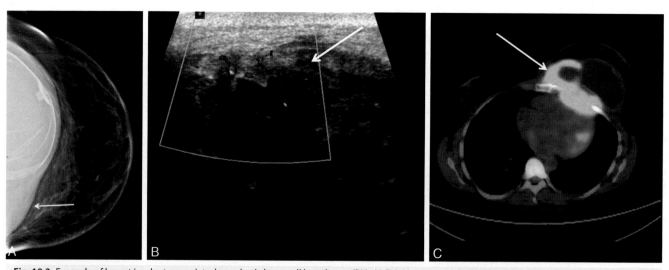

Fig. 18.3 Example of breast implant–associated anaplastic large cell lymphoma (BIA-ALCL). Mammography (A) demonstrates asymmetry (*arrow*) in the medial left breast adjacent to the implant. Sonography (B) shows a heterogeneous mass (*arrow*) with additional peri-implant fluid seen at time of real-time imaging. Positron emission tomography–computed tomography (PET-CT) (C) shows a fluorodeoxyglucose (FDG) avid mass (*arrow*) with fluid more centrally. Large fluid collections with or without the presence of a capsular masses are characteristic findings associated with BIA-ALCL.

For simple seromas without evidence of infection, the necessity of aspiration usually involves discussion with the surgeon. Ultrasound remains the imaging modality of choice for both detection and aspiration guidance because small- to moderate-sized seromas may be difficult to identify on mammography. MRI is not typically recommended for detection or diagnosis but may be useful in some cases to assess the overall size and extent of the collection along with presence or absence of an associated mass or focal abscess (Fig. 18.4).

An implant-associated hematoma may clinically present with focal pain and/or swelling of the affected breast and usually occurs immediately after surgery as a result of postoperative bleeding. Most collections are small and will resolve gradually over time. On mammography, small hematomas may be occult while larger collections may present as a nonspecific mass along the implant margin, which may calcify over time. Ultrasound, the best imaging tool for early assessment, will demonstrate an oval, circumscribed, avascular mass with variable internal echogenicity depending on the age of blood products (Fig. 18.5A). These imaging features are often nonspecific; thus, close clinical and imaging follow-up, aspiration, or biopsy may be required to exclude a breast abscess or malignancy. MRI may demonstrate an oval, circumscribed, nonenhancing mass with variable internal signal, depending on the age of hemorrhage, type of hemoglobin, and imaging sequence (Fig. 18.5B–D). Delayed hematomas are very rare but may occur years after implant placement as a result of fracture or erosion of capsular vessels from trauma, inflammation, or corticosteroid use leading to chronic leakage and pooling of blood.

LATE IMPLANT COMPLICATIONS

Late complications of implants most commonly include capsular contracture and implant rupture. Capsular contracture occurs when the collagen fibrous capsule that surrounds the implant thickens and compresses the prosthesis resulting in pain, increased firmness, and distortion of the affected breast. The etiology is unclear, but some theories suggest that genetic susceptibility in combination with subclinical infection or subtle implant leaks in the intraoperative setting may result in marked inflammatory

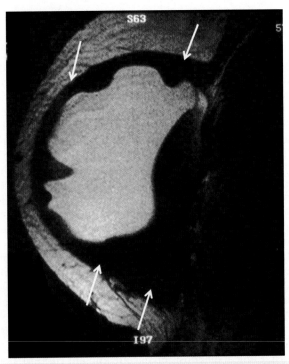

Fig. 18.4 Sagittal T2-weighted implant magnetic resonance imaging (MRI) with water saturation demonstrates a large seroma surrounding a silicone implant (*arrows*). Note the undulating contour of the silicone implant shell, which suggests abnormal compression from the surrounding fluid. Aspiration is recommended to due to the risk of infection.

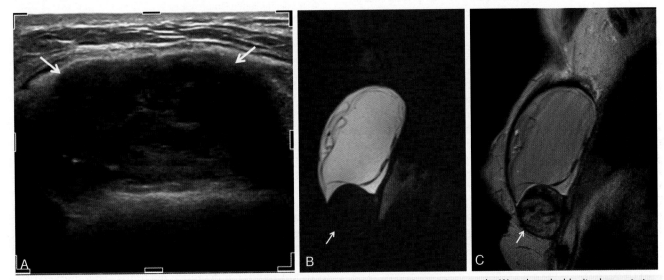

Fig. 18.5 Older adult patient presented with a palpable mass following minor trauma to her breast. Sonography (A) at the palpable site demonstrates an avascular, solid-appearing mass. Sagittal noncontrast breast magnetic resonance imaging (MRI) demonstrates a ruptured implant with a large hematoma at the inferior aspect of the implant (*arrows*). Note that the hematoma is hypointense on the silicone selective sequence (B) and demonstrates mixed signal on T1-weighted imaging, consistent with evolving stages of blood products. A hematoma will not enhance with contrast.

change and exuberant scar reaction around the implant, leading to contractures and distortion. Capsular contracture is a clinical diagnosis and is difficult to detect with certainty on any imaging modality. Associated findings described on imaging include a round or spherical rather than oval shape of the implant, the presence of capsular calcifications on mammography, or multiple radial folds on MRI; however, these findings are nonspecific, as they are frequently visualized with normal implants. Severe contracture may require surgical intervention, which involves resection of the capsule (i.e., capsulectomy) and implant removal followed by implant replacement (Box 18.4).

Implant rupture is a commonly recognized delayed complication of implant placement. The risk increases with implant age, with most ruptures occurring 10 to 15 years after implantation.[6] Saline implant ruptures are usually clinically obvious and do not require imaging for diagnosis because a tear in the saline implant shell will lead to rapid deflation of the implant and a decrease in size of the affected breast. Clinical diagnosis of silicone implant rupture, however, is challenging, as most ruptures are either asymptomatic or associated with nonspecific symptoms. The most common signs and symptoms include a change in breast shape, focal or nonfocal pain, palpable lump, or asymmetry. However, clinical findings may be absent in up to 50% of cases[6]; therefore, imaging is usually necessary for accurate diagnosis of silicone implant rupture.

There are two types of implant rupture: intracapsular and extracapsular.

An intracapsular rupture occurs when the implant elastomer shell tears but silicone remains contained within the collagen fibrous capsule formed by the breast. This type of rupture is difficult to detect clinically or on mammography where the contour of the implant will typically appear normal. On ultrasound, a characteristic and reliable sign of intracapsular rupture is the "step ladder" sign, which presents as discontinuous, echogenic, parallel lines reflecting from a collapsed implant elastomer shell with the surrounding silicone gel contained by an intact fibrous capsule (Fig. 18.6). However, this sonographic sign is not sensitive and will not be apparent unless there is a larger tear with complete collapse of the implant shell. Small, focal defects and early, noncollapsed intracapsular rupture are difficult to detect with sonography and usually only identified by MRI (Box 18.5).

Intracapsular rupture can progress to extracapsular rupture when free silicone extrudes through the collagen fibrous capsule into the surrounding breast parenchyma,

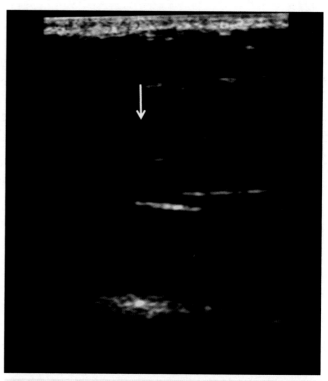

Fig. 18.6 Sonographic appearance of intracapsular rupture: Ultrasound image demonstrates the step ladder sign with multiple parallel, echogenic lines (*arrow*), analogous to a ruptured and collapsed implant shell floating within a viscous silicone gel matrix, but still contained within an intact collagen fibrous capsule.

occasionally traveling to the lymphatic system. Small, localized extracapsular leaks may be undetectable on mammography. Larger extracapsular rupture may present as a new focal contour irregularity, focal high-density free silicone within the breast parenchyma, or, in the advanced stages, a larger global asymmetry (Fig. 18.7A–C). If the findings are inconclusive on mammography, sonography performed with a high-frequency linear transducer (7–12 MHz) is a useful tool for a definitive diagnosis. The characteristic sign associated with extracapsular rupture on ultrasound is the "snow storm sign," a heterogeneous, echogenic artifact caused by silicone droplets interspersed within breast

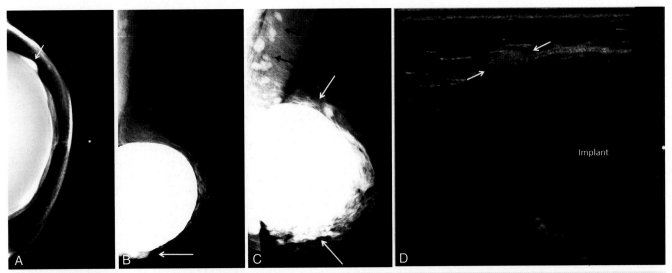

Fig. 18.7 Examples of extracapsular rupture on mammography and ultrasound. (A) Craniocaudal implant view demonstrates a subtle focal contour irregularity (*arrow*). A mediolateral oblique (MLO) view in a different patient (B) demonstrates irregularity at the inferior aspect of the implant with discontinuity of the implant shell (*arrow*). A third patient (C) with extensive free silicone throughout the parenchyma (*arrowheads*) with uptake into the axillary lymph nodes (*arrows*). Ultrasound imaging in a different patient (D) demonstrates the classic "snowstorm" sign along the surface of the implant (*arrow*), consistent with the presence of extracapsular silicone.

Box 18.6   Imaging Findings of Intracapsular Rupture

- Mammography
  - Frequently normal
- Ultrasound
  - "Step ladder" sign
- Breast magnetic resonance imaging (MRI)
  - "Inverted teardrop," "noose," or "keyhole" sign
  - "Droplet sign"—nonspecific
  - "Subcapsular line" sign
  - "Linguine" sign

---

tissue (Fig. 18.7D). This is a specific and highly reliable sign of implant rupture. Of note, the presence of extracapsular silicone or a silicone granuloma within the breast parenchyma does not necessarily indicate rupture of the current implant but may denote residual silicone from a prior implant rupture in a patient who has since undergone implant exchange. Therefore a careful history from the patient and comparison with prior imaging studies is essential to ensure an accurate diagnosis. If there is any diagnostic uncertainty regarding silicone implant integrity, breast MRI can be performed (Box 18.6).

Breast MRI without intravenous contrast is considered the gold standard for evaluation of implant integrity with sensitivity for a rupture estimated at between 80% and 90% and specificity between 90% and 97%.[7] In asymptomatic patients, the FDA currently recommends breast MRI to screen for silent rupture 5 to 6 years after implant placement followed by every 2 to 3 years thereafter.[8] In contrast, the American College of Radiology Appropriateness Criteria states that imaging is "usually not appropriate" to evaluate silicone implants in asymptomatic women but that MRI should be performed for those with suspected implant complications. MRI's high accuracy for detection of implant rupture extends from its ability to selectively suppress or enhance signal intensities of water, fat, and silicone. Breast MRI is best performed with patient in a prone position using a dedicated breast coil for high spatial resolution, which is necessary to characterize small implant defects. The preferred magnet strength is 1.5 Tesla or greater. Protocols may vary, but generally include a T1-weighted sequence to better define breast anatomy. Most importantly, the MRI must include silicone-selective bright fluid sequence, commonly a STIR sequence with water suppression or alternatively a T2-weighted fast spin echo with fat and water suppression in order to emphasize the signal from silicone (i.e., silicone hyperintense, water suppressed). This may also be supplemented with silicone-suppressed sequences. Silicone-specific sequences allow for detection of intracapsular rupture and for identification of small free silicone deposits or silicone granulomas in the breast parenchyma, which are diagnostic of extracapsular rupture. Multiplanar imaging or reformatting in the axial, sagittal, and coronal planes is useful for differentiating subtle focal ruptures from surface folds. On MRI, normal implants, regardless of type, should have a smooth outer contour.

MRI is never indicated for the evaluation of saline implants. If unintentionally imaged, intact saline implants would appear dark on silicone-selective water-suppressed sequences. An injection port or fill valve will be readily apparent along the surface of saline but absent in silicone implants.

Intracapsular rupture is frequently only visible on breast MRI. There are a number of characteristic signs that are important to recognize, which help determine not only the extent of rupture but also the degree of implant shell collapse (Table 18.1). The earliest sign of intracapsular rupture is a focal tear within the cusp of an implant fold resulting in a focal, contained leak of silicone resembling a "noose," "inverted teardrop," or "keyhole." This occurs when there is a small tear within the invagination of an implant fold, the weakest portion of the implant shell (Fig. 18.8). If a tear occurs along the margin of the implant shell, the viscous silicone gel may migrate through the defect and collect between the shell and fibrous capsule. The resulting partial inward collapse of the shell produces a curved or wavy, dark line parallel to the fibrous capsule and contiguous with the rest of the implant shell, referred to as the "subcapsular line sign" (see Fig. 18.8). Finally, if the implant shell completely ruptures and collapses, multiple dark serpiginous lines may be identified floating within the viscous silicone gel; this appearance is called the "linguine sign" (Fig. 18.9), analogous to the "step ladder sign" seen on ultrasound. A less common sign associated with rupture is the droplet sign, which is the presence of an air or water droplet within the implant lumen.[9] This is not a reliable sign of rupture on its own and may be seen as an inclusion in normal implants. However, the presence of a droplet sign should prompt careful interrogation of the implant to look for other subtle signs of rupture.

Radial folds are normal intact folds along the surface of an implant and should not be misdiagnosed as small intracapsular tears. On the silicone-sensitive sequence, a radial fold appears as a dark line extending inward from the periphery of the implant and ending blindly. These folds are closely apposed surface invaginations of the implant shell and do not contain silicone within the cusp of the fold and therefore should be easily distinguished from the "noose" or "keyhole" signs associated with intracapsular rupture (Fig. 18.10).

As implants age, the risk of gel bleed, a unique complication of viscous silicone gel implants, increases. Gel bleed occurs when microscopic amounts of viscous silicone gel seep through an intact silicone shell, which acts as a semipermeable membrane. On MRI, a small "keyhole," "teardrop," or "noose" sign may be present, thus mimicking a

Table 18.1 Magnetic Resonance Imaging (MRI) Signs of Intracapsular Rupture

MRI Sign	Size of Implant Tear	Degree of Implant Shell Collapse
"Keyhole" sign	Small, focal	Minimal to none
"Inverted teardrop" sign		
"Noose" sign		
"Subcapsular line" sign	Moderate	Partial
"Linguine" sign	Large	Complete

Adapted from Seiler SJ, Sharma PB, Hayes JC, Ganti R, Mootz AR, Eads ED, Teotia SS, Evans WP: Multimodality imaging-based evaluation of single-lumen silicone breast implants for rupture, *RadioGraphics* 37:2, 366–382, 2017.

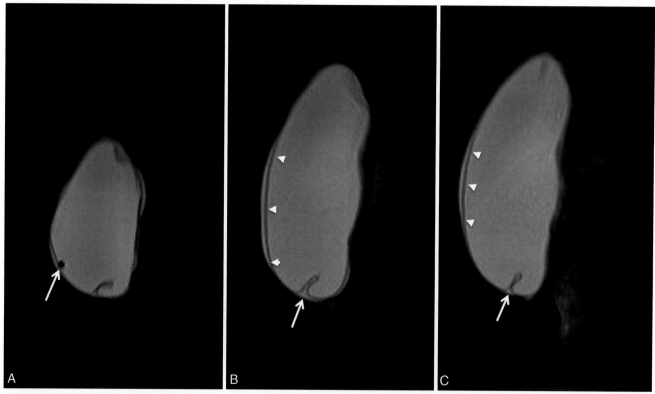

Fig. 18.8 Magnetic resonance imaging (MRI) signs of intracapsular rupture. Silicone-selective sagittal images in a young patient with implants (A) demonstrates a small water droplet, referred to as the "droplet sign" (*arrow*). A (B) "keyhole sign" is also visible in the inferior aspect of this implant (*arrow*). Note the presence of silicone within the apex of the keyhole, as well as outside of the implant shell. A thin, hypointense line (implant shell) is identified anteriorly, parallel to the surface of the implant shell consistent with a "subcapsular line" sign. Note the line extends from surface to surface of the collagen fibrous capsule (*arrowheads*) and silicone is seen on either side of it. An (C) inverted "teardrop" or a "noose" sign is also identified along the inferior aspect of this implant (*arrow*) along with the "subcapsular line" sign (*arrowheads*). The implant shell is closely apposed in the area of the "inverted teardrop," which differs from the keyhole sign. Note the presence of silicone within the "teardrop," as well as outside of the implant shell.

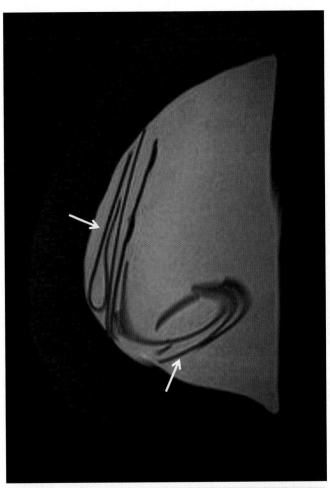

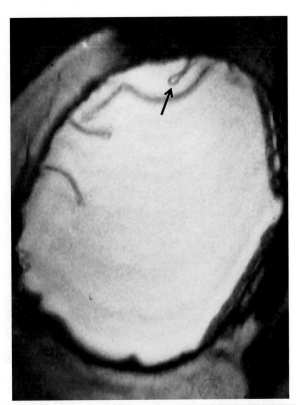

Fig. 18.11 Sagittal T1-weighted magnetic resonance imaging (MRI) demonstrates a single "inverted teardrop" sign (*arrow*) with an otherwise intact implant. The presence of a solitary imaging sign of a focal tear should prompt a differential diagnosis of gel bleed versus intracapsular rupture. Surgical excision revealed an intact implant.

Fig. 18.9 Intracapsular rupture on magnetic resonance imaging (MRI) with complete collapse of the implant shell. Sagittal silicone-selective image demonstrates serpiginous hypointense lines (*arrows*) floating within the viscous silicone gel but still contained within the fibrous collagen capsule.

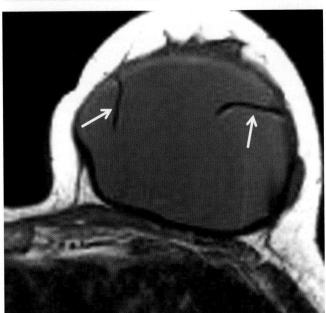

Fig. 18.10 Axial T1-weighted magnetic resonance imaging (MRI) demonstrates normal implant surface folds referred to as "radial folds" (*arrows*). Note the lack of silicone within these surface invaginations which distinguish them from "keyhole" or "inverted teardrop" signs. They also do not extend from surface to surface of the implant shell like the "subcapsular line" sign.

focal intracapsular tear (Fig. 18.11). If only a single site of a possible focal tear is identified on MRI, with an otherwise completely intact implant, the differential diagnosis should include gel bleed versus focal intracapsular rupture. With prolonged and larger gel bleeds, silicone may enter the lymphatics and travel to the axillary, internal mammary, or even mediastinal lymph nodes or to other parts of the body.

Long-term integrity of the newest generation of cohesive gel (commonly known as "gummy") implants is still unknown, but existing data indicate a lower incidence of rupture, likely the result of a thicker, more durable outer shell. The semisolid gel matrix is also unlikely to migrate into adjacent tissue or leak through an intact shell as seen with the earlier generation of viscous silicone gel implants; thus, rupture is difficult to detect on conventional mammography or ultrasound. On MRI, heterogeneous signal within the gel matrix, particularly the presence of multiple large water droplets, indicates focal degeneration of the gel matrix, which may be the earliest sign of implant compromise (Fig. 18.12A–B). When cohesive gel implants rupture, the implant shell will tear and gel matrix will fracture, producing a hypointense fracture line on MRI, a sign of intracapsular rupture. If the fracture line is associated with a contour abnormality and heterogeneous signal within the lumen is present from admixture of silicone and serous fluid, extracapsular rupture should be suspected. These larger ruptures frequently compromise the shape and appearance of the affected breast and thus are often diagnosed clinically without the need for imaging confirmation.[7]

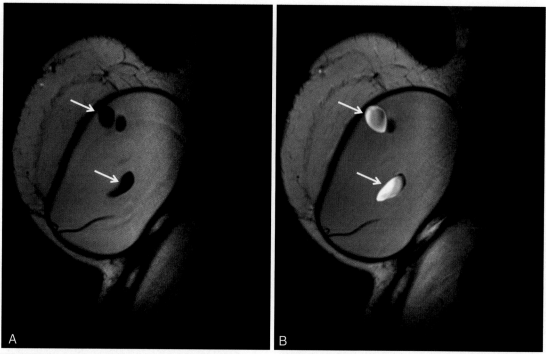

Fig. 18.12 T2-weighted sagittal magnetic resonance imaging (MRI) without and with water saturation of a left cohesive gel implant. Note the presence of multiple large water droplets (*arrows*) within the left breast implant, which are dark on image with water saturation (A) and hyperintense without water saturation (B). These findings are suggestive of early gel matrix degeneration.

Breast Reconstruction After Mastectomy

Breast reconstruction uses specialized plastic surgery techniques to restore the shape of the breast to a near-normal appearance following surgery for breast cancer. After mastectomy, the breast may be reconstructed by using implants, autologous tissue flaps, or a combination of both.

Implant reconstruction is the most common reconstruction method in the United States. This standard surgical technique involves a two-stage approach. In the first stage, a tissue expander is placed in the mastectomy bed, typically deep to the pectoralis muscles. The expander is then gradually filled with saline through a port over 3 to 6 months to create space for the implant. This port is usually ferromagnetic; therefore MRI should not be performed while the expander is in place. In the final stage, the expander is exchanged for a breast prosthesis.

Breast ptosis and capsular contracture are two challenges encountered with implant reconstruction after mastectomy. In recent years, the increasing use of acellular dermal matrix (ADM), a mesh-like sheet of material derived from animal or human cadaveric skin, has been successful in alleviating these complications and improving cosmesis. The purpose of ADM is to create a sling along the superior-lateral and inferior aspect of the prosthesis in order to stabilize implant position and redefine the inframammary fold for a more natural and symmetric cosmetic outcome. Complete coverage of the implant with ADM also provides an additional layer of cushion between the skin and implant, which decreases the risk of capsular contracture

(Fig. 18.13A). ADM is usually not discernible on clinical examination or mammography. On occasion, it may present as a palpable lump at the lateral or inferior aspect of the implant. ADM should not be mistaken for implant rupture on imaging. The presence of a vague horizontally oriented hypoechoic mass adjacent to the implant margin on ultrasound is suggestive of ADM, not rupture (Fig. 18.13B). On MRI, ADM will commonly present as a nonenhancing plaque-like mass abutting the implant, demonstrating low signal on silicone-selective sequences and intermediate signal similar to breast tissue on T1-weighted imaging (Fig. 18.13C–D).

In recent years, improvements in microsurgical techniques have led to increased use of autologous flaps for breast reconstruction. The most commonly harvested autologous flaps are the transverse rectus abdominis myocutaneous (TRAM), latissimus dorsi (LD), or deep inferior epigastric perforator (DIEP) flap, all of which have unique features on imaging (Box 18.7).

The TRAM flap, either pedicled or free, was initially the most commonly executed autologous myocutaneous flap (AMF). With a pedicled TRAM flap, an elliptical incision is made along the lower abdominal wall. The skin, underlying fat, and contralateral rectus abdominis muscle are then mobilized along with their blood supply, the superior epigastric artery, and vein (Fig. 18.14A). The skin of the harvested tissue is then de-epithelialized and the flap is rotated and tunneled subcutaneously at the mastectomy site to form the mound of the breast. A free TRAM flap is created similarly; however, instead of mobilizing the entire contralateral rectus abdominis muscle, only a small portion of the muscle is harvested along with its blood supply,

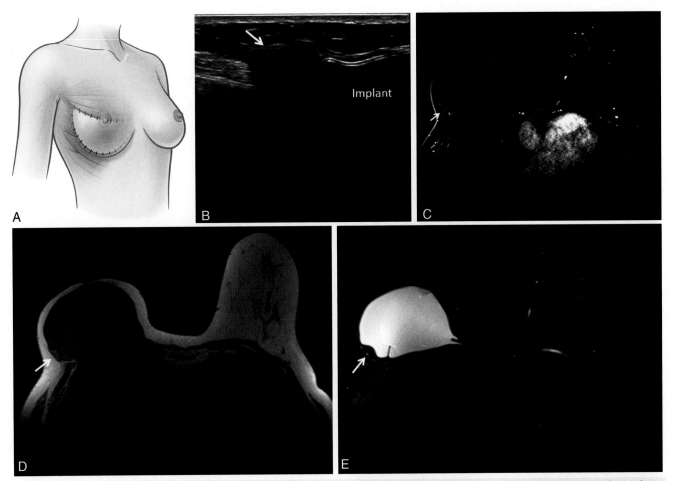

Fig. 18.13 (A) Illustration of an acellular dermal matrix (ADM) sling. Note the shaded area shows the location of the sling containing the implant. (B) Sonography of a palpable lump in a patient status post implant reconstruction demonstrates a hypoechoic mass along the lateral aspect of the implant (*arrows*). The location and appearance are consistent with an ADM sling. Note that unlike rupture, there is no evidence of a "snow storm sign" artifact. This same ADM sling (C–E) is redemonstrated on magnetic resonance imaging (MRI) (*arrows*). Note that it does not enhance with contrast, is similar in signal to the breast parenchyma on non-fat-suppressed images, and is hypointense on silicone-selective sequences.

Box 18.7   Most Commonly Performed Autologous Flaps

- Myocutaneous flaps
  - Transverse rectus abdominus myocutaneous (TRAM) (pedicled)
  - TRAM (free)
  - Latissimus dorsi (LD)
- Perforator flaps
  - Deep interior epigastric perforators (DIEP)
  - Superficial inferior epigastric artery (SIEA)

the inferior epigastric artery, and vein (Fig. 18.14B). The artery and vein are subsequently anastomosed to either the internal mammary, thoracodorsal, or subscapular vessels using microsurgical techniques. Advantages of the free flap include a more robust blood supply from the inferior epigastric vessels and a decreased risk of abdominal wall hernias because less muscle tissue is excised.[10] Both flaps have a similar appearance on imaging. On mammography, dense vertical and rounded muscle fibers may initially be

visualized along the posterior aspect of the mammogram on both the CC and MLO views (Fig. 18.15A). Over time, the muscle often atrophies and becomes replaced with fat; therefore it may no longer be visible on mammography (Fig. 18.15B). On breast MRI, TRAM flaps will demonstrate a characteristic, triangular-shaped muscle at the posterior central aspect of the reconstructed breast (Fig. 18.16A). The anastomotic site of the free TRAM is frequently identifiable on MRI by the presence of signal void artifact emanating from surgical clips (Fig. 18.16B).

The LD flap is another pedicled flap harvested from the upper back by mobilizing the latissimus dorsi muscle, skin, and subcutaneous fat and rotating the tissue forward to reform the breast at the ipsilateral mastectomy site (Fig. 18.17A). This flap alone may not provide sufficient tissue to create the appropriate volume necessary for symmetry; therefore it is frequently combined with an implant (Fig. 18.17C). On MRI, the LD muscle will be visualized extending from its lateral origin toward the anterior chest wall to form the mound of the breast and will be a rounder, rather than a triangle-shaped, configuration (Fig. 18.17B).

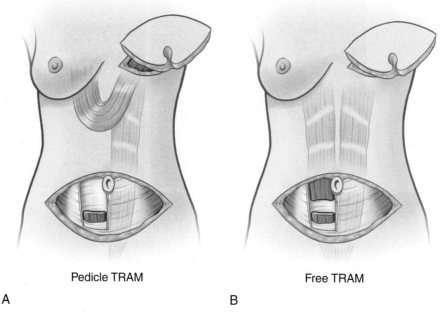

Pedicle TRAM

Free TRAM

A   B

Fig. 18.14 Pedicled and free transverse rectus abdominis myocutaneous (TRAM) flap technique is illustrated. With the pedicled TRAM flap (A), the entire contralateral muscle along with the skin, subcutaneous fat and blood supply is mobilized to reconstruct the breast. In contrast, the free TRAM flap technique (B) only removes a small portion of the rectus abdominis muscle along with the skin, subcutaneous fat, and inferior epigastric blood vessels.

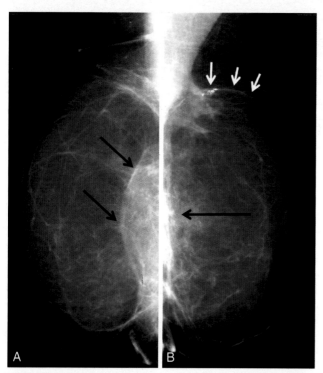

Fig. 18.15 Bilateral digital mammogram mediolateral oblique (MLO) views (A) from pedicled transverse rectus abdominis myocutaneous (TRAM) flap reconstruction demonstrates dense, curvilinear rectus abdominus muscle fibers posteriorly on the right breast (*black arrows*). The flap muscle frequently atrophies over time and becomes replaced with fat (B), and thus may no longer be visible on mammography, as demonstrated on the left side (*black arrow*). Note the thin, dense line visible at the periphery of the flap (*white arrows*). This represents the de-epithelialized skin of the abdominal flap, sometimes referred to as the "contact line." Residual breast tissue is present superficial to this line where most recurrences will occur.

The DIEP flap is the most common type of perforator flap where donor skin and fat are transferred from the lower abdomen without mobilizing any portion of the muscle. Instead, the deep inferior epigastric perforator vessels are dissected and anastomosed to either the internal mammary or thoracodorsal vessels using microsurgical techniques. It is easily distinguished from muscular flaps due to the lack of muscle seen within the reconstructed breast on MRI (Fig. 18.18A–B). Another variation of the DIEP perforator flap is the superficial inferior epigastric artery (SIEA) flap, which relies on blood supply from the superficial inferior epigastric vessels. The technique for harvesting the SIEA flap is less invasive than a DIEP, which is a distinct advantage. However, the blood supply from these superficial vessels is frequently less robust; thus, this technique is not as commonly performed (Box 18.8).

When sufficient lower abdominal tissue is not available for use, other options for reconstruction include buttock or thigh flaps such as a gluteal artery perforator (GAP), transverse upper gracilis (TUG) flaps, and others. Because these techniques are less commonly used, they will not be discussed in detail in this chapter.

The final phase of breast reconstruction, if the native nipple has not been spared, is nipple-areolar reconstruction, which involves reforming the nipple-areolar complex using nipple-sharing grafts, autologous flaps, intradermal tattoos, or a combination of these techniques. Most of these reconstruction methods have nonspecific findings on imaging, namely just surgical scars along the nipple or areolar margin. However, nipple tattoos may present with unique imaging findings. On mammography, intradermal tattoos, which contain microscopic metallic fragments, may mimic skin calcifications along the confines of the reconstructed

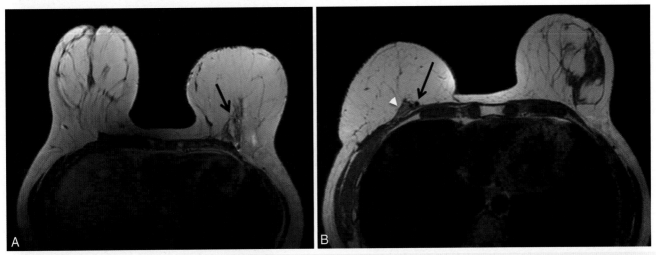

Fig. 18.16 A pedicled transverse rectus abdominis myocutaneous (TRAM) flap (A) on T1-weighted magnetic resonance imaging (MRI) demonstrates the typical appearance of a triangular shaped rectus abdominis muscle posteriorly (*arrow*). A free TRAM flap (B) has a similar appearance with a portion of the muscle (*arrowhead*), as well as signal void from surgical clip artifact at the anastomotic site medially (*arrow*). This is the site of anastomoses of the inferior epigastric artery and vein to perforator branches from the internal mammary vessels.

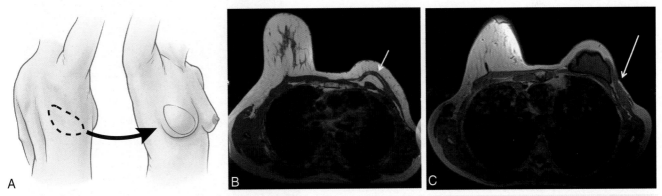

Fig. 18.17 Illustration of the latissimus dorsi (LD) flap technique (A). The LD flap is a pedicle flap rotated from the upper back forward to reconstruct the breast. T1-weighted axial magnetic resonance imaging (MRI) (B) demonstrates the lateral extension of the muscle with a rounded appearance posteriorly (*arrowheads*) in contrast to the triangular shape of the transverse rectus abdominis myocutaneous (TRAM) flap. The LD flap is sometimes combined with an implant (C) for reconstruction. Again, note how the muscle is rotated from the lateral aspect (*arrows*) to cover a portion of the implant.

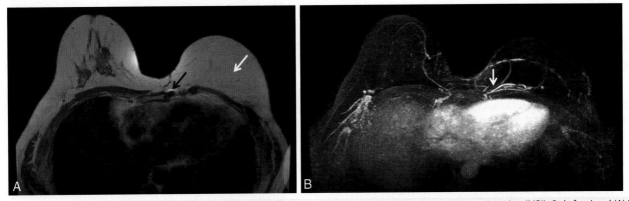

Fig. 18.18 A deep inferior epigastric perforator (DIEP) flap on contrast-enhanced T1-weighted magnetic resonance imaging (MRI). Only fat signal (A) is identified in the reconstructed breast with no muscular tissue present (*white arrow*). Peristernal signal void is identified at the site of microsurgical vascular anastomoses (*black arrow*). On maximum-intensity projection (MIP) image (B), the site of vascular anastomoses is nicely demonstrated (*white arrow*).

nipple (Fig. 18.19). Otherwise, imaging findings of a reconstructed nipple are nonspecific and may be difficult to differentiate from the normal nipple.

Following breast reconstruction, autologous fat grafting or lipografting is increasingly being offered to improve aesthetic outcome. This technique transfers free fat from the lower abdomen or thigh to areas of contour deformities along the periphery of the reconstructed breast or within nipple to improve cosmesis and symmetry. The fat is harvested using a liposuction technique and centrifuged to isolate the pure adipocytes (Fig. 18.20A). This liquefied fat is then reinjected into areas of soft tissue defects where it relies on the wound bed to grow vessels for survival. Not all of the injected fat survives. Nonviable fat results in superficial, focal areas of fat necrosis or oil cysts that are usually easily palpable. On mammography, oil cysts may present as thin-walled lucent masses (Fig. 18.20B). On sonography, an oil cyst at a site of lipoinjection can have variable appearances, including a cystic lesion or a circumscribed round or oval hypoechoic solid mass (Fig. 18.20C). However, care must be taken to ensure that the mass meets all imaging features of benignity. Any morphologic feature suggestive of malignancy should warrant a biopsy, as recurrences commonly occur in a similar location in the superficial residual breast tissue.

Breast Reconstruction Risks and Complications

After breast reconstruction, typical postsurgical complications, such as hematoma or seroma formation and infection or implant deflation/rupture, are not uncommon and were discussed in detail earlier in the chapter. There are, however, a number of unique imaging findings and complications associated with autologous tissue reconstruction, such as skin thickening or fibrosis, epidermal inclusion cysts, fat necrosis, or recurrent malignancy, that are important for a radiologist to recognize.

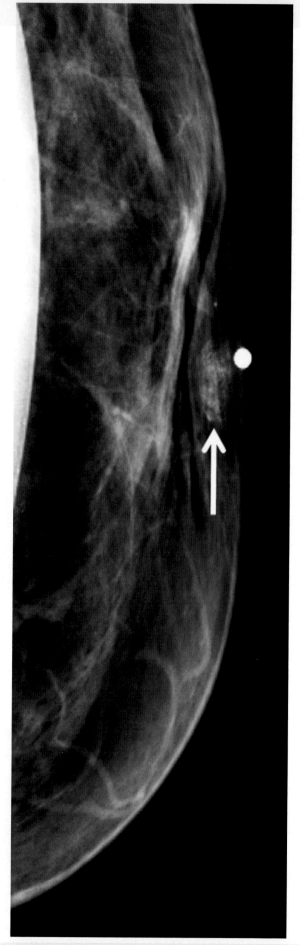

Fig. 18.19 Left mediolateral oblique (MLO) digital mammogram of a reconstructed breast demonstrates punctate densities mimicking calcifications in a circular distribution within the skin (*arrow*), consistent with a nipple-areolar tattoo.

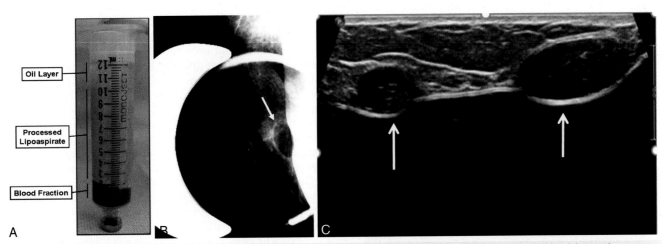

Fig. 18.20 Centrifugation of lipoaspirate (A) obtained from the lower abdomen separates the liquefied fat from other cellular debris and enzymes. The pure liquid fat can then be injected into areas where additional volume is needed. Injected fat (B) that does not survive may present as thin-walled radiolucent oil cysts on mammography (*arrow*), or (C) circumscribed hypo- or isoechoic oval masses on ultrasound (*white arrows*).

Skin thickening or fibrosis is common after breast reconstruction, usually the result of surgery and radiation therapy, both of which can affect venous and lymphatic drainage. Benign skin thickening and fibrosis are difficult to differentiate from inflammatory cancer on conventional imaging (Fig. 18.21) or ultrasound, and MRI may not yield additional diagnostic information. On MRI, both benign and malignant changes may appear hyperintense on T2-weighted imaging and can enhance with contrast, although the enhancement pattern is usually more intense with inflammatory cancer. Skin punch biopsy is often required for definitive diagnosis.

An epidermal inclusion cyst (EIC) is a benign mass lined with squamous epithelium, usually located within the dermal layer of the skin. EIC formation is generally the result of a traumatic insult to the skin, which is thought to incite an inflammatory response, leading to downward epithelial proliferation at the site. This uncommon lesion may develop on the surface of the tunneled portion of the flap if de-epithelialization of the skin is incomplete. Any residual epithelial remnants may undergo cellular proliferation and trigger cyst formation. An EIC commonly occurs at the periphery of the flap near the surgical scar and will typically present with benign morphologic features on imaging such as circumscribed margins and lack of posterior shadowing on sonography (Fig. 18.22A–B). No enhancement will be seen on MRI. If not definitively benign on ultrasound, tissue sampling may be necessary for diagnosis.

The most common complication associated with breast reconstruction is fat necrosis, occurring in up to 35% of postoperative patients.[11,12] It typically occurs at the periphery of a flap where perfusion is limited. For any new palpable lump following mastectomy with or without reconstructive surgery, the American College of Radiology Appropriateness Criteria currently recommends ultrasound as the initial imagining modality. However, sonographic findings of fat necrosis are often nonspecific and may range from vague, focal echogenic masses to anechoic oil cysts to complex cystic masses or solid shadowing masses with or without calcifications. Mammography is often more helpful to look for typical features of benign fat necrosis such as coarse, dystrophic, or rim calcifications or radiolucent oil cysts. If diagnosis is uncertain on conventional imaging, a tissue biopsy is recommended for confirmation.

Fat necrosis may present with a spectrum on findings on MRI (Fig. 18.23A–B). The most common presentation is a nonenhancing or rim-enhancing mass with internal fat signal. The central fat is best appreciated on a T1-weighted non-fat-suppressed sequence. Enhancement, if present, is typically thin and peripheral with persistent or plateau enhancement kinetics. Biopsy should be considered for any enhancing mass without central fat signal.

Breast Cancer Recurrence After Mastectomy

The risk of locoregional recurrence or second primary malignancy in the reconstructed breast is low, estimated at 4% to 15%.[13] Majority of cancers recur within the subcutaneous residual breast tissue anterior to the abdominal flap where they may be easily palpable.[14] On mammography and MRI, recurrent breast cancer commonly presents in residual breast tissue superficial to a thin, dense line representing the de-epithelialized skin of the tunneled portion of the abdominal flap (Fig. 18.24A–C). The second most common site of recurrence is the chest wall where recurrence may present as a palpable lump, may present as focal pain, or may be clinically silent. Regardless of the location, recurrent tumors resemble primary breast malignancies on imaging. Mammography or sonography may demonstrate an irregular mass, with or without posterior shadowing, or less commonly suspicious calcifications or architectural distortion. Detection of chest wall recurrences, deep to the flap or implant, is particularly challenging on conventional imaging; thus, breast MRI is frequently necessary

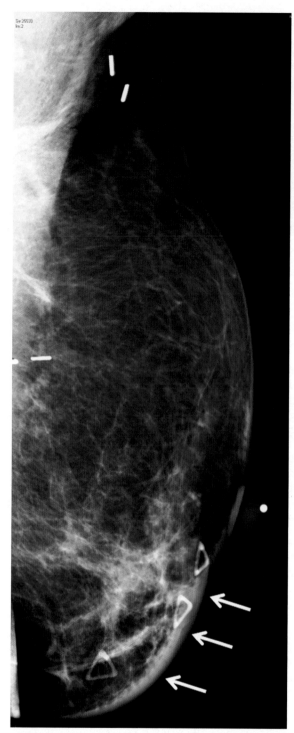

Fig. 18.21 Left breast digital mammogram mediolateral oblique (MLO) view demonstrates benign skin thickening and fibrosis (*arrowheads*) in a patient status post free transverse rectus abdominis myocutaneous (TRAM) flap reconstruction and radiation therapy.

Routine imaging surveillance of the asymptomatic reconstructed breast remains controversial. Screening has historically not been recommended in this population because recurrences are rare and usually easily palpable; fat necrosis is common, which may lead to false-positive findings and unnecessary biopsies.[15] Similarly, the use of breast MRI to screen for chest wall recurrence is also not a common practice, as chest wall recurrences are very rare and are frequently associated with metastatic disease; thus, prognosis may not be improved with early detection. One recent imaging study found that screening mammography in women following AMF reconstruction may be beneficial for detecting clinically silent recurrences.[16] Additional long-term studies are needed to determine the true benefit of surveillance after breast reconstruction. Until then, there are no clear guidelines for screening in this population.

Reduction Mammoplasty

Reduction mammoplasty is a surgical technique designed to reduce the size and volume of breast tissue. It is frequently requested to either improve cosmetic appearance or alleviate back, shoulder, or arm pain—symptoms that are sometimes associated with an excessive volume of breast tissue. Surgical techniques for reduction vary; however, all methods involve repositioning of the nipple and removal of glandular tissue. The inverted T incision with removal of the inferior pedicle is the most common technique, where an incision is made around the areolar margin and extended vertically to the inframammary fold, followed by a horizontal incision along the inframammary fold. The vertical "lollipop" technique is similar but does not include the horizontal inframammary incision (Fig. 18.26A). The resulting scars produce characteristic findings on mammography such as periareolar dermal calcifications, skin thickening, or parenchymal redistribution with inferior displacement of glandular tissue (Fig. 18.26B). These changes may be more subtle with the vertical technique, which produces less scarring. Additional typical postsurgical findings include oil cysts or coarse dystrophic calcifications from fat necrosis.

Explantation

Implant removal or explantation is typically performed to address implant-associated discomfort or complications. Typical mammographic findings after explantation include architectural distortion from surgical scarring, fat necrosis, dystrophic calcifications, or residual free silicone within the breast tissue or axillary lymph nodes (Fig. 18.27A). Silicone granulomas will present as focally dense masses on mammography, mimicking a foreign body, and thus usually are easily distinguishable from benign or malignant breast masses.

The explantation technique usually involves removing both the implant and its surrounding fibrous capsule. If, however, the capsule is not removed, findings of a collapsed fibrous capsule with associated coarse calcifications may be encountered on mammography, typically in a

for diagnosis and for determining the extent of disease. Recurrences on MRI may present as either a mass or focal non-mass enhancement, typically with fast early enhancement and delayed plateau or washout kinetics (Fig. 18.25; Box 18.9).

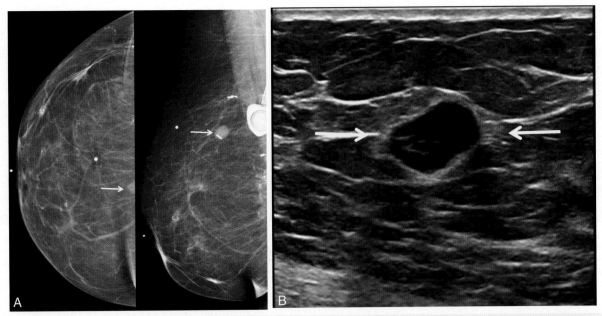

Fig. 18.22 Epidermal inclusion cyst after autologous myocutaneous flap (AMF) reconstruction. Right breast digital mammogram (A) in a patient status post free transverse rectus abdominis myocutaneous (TRAM) reconstruction demonstrates a circumscribed oval mass posteriorly on craniocaudal (CC) and mediolateral oblique (MLO) views (*arrows*). On sonography (B) the mass is circumscribed and hypoechoic. Biopsy revealed epidermal inclusion cyst, which developed in the tunneled portion of the skin of the AMF.

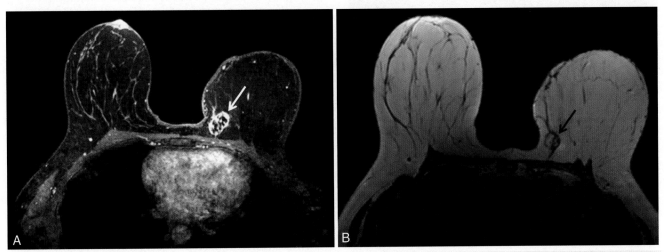

Fig. 18.23 Fat necrosis on magnetic resonance imaging (MRI) may have variable appearances. Contrast-enhanced T1-weighted axial subtraction MRI (A) in this patient status post pedicled transverse rectus abdominis myocutaneous (TRAM) flap reconstruction demonstrates a complex enhancing mass at site of palpable lump (*white arrow*). Non-fat-suppressed image (B) demonstrates fat signal within the mass (*black arrow*), which is diagnostic of benign fat necrosis.

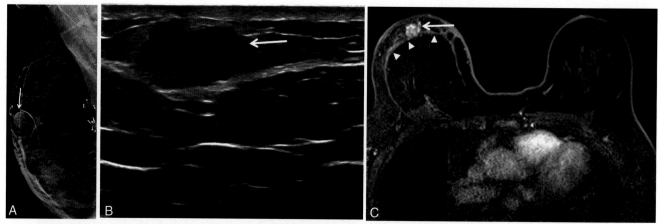

Fig. 18.24 Example of breast cancer recurrence in a reconstructed breast. This patient, status post free transverse rectus abdominis myocutaneous (TRAM) reconstruction, presented with a palpable mass. Mammography (A), sonography (B), and magnetic resonance imaging (MRI) (C) demonstrate a superficial, irregular mass at the palpable site (*arrows*). Note how this recurrence has occurred within the residual breast tissue just superficial to the de-epithelialized layer of the abdominal flap (*arrowheads*).

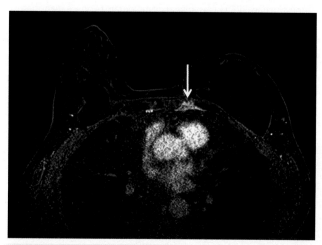

Fig. 18.25 Chest wall recurrence. Dynamic contrast-enhanced magnetic resonance subtraction image demonstrates focal non-mass enhancement involving the left medial intercostal muscles and adjacent subcutaneous tissues (*arrow*) consistent with chest wall recurrence.

Box 18.9   Complications of Autologous Flap Breast Reconstruction

- Benign
  - Skin thickening/fibrosis
  - Epidermal inclusion cysts
  - Fat necrosis
  - Seroma/hematoma
  - Infection

---

posterior-central location (Fig. 18.27B). A retained, intact fibrous capsule may form a potential space within the breast tissue, where rarely blood or fluid can accumulate, creating the appearance of a "pseudoimplant" on mammography. This unusual complication may occur at any time following implant removal. Patients may present with a history of minor trauma with associated pain and swelling of the affected breast (Fig. 18.27C). These complications are less likely to occur today, as modern surgical explanation techniques recommend a partial or complete capsulectomy at the time of implant removal.

KEY POINTS

- Implant displaced views are required in addition to routine mammographic views for cancer screening.
- Breast magnetic resonance imaging (MRI) has the highest sensitivity and specificity for both intracapsular and extracapsular silicone implant rupture.
- Signs of intracapsular rupture include the "step ladder" sign on ultrasound and the "linguine," subcapsular line, "noose," "teardrop," and "keyhole" signs on MRI.
- Signs of extracapsular rupture include free silicone in the breast parenchyma on MRI and mammography and the "snow storm" sign on ultrasound.
- Saline implant rupture is often clinically evident and usually does not require imaging.
- Breast implant–associated anaplastic large cell lymphoma (BIA-ALCL) is a rare T-cell lymphoma that usually presents with a large peri-implant fluid collection.
- After mastectomy, breast reconstruction options include implants, autologous flaps, or a combination of both.
- The most common autologous reconstructions include the transverse rectus abdominis myocutaneous (TRAM) flap and deep inferior epigastric perforator (DIEP) flap.
- Fat necrosis is the most commonly encountered complication after reconstruction surgery.
- Following breast reconstruction surgery, recurrent breast cancer most commonly occurs in a superficial location within the residual breast tissue.
- Periareolar skin calcifications, parenchymal redistribution, oil cysts/fat necrosis, and dystrophic calcifications are typical imaging findings encountered after reduction mammoplasty.

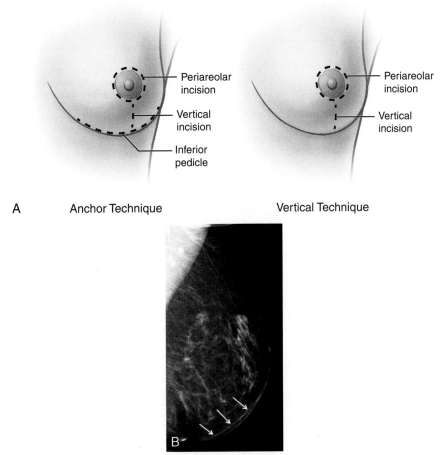

Fig. 18.26 Reduction mammoplasty. Illustration showing the two most common techniques: (A) "inverted T" or "anchor" method (B) or vertical method with the characteristic incision scars. Digital mammogram mediolateral oblique (MLO) view (C) demonstrates the classic vertical incision scar (*arrowheads*).

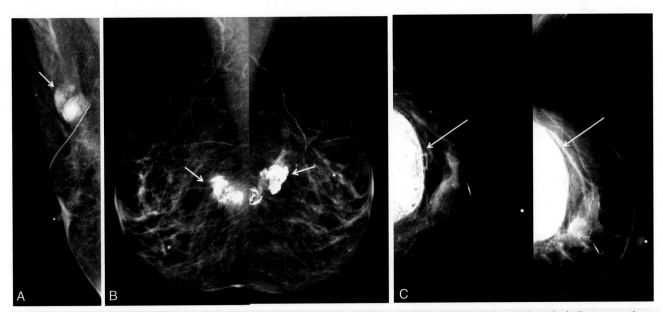

Fig. 18.27 Explantation findings on mammography. Right digital mediolateral oblique (MLO) mammogram shows (A) residual silicone granuloma (*arrow*) after extracapsular rupture of silicone implant. (B) Bilateral digital mammogram demonstrates coarse calcifications in a posterior, central distribution (*arrows*). This is characteristic of a collapsed fibrous capsule with capsular calcifications after implant removal. (C) A patient who had an implant removed years ago presented with rapid "swelling" of the left breast after an intense physical therapy session. Left breast digital mediolateral oblique (MLO) view demonstrates a large seroma/hematoma (*arrows*) accumulated within the residual fibrous capsule mimicking the appearance of a retro-pectoral implant.

References

1. Peters W, Smith D. Calcification of breast implant capsules: incidence, diagnosis and contributing factors. *Ann Plast Surg.* 1995;34(1):8–11.
2. Janowsky EC, Kupper LL, Hulka BS. Meta-analyses of the relation between silicone breast implants and the risk of connective-tissue diseases. *N Engl J Med.* 2000;342:781.
3. Hölmich LR, Lipworth L, McLaughlin JK, Friis S. Breast implant rupture and connective tissue disease: a review of the literature. *Plast Reconstr Surg.* 2007;120:62S.
4. U.S. Food and Drug Administration. Medical Devices. Breast Implants. https://www.fda.gov/medical-devices/implants-and-prosthetics/breast-implants.
5. De Boer M, van Leeuwen FE, Hauptmann M, et al. Breast implants and the risk of anaplastic large-cell lymphoma in the breast. *JAMA Oncol.* 2018;4(3):335–341.
6. Juanpere S, Perez E, Huc O, Motos N, Pont J, Pedraza S. Imaging of breast implants-a pictorial review. *Insights Imaging.* 2011;2(6):653–670. https://doi.org/10.1007/s13244-011-0122-3.
7. Seiler SJ, Sharma PB, Hayes JC, et al. Multimodality imaging-based evaluation of single-lumen silicone breast implants for rupture. *RadioGraphics.* 2017;37(2):366–382.
8. U.S. Food and Drug Administration. Update on the Safety of Silicone Gel-Filled Breast Implants (2011)- Executive Summary. https://www.fda.gov/medical-devices/breast-implants/update-safety-silicone-gel-filled-breast-implants-2011-executive-summary.
9. BI-RADS Committee   *ACR BI-RADS Atlas.* 5th ed. Reston, VA: American College of Radiology; 2013.
10. Pinel-Giroux FM, El Khoury MM, Trop I, Bernier C, David J, Lalonde L. Breast reconstruction: review of surgical methods and spectrum of imaging findings. *RadioGraphics.* 2013;33(2):435–453.
11. Baumann DP, Lin HY, Chevray PM. Perforator number predicts fat necrosis in a prospective analysis of breast reconstruction with free TRAM, DIEP, and SIEA flaps. *Plast Reconstr Surg.* 2010;125(5):1335–1341.
12. Bilgen IG, Ustun EE, Memis A. Fat necrosis of the breast: clinical, mammographic and sonographic features. *Eur J Radiol.* 2001;39(2):92–99.
13. Pinel-Giroux FM, El Khoury MM, Trop I, Bernier C, David J, Lalonde L. Breast reconstruction: review of surgical methods and spectrum of imaging findings. *RadioGraphics.* 2013;33(2):435–453.
14. Patterson SG, Teller P, Iyengar R, et al. Locoregional recurrence after mastectomy with immediate transverse rectus abdominis myocutaneous (TRAM) flap reconstruction. *Ann Surg Oncol.* 2012;19:2679.
15. Freyvogel M, Padia S, Larson K, et al. Screening mammography following autologous breast reconstruction: an unnecessary effort. *Ann Surg Oncol.* 2014;21:3256.
16. Parikh RP, Doren EL, Mooney B, Sun WV, Laronga C, Smith PD. Differentiating fat necrosis from recurrent malignancy in fat-grafted breasts: an imaging classification system to guide management. *Plast Reconstr Surg.* 2012;130(4):761–772.

Suggested Readings

De Boer M, van Leeuwen FE, Hauptmann M, et al. Breast Implants and the Risk of Anaplastic Large-Cell Lymphoma in the Breast. *JAMA Oncol.* 2018;4(3):335–341.

Juanpere S, Perez E, Huc O, Motos N, Pont J. Pedraza S. Imaging of breast implants—a pictorial review. *Insights Imaging.* 2011;2(6):653–670.

Mauro S, Eugenio F, Roberto B. Late recurrent capsular hematoma after augmentation mammoplasty: case report. *Aesthetic Plast Surg.* 2006;29:10–12.

19 Special Populations in Breast Imaging

JULIE GIBBONS, DAKOTA ORVEDAL AND PETER R. EBY

OVERVIEW *This chapter covers breast imaging in special patient populations, including the young, pregnant, lactating, male, transgender, or combinations thereof. This includes management guidelines, common imaging findings, and pathologies that breast radiologists should be familiar with.*

The Breast Imaging Reporting and Data System (BI-RADS) Atlas comprises a thorough and evidence-based guide for accurate image interpretation and management of most common clinical scenarios encountered in women 40 years and older. However, radiologists must also address the less common signs, symptoms, and concerns of unique populations, such as those who are younger, pregnant, lactating, male, or transgender. This chapter will outline a framework for navigating and meeting the needs of these special populations. The framework is derived from nearly all of the rules of image interpretation presented in the BI-RADS Atlas. Case examples are provided along with pearls and pitfalls to ensure imaging and management success. Supplemental evidence from the literature, along with special consideration of disease incidence relative to age, gender, and pregnancy, is incorporated to clarify best management practices.

The first consideration when approaching a concerned patient, particularly if they are younger, male, or a transgender woman, is the lower likelihood of breast cancer compared with female patients 40 years and older. Simply stated, a benign cause is more likely than breast cancer in these patients. The consequences, however, of missing a breast cancer in a young or male patient can be devastating. Uncommon clinical encounters combined with infrequent but serious diagnoses can elevate stress levels for everyone. The first rule for the radiologist is this: Do not panic. The second rule for the radiologist is this: Do not panic. The third rule for the radiologist is to listen to the patient. The fourth rule for the radiologist is to use the BI-RADS Atlas to correctly classify all imaging findings, and the fifth rule for the radiologist is to apply the appropriate differential diagnosis for the unique patient.

Young

How young is young? For the purposes of this chapter, we will consider any woman under 30 years to be young. The vast majority present with clinically or self-detected signs or symptoms; however, there is also a subset of the young population who are asymptomatic and present with screen-detected abnormalities. These are women with a greater than average lifetime risk of developing breast cancer who have initiated screening with mammography, ultrasound, and/or magnetic resonance imaging (MRI) before the age

of 40. Please see Chapter 11 for details about screening high-risk women.

YOUNG: DIFFERENTIAL CONSIDERATIONS

The top differential diagnoses for young patients presenting with a focal symptom, such as a palpable abnormality or pain, include normal tissue, simple and complicated cysts, and fibroadenomas (Box 19.1). Phyllodes tumors, papillomas, abscess or mastitis, tumoral pseudoangiomatous stromal hyperplasia (PASH), and breast cancer are also possible but less likely. In patients under 19, fibroadenomas account for 91% of the masses that are visible on ultrasound (Fig. 19.1), and breast cancer is exceedingly rare.

YOUNG: IMAGING MANAGEMENT

For women under 30 with a focal breast sign or symptom, the first step in evaluation is a breast ultrasound targeted to the site of clinical concern. This choice of initial imaging test is guided by the incidence of cancer by decade, as the risk changes significantly over time (Table 19.1 and Box 19.2). Whereas only 1 out of 1681 women in their 20s will develop cancer before turning 30, 1 out of 232 women in their 30s will develop breast cancer before turning 40, and 1 out of 69 women in their 40s will develop breast cancer before turning 50.

The dramatic increase in risk explains the recommendation to start screening at age 40, as well as the recommendation to use ultrasound as the first test in symptomatic women under 30 years. Mammography is not routinely performed in women under 30 due to the very low likelihood

---

Box 19.1 Young Women (<30 Years Old): Differential Considerations for Palpable Breast Lumps

- Normal breast tissue
- Cyst and fibrocystic changes
- Fibroadenoma
- Phyllodes tumor
- Pseudoangiomatous stromal hyperplasia
- Papilloma
- Breast cancer
- Other: hematoma, abscess, fat necrosis

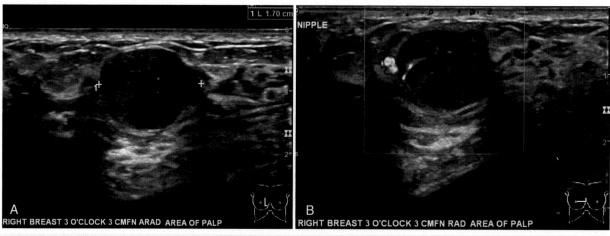

Fig. 19.1 A 15-year-old girl presented with a new palpable lump in the right breast. Targeted ultrasound (A) of the palpable lump demonstrates a circumscribed hypoechoic parallel oval mass with a gentle lobulation. Doppler imaging (B) confirms a small amount of internal flow within the mass. The findings were assessed as BI-RADS 3 (probably benign), and short-term follow-up with ultrasound was scheduled. The patient was also encouraged to monitor the palpable finding and return early if she was concerned about any changes. After 2 years, the finding was stable and assessed as BI-RADS 2 (benign). This most likely represented a juvenile fibroadenoma.

Table 19.1   The Risk of Breast Cancer in Women Increases With Age

Age	Risk of Malignancy in the Next Decade	American College of Radiology (ACR) Appropriateness for Initial Evaluation of Palpable Lumps	
		Mammogram First	Ultrasound First
20	1:1681	3	9
30	1:232	8	8
40	1:69	9	4

Ultrasound is the first imaging test recommended for women in their 20 s, because the likelihood of cancer is low and the sensitivity of mammography is lower in younger patients with relatively denser breast tissue.
ACR Appropriateness Rating scale: 1–3 (usually not appropriate); 4– 6 (may be appropriate); 7– 9 (usually appropriate)

Box 19.2   Imaging Evaluation of Suspicious Symptoms in Young Women (<30 Years Old)

- Incidence of breast cancer is very low among young women at average risk.
- Sensitivity of mammography is limited by relatively denser tissue in younger women.
- Ultrasound is recommended as the initial imaging modality.
- Mammography is not contraindicated and may be considered when a suspicious ultrasound finding is identified.
- If performing mammography, get mediolateral oblique (MLO) and craniocaudal (CC) views of the contralateral asymptomatic breast to assess for asymmetries.

of breast cancer and the lower yield of mammography in younger patients with relatively denser breasts. There is also a desire to avoid unnecessary radiation, albeit a very low dose, in younger and more radiosensitive patients. However, while mammography is rarely used in women under 30, it is not contraindicated. If the sonographic findings are suspicious or do not explain the patient's symptoms, mammography may be appropriate in some cases (Box 19.3).

Box 19.3   Mammography in Women Younger Than 30 Years

- Not routinely performed, but not contraindicated.
- If ultrasound finding might represent fat necrosis or other benign calcification, mammography can help establish benignity.
- If ultrasound finding is highly concerning for malignancy, mammography can further characterize and assess extent of disease.
- If ultrasound is negative but clinical examination is highly suspicious, mammography should be considered for further evaluation.
- Bilateral mammogram should be performed in any women with proven cancer.
- Mammography can provide guidance for preoperative localization.
- Mammography can be used to assess response to therapy.
- Have a lower threshold to perform mammography in high-risk patients.

YOUNG: MANAGEMENT OF BREAST MASSES

The same imaging features, assessment structure, and classification system used to guide the management of breast masses in patients 40 years and older are used to guide the management of breast masses in younger patients. The lower incidence of breast cancer in this population means that the majority of breast masses will fall into the benign (BI-RADS 2) or probably benign (BI-RADS 3) categories.

YOUNG: PROBABLY BENIGN

Masses with imaging features meeting criteria for BI-RADS category 3 can be safely monitored with ultrasound and physical examination (Fig. 19.2 and Box 19.4). Masses that remain stable for 2 to 3 years can be deemed benign and require no additional follow-up (Box 19.5). Image-guided biopsy of a BI-RADS 3 mass may also be performed at any time if the patient prefers not to wait for the short-interval follow-up for example, if the patient is too anxious or if there is concern of not returning for follow-up.

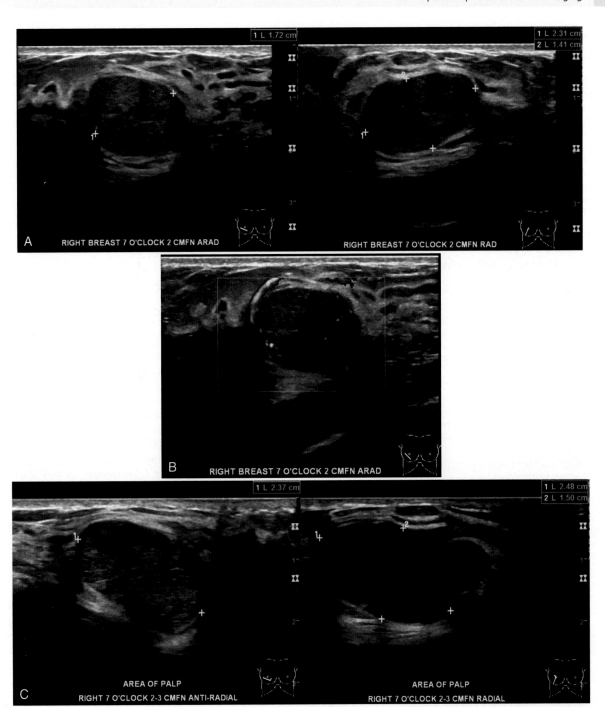

Fig. 19.2 A 20-year-old woman presented with a new palpable lump in the right breast. Targeted ultrasound (A) of the palpable lump demonstrates a circumscribed hypoechoic parallel oval mass. Doppler imaging (B) confirms a small amount of internal flow within the mass. The findings were assessed as BI-RADS 3, and short-term follow-up with ultrasound was scheduled. The patient was also encouraged to monitor the palpable finding and return early if she was concerned about any changes. The patient returned 6 months after the initial visit and reported that the lump had grown. Ultrasound (C) confirmed increased size of the mass in both length and volume by greater than 20%. This mass was assessed as BI-RADS 4A and a biopsy was recommended. Pathology yielded benign fibroadenoma.

If the physical examination of a BI-RADS 3 mass changes (e.g., grows) on palpation, the patient should return immediately for imaging reassessment. Although most of these masses are fibroadenomas, it is nearly impossible to distinguish them from phyllodes tumors using ultrasound alone. Tissue sampling should be recommended if the mass volume or largest dimension increases more than 20% in 6 months, as this increases the likelihood of phyllodes tumor (see Fig. 19.2, Box 19.6, and Table 19.2). If pathology

demonstrates phyllodes tumor, complete excision with clear margins should be performed. Phyllodes tumors and fibroepithelial lesions are covered in Chapter 9.

Biopsy should be performed for masses with one or more suspicious imaging features (Fig. 19.3 and Box 19.5). Extra vigilance is needed when evaluating solid masses that are circumscribed and homogeneously hypoechoic but are antiparallel, round, or have increased in size. Solid masses that are round can represent high-grade, fast-growing,

Box 19.4   Differential Diagnosis of Probably Benign Masses (BI-RADS 3)

- Fibroadenoma (most common)
- Phyllodes tumor
- Tumoral pseudoangiomatous stromal hyperplasia (PASH)
- Complicated cyst
- Papilloma
- Rarely cancer: Beware this potential pitfall!
  - Probably benign masses MUST be parallel, oval, and circumscribed.
  - Any mass that is round (unless meeting criteria of a complicated cyst or simple cyst) is suspicious and may represent a rapidly growing high-grade invasive carcinoma.

Box 19.5   Management of Probably Benign Breast Masses

- Safety of monitoring palpable lumps with BI-RADS 3 features with ultrasound and physical examination:
  - If it is stable for 2–3 years, it can be assessed as benign and no additional follow-up required.
  - If it changes/grows on physical examination, return for follow-up imaging immediately.
- When should percutaneous sampling be performed?
  - The patient is too anxious to wait 6 months, requires a more urgent answer (e.g., planning to get pregnant, organ transplant candidate), or could be lost to follow-up.
  - Volume or largest dimension of the mass increases by >20% in 6 months.
  - Develops suspicious features at follow-up, no longer meeting probably benign criteria.
- Excisional biopsy should be performed if
  - Percutaneous sampling demonstrates phyllodes tumor (or fibroepithelial lesion with features concerning for phyllodes tumor).
  - Percutaneous sampling demonstrates fibroadenoma, but it grows by >20% at follow-up.
  - Percutaneous sampling demonstrates fibroadenoma, but the patient desires excision, because the mass is large and symptomatic.

Box 19.6   Fibroadenoma Versus Phyllodes

- Both are fibroepithelial lesions and have similar imaging characteristics.
- Phyllodes tumor mean age at diagnosis: 40–49.
- Fibroadenoma mean age at diagnosis: 30–39.
- Phyllodes tumors are faster growing with potential for local recurrence.
- Approximately 25% of phyllodes tumors are malignant.
- Wide surgical excision is recommended for all phyllodes tumors.
- Fibroadenomas are benign and generally do not require excision.
- Most phyllodes tumors are very large at presentation.
- Larger size and rapid growth increase likelihood of phyllodes.

Table 19.2   Mass Size Measurements Corresponding to Fig. 19.2

	December	June	Difference
Length	1.7 cm	2.4 cm	41%
Width	2.3 cm	2.5 cm	9%
Height	1.4 cm	1.5 cm	7%
Volume	2.7 cm^3	4.5 cm^3	67%

The largest measurement and the volume of the mass increased by more than 20% in 6 months, upgrading the mass from a BI-RADS 3 (probably benign) to a BI-RADS 4 (suspicious) with a recommendation for biopsy.

benign fat necrosis) of the patient or biopsy plan (e.g., segmental fine pleomorphic calcifications extending beyond the palpable mass) (Fig. 19.4).

YOUNG: MANAGEMENT OF THE PATHOLOGIC NIPPLE

Systemic hormonal influences explain the majority of bilateral milky spontaneous or expressed discharge in young women. Bilateral discharge does not require diagnostic imaging evaluation. However, when a young patient under 30 presents with suspicious nipple symptoms, including pathologic nipple discharge (i.e., unilateral, clear or bloody, and spontaneous), targeted ultrasound should be the initial modality used. Ultrasound should be directed to the subareolar region of the affected breast. Mammography may be complementary, especially for the detection of subtle calcifications. If initial imaging does not demonstrate a correlation with the patient's symptoms, breast MRI or, less commonly, ductography could be considered. Symptom evaluation of the nipple is covered in depth in Chapter 14.

Papilloma is uncommon in patients younger than 30, but can be considered when presenting with unilateral suspicious nipple discharge and one or more intraductal masses on ultrasound (Fig. 19.5). Solitary and multiple papillomas are covered in greater detail in Chapter 9. In contrast to papillomas, juvenile papillomatosis (also known as "Swiss cheese disease") is a benign mass seen in patients younger than 30, which typically presents as a mobile palpable lump without discharge (Box 19.7). Ultrasound most commonly shows a complex mass with multiple small cystic components.

YOUNG: SPECIAL CONSIDERATIONS FOR PATIENTS UNDER 18

Providing care to minors requires additional special consideration. In some cases, it may be appropriate to have a parent present for the examination and discussion. Physical and emotional maturity are highly variable in adolescence, and care should be taken to respect the individual preferences of the patient. Some young women may be embarrassed or reluctant to let a physician see her breast or to discuss their symptoms. Be mindful of the patient's signals. In addition, a legal guardian's consent is generally required for any biopsies performed.

Fortunately, breast cancer is extremely rare in the pediatric and adolescent population, comprising less than 0.1% of all breast cancers with an incidence of less than 1 per 100,000 among females under 19. Imaging and clinical

invasive breast cancer. If any suspicious features are identified, ultrasound-guided biopsy should be recommended. Diagnostic mammography is not contraindicated and may be considered in a patient with a suspicious sonographic finding (Table 19.3). The mammogram may show additional features that change the management (e.g., classic

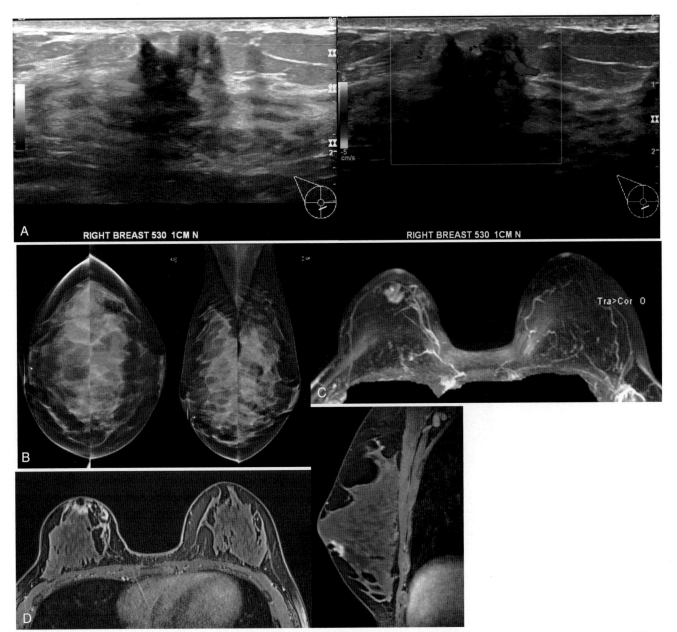

Fig. 19.3 An 18-year-old woman presented with a new palpable lump in the right breast. Ultrasound (A) was appropriately performed first and demonstrated a hypoechoic, irregular mass with noncircumscribed angular margins, posterior shadowing, and internal vascularity. The mass was assessed as BI-RADS 4, and biopsy was recommended. Pathology demonstrated invasive ductal carcinoma. A bilateral diagnostic craniocaudal (CC) and mediolateral oblique (MLO) mammogram (B) was performed to evaluate for additional suspicious findings in both breasts. The mammogram showed extremely dense breast tissue without any other abnormalities. MRI was performed to evaluate the extent of disease. Subtraction maximum intensity projection (MIP) (C) as well as axial and sagittal postcontrast T1 fat-suppressed (D) magnetic resonance images show an enhancing irregular subareolar mass with susceptibility artifact from the biopsy marker. Findings were consistent with unifocal carcinoma. No other suspicious findings were present.

Table 19.3 Ultrasound characterisitcs of benign, probably benign, and suspicious masses

	BI-RADS 2	BI-RADS 3	BI-RADS 4
Margin	Circumscribed	Circumscribed	Angular, indistinct, microlobulated, or spiculated
Shape	Oval	Oval	Round or irregular
Orientation	Parallel	Parallel	Not parallel
Echogenicity	Anechoic	Hypoechoic or isoechoic	Heterogeneous, hypoechoic, or complex cystic and solid
Posterior features	Enhancement	Enhancement or none	Shadowing
What is it?	Simple cyst	Probably fibroadenoma	Suspicious

If the ultrasound finding has any feature that cannot be classified as BI-RADS 2 or 3, ultrasound-guided tissue sampling is warranted. It may be appropriate to either proceed directly to the biopsy or first perform a mammogram for further characterization of the suspicious sonographic finding.

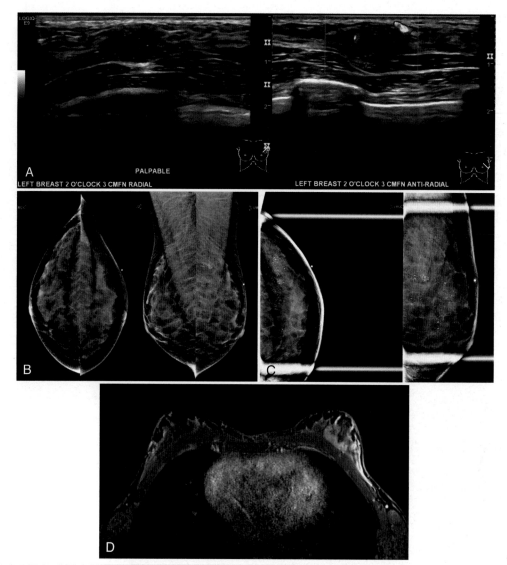

Fig. 19.4 A 28-year-old woman presented with a new palpable lump in the left breast. Ultrasound was appropriately performed first and demonstrated a hypoechoic, irregular mass with angular margins, internal vascularity, and associated hyperechoic foci. (A) A bilateral diagnostic craniocaudal (CC) and mediolateral oblique (MLO) mammogram (B) was performed because of the suspicious features of the mass. The mammogram showed extremely dense breast tissue and microcalcifications at the site of the palpable abnormality in the upper outer quadrant of the left breast. The right breast was negative. Magnification views better demonstrate the fine pleomorphic and coarse heterogeneous calcifications extending over a considerably larger area than the sonographic mass (C). An assessment of BI-RADS 5 (highly suggestive of malignancy) was given. Pathology from ultrasound-guided biopsy of the mass yielded invasive ductal carcinoma and ductal carcinoma in situ with associated calcifications. MRI demonstrated segmental non-mass enhancement abutting the pectoralis in the upper outer quadrant of the left breast corresponding to the mammographic extent of calcifications (D).

follow-up is reasonable for the vast majority of children and adolescents presenting with breast masses, as nearly all in this population are benign, with fibroadenoma being the most common. While some patients or their parents may insist on biopsy or surgical excision in response to fear, a noninvasive approach is generally preferred, as it is less traumatic and reduces the risk of damage to the undeveloped or underdeveloped breast tissue. Damage to a normal developing breast bud can result in permanent partial or total failure of breast development.

Although exceedingly rare, there are case reports of pediatric breast carcinomas in the literature, most commonly secretory carcinoma, a slow-growing tumor with favorable prognosis. There are also rare benign lesions in children/adolescents that may require surgical consultation due to large size and progressive growth (e.g., phyllodes tumor, giant pseudoangiomatous stromal hyperplasia, and giant

juvenile fibroadenoma). Lastly, there are developmental variants, such as a breast bud or asymmetric developing breast tissue in a child/adolescent or breast tissue in a neonate related to maternal hormones, that can present with a palpable finding. In these cases, imaging can sometimes be useful to establish benignity (Box 19.8).

YOUNG: SUMMARY

- Cancer is an unlikely diagnosis in this population.
- For diagnostic imaging evaluation of focal symptoms in patients under 30 years, start with ultrasound.
- If there are imaging features that deviate from benign or probably benign, biopsy should be recommended.
- Mammography is not contraindicated for women in their 20s and may be appropriate after ultrasound in some scenarios.

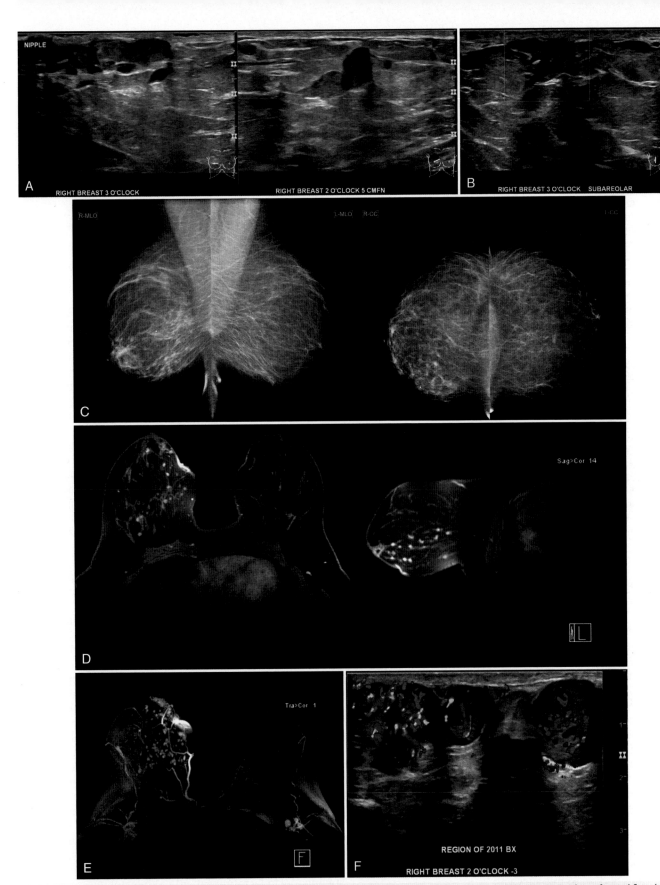

Fig. 19.5 A 22-year-old woman presented with spontaneous right breast bloody nipple discharge. Ultrasound (A) appropriately performed first demonstrates multiple small oval hypoechoic periareolar masses with internal vascularity (B). Closer inspection confirmed these masses to be within dilated ducts. Biopsy was recommended and performed of two representative masses (one central and one peripheral). Pathology demonstrated papilloma at both sites. Bilateral mediolateral oblique (MLO) and craniocaudal (CC) mammographic images show numerous small oval circumscribed masses in the lower inner quadrant of the right breast, including two with the biopsy markers (C). Magnetic resonance imaging (MRI) was ordered to evaluate the full extent of the findings and screen the contralateral breast. Axial and sagittal postcontrast fat-saturated T1 MRI images demonstrate numerous small circumscribed oval enhancing masses throughout the lower inner quadrant of the right breast, with minimal background parenchymal enhancement (D). Subtraction maximum-intensity projection also demonstrates the numerous enhancing masses (E). A diagnosis of papillomatosis was made, and surgical consultation was advised to discuss excision. The patient declined the recommended surgery. Ultrasound images (F) obtained 3 years later show progression, with multiple enlarging periareolar intraductal masses with internal vascularity.

Box 19.7   Juvenile Papillomatosis (also Known as "Swiss Cheese Disease")

- Mean age of diagnosis is 23 years.
- Clinical presentation
  - Palpable, mobile, discrete mass.
- Imaging appearance
  - Mammogram rarely performed
  - Ultrasound: variable cysts/masses.
- Pathology appearance
  - Multiple small cysts within dense stroma ("Swiss cheese" appearance).
- Management
  - Complete excision is usually performed.
- Cancer risk
  - Juvenile papillomatosis is benign but may be a risk marker for familial breast cancer.
  - Slightly increased lifetime risk of cancer suggested but not confirmed.

Box 19.8   Special Considerations for Patients Under 18

- It may be appropriate to have a parent or guardian in the room during the examination and/or to discuss results.
- Always ask the patient's preference.
- Be sensitive to the embarrassment or self-consciousness of adolescence.
- Cancer is extremely rare.
- A noninvasive approach is appropriate in the vast majority of cases.
- Avoid damage to the undeveloped/underdeveloped breast.
- Do not biopsy or excise the breast bud, as this can result in permanent disruption of normal breast development.

Box 19.9   Pregnant and Lactating: Differential Considerations for a Palpable Lump

- Normal
- Cyst
- Mastitis, abscess
- Galactocele
- Fibroadenoma
- Lactating adenoma
- Phyllodes tumor
- Cancer

Pregnant or Lactating

Pregnant and lactating patients share many of the same diagnoses and management strategies as the young women described above. There are a few additional common clinical entities unique to the pregnant or lactating patient, however, such as pregnancy-associated breast cancer (PABC), lactating adenomas, and galactoceles. Mastitis is also more common in the lactating patient (Box 19.9). Pregnant and lactating patients also raise some unique clinical management issues that must be addressed, including concerns regarding radiation exposure, the contraindication to administering gadolinium agents during pregnancy, and the risk of developing a milk fistula following percutaneous image-guided biopsy. However, when a pregnant or lactating patient presents with suspicious breast signs or symptoms, such as a palpable lump, diagnostic imaging should never be deferred, as a delay in breast cancer diagnosis can be particularly devastating in this population with already higher mortality rates and lower rates of disease-free survival.

PREGNANT OR LACTATING: IMAGING SAFETY AND EXPECTED IMAGING APPEARANCES

Understanding the effects of pregnancy and lactation on imaging sensitivity and the risks each modality presents is essential not only to guide image management but also to have informed discussions with referring providers and patients when they present for breast imaging.

The American College of Radiology (ACR) Appropriateness Criteria recommends breast ultrasound as the first-line imaging modality for evaluation of focal breast symptoms in pregnant and lactating women regardless of age. The sensitivity and negative predictive value of ultrasound for cancer detection in symptomatic pregnant and lactating patients are nearly 100%. If the sonographic findings are suspicious or do not explain the patient's symptoms, mammography should be performed.

Mammography is safe for pregnant and lactating patients and is not contraindicated. There is no scientific evidence to indicate risk to a developing fetus or risk to the rapidly proliferating breast epithelium. While the procedure is safe, the increase in breast density during pregnancy and lactation can limit mammographic sensitivity. Therefore digital breast tomosynthesis (DBT) may be particularly useful in this population. Breast feeding or pumping prior to mammography is also recommended, not only to improve tissue compliance with compression and decrease overall breast density but also to make the examination more comfortable for the patient (Box 19.10).

Ultrasound is safe during pregnancy and lactation and, as described above, should be used as the first-line diagnostic tool for symptom evaluation. However, there are no studies evaluating whole-breast ultrasound for screening in pregnant or lactating patients. The ACR Appropriateness Criteria state that while ultrasound may be considered for supplemental screening in intermediate and high-risk patients, it can increase false positives, prompting potentially unnecessary biopsies and increasing the risk of milk fistula in lactating women. The expected sonographic appearance of the breast tissue during pregnancy and lactation includes increased fibroglandular tissue and, in lactating patients in particular, a diffuse increase in echogenicity secondary to increased fat in the tissue from milk in lobules and within dilated ducts.

While MRI with gadolinium is relatively contraindicated during pregnancy, it is safe for use during lactation. It may be used for high-risk screening and as a diagnostic and staging tool in lactating patients. While not necessary, milk can be pumped and discarded for 24 hours following contrast administration if a patient has concerns about passing gadolinium to her breast-feeding child. The expected MRI appearance of the breast during lactation includes increased fibroglandular tissue, increased background parenchymal enhancement, increased vascularity, and increased signal on the T2 weighted images (Box 19.11).

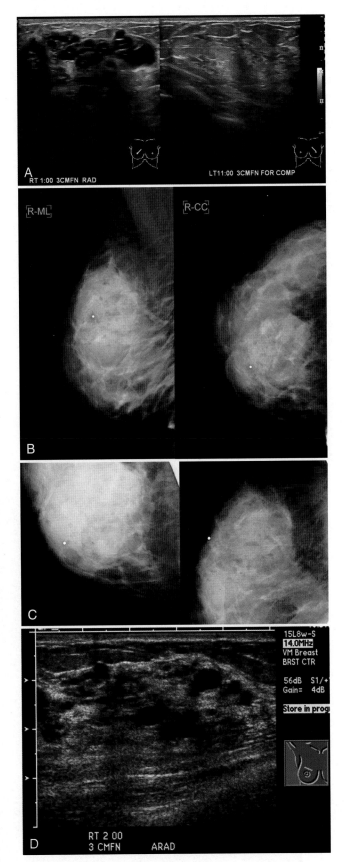

Fig. 19.6 A 26-year-old lactating woman presented with a palpable lump in the upper inner quadrant of the right breast. She denied fever, erythema, or tenderness. Ultrasound was appropriately performed first (A). In the area of clinical concern at 1 o'clock in the right breast there is a complex cystic and solid mass versus multiple complicated cysts. This lesion is composed predominantly of small anechoic cystic components with interspersed septations and possible interspersed solid components. Ultrasound was also performed of the left breast upper inner quadrant at 11 o'clock for comparison. The left side reveals homogeneous fibroglandular tissue. A diagnostic mammogram (B) was then obtained to assist the evaluation. These images reveal extremely dense breast tissue. Spot compression views (C) in the area of clinical concern demonstrate fat density areas that are round and oval on the craniocaudal (CC) projection but convert to fluid-fluid levels on the mediolateral (ML) projection. The sonographic and mammographic findings together confirm a diagnosis of galactocele, and biopsy was avoided. Follow-up ultrasound (D) after cessation of lactation demonstrates interval near resolution of the mass.

Box 19.10 Mammograms in the Pregnant or Lactating Patient

- Mammography is not routinely performed in the diagnostic setting, but it is not contraindicated.
- Mammographic density is increased.
- Mammographic sensitivity is lower than ultrasound for masses but better for calcifications.
- Radiation risks:
  - There is no scientific evidence to indicate any risk to a developing fetus.
  - No teratogenic effects have been reported below 0.05 Gy.
  - Mammography can be safely performed with abdominal shielding.
  - There is no evidence of increased risk to the rapidly proliferating breast epithelium.
- Patients should pump or breastfeed before mammography to improve tissue compliance with compression and decrease overall density.

Box 19.11 Magnetic Resonance Imaging (MRI) in the Pregnant or Lactating Patient

- Gadolinium administration is contraindicated during pregnancy.
- MRI screening for high-risk patients should be performed before or after pregnancy.
- MRI with gadolinium can be performed safely in lactating women.
- MRI may be considered to evaluate extent of disease for pregnancy-associated breast cancer in the postpartum or lactating patient.
- Background parenchymal enhancement in lactating women is usually marked.
- While not necessary, patients can pump and discard breast milk for 24 hours following gadolinium administration.

PREGNANT OR LACTATING: BENIGN MASSES

During pregnancy, fibroadenomas are the most commonly encountered solid masses. Similar to nonpregnant patients, fibroadenomas are usually oval or round, circumscribed, hypoechoic, and parallel. Because they are hormone dependent, growth during pregnancy is common. If growth is rapid, fibroadenomas can infarct, causing the presentation of focal pain or a tender palpable abnormality and demonstrating internal cystic spaces and indistinct margins on imaging.

During lactation, galactoceles are one of the most commonly encountered benign masses (Fig. 19.6 and Box 19.12). They represent retention cysts from occluded lactiferous ducts and contain all the components of normal breast milk: water, fat, protein, and calcium. The concentrations of each component are variable, and therefore galactoceles can have multiple different imaging appearances, including that of a simple cyst, complicated cyst (with fat-fluid level), complex solid and cystic mass, and solid mass (including pseudolipoma or pseudohamartoma). Ultrasound may demonstrate mobility of the fat-fluid level or other components to confirm that it is a galactocele. Doppler should also be used to ensure there is no internal vascularity. If a finding demonstrates the classic appearance of a galactocele with a fat-fluid level, this can be assessed as benign (BI-RADS 2) and no further imaging workup is required. Aspiration is indicated if imaging features are equivocal or for symptom relief. Milky aspirate is diagnostic.

Box 19.12   Galactocele

- Common benign mass during lactation
- Retention cyst from occluded lactiferous duct containing milk-like fluid
- Appearances
  - Cyst with fat-fluid level (pathognomonic, assessed as BI-RADS 2)
  - Complex cystic and solid mass
  - Solid mass (including appearance of pseudolipoma or pseudohamartoma)

Lactating adenomas most commonly occur during the third trimester or postpartum during lactation (Fig. 19.7). Their clinical presentation and imaging appearance are similar to fibroadenomas, although they may demonstrate microlobulated margins or cystic components. Like fibroadenomas, lactating adenomas can also infarct. Due to the nonspecific imaging appearance, lactating adenomas often require percutaneous tissue sampling for diagnosis. Benign concordant pathology demonstrating lactating adenoma requires no further clinical management. Once lactation has stopped, these masses usually regress as the breast parenchyma returns to its prelactational state.

PREGNANT OR LACTATING: MASTITIS AND BREAST ABSCESSES

During lactation, bacteria, most commonly staphylococcus and streptococcus, originating from the skin or the baby's mouth can be introduced through the ducts or disrupted dermis of the nipple/areola. Stagnant milk within the breast, from either a blocked duct or infrequent emptying, further increases the risk of infection. If attempts to manage mastitis clinically, such as with warm compress and antibiotics, are unsuccessful, then sonographic interrogation is recommended to determine whether there is an underlying abscess that may require percutaneous aspiration or drain placement. Aspiration can be both therapeutic and diagnostic, as

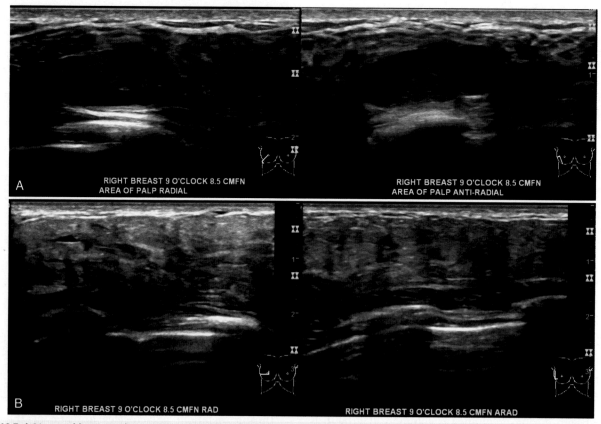

Fig. 19.7 A 21-year-old patient who was 5 months pregnant presented with a palpable right breast lump. Ultrasound (A) confirmed an oval, parallel, circumscribed, homogeneously hypoechoic mass with posterior enhancement. A fibroadenoma or lactating adenoma was suspected. Given the probably benign features, this mass was assessed as BI-RADS 3. She returned 7 months later when she was postpartum and lactating. Follow-up ultrasound (B) showed resolution of the mass.

the fluid is typically sent for culture and sensitivities. The sonographic appearance of an abscess can, however, sometimes mimic malignancy. Doppler evaluation can be helpful in these cases (Fig. 19.8). Typically, if the finding demonstrates peripherally increased vascularity it likely represents infection, while internal vascularity is more indicative of a solid mass. Clinical presentation of fever, local erythema, and tenderness can also be helpful in establishing an infectious diagnosis. Follow-up ultrasound can be performed to assess for improvement or resolution of an abscess after appropriate treatment, but it is not necessary.

PREGNANCY-ASSOCIATED BREAST CANCER

Any breast cancer diagnosed during pregnancy, lactation, or within 12 months postpartum meets the definition of PABC (Fig. 19.9 and Box 19.13). Although an unlikely diagnosis in a pregnant or recently postpartum patient, PABC must be considered, as it is often high grade and may be stimulated by increased levels of circulating endogenous hormones. Limited data suggest PABC is more often larger, node positive, and metastatic at the time of diagnosis than non-PABC in age-matched peers. Therefore even a short delay in diagnosis can adversely affect prognosis in these patients.

PERCUTANEOUS PROCEDURES IN LACTATING PATIENTS

If initial diagnostic imaging demonstrates a suspicious mass, percutaneous tissue sampling is indicated to avoid delay in cancer diagnosis. A unique consideration for lactating patients, however, is the risk of developing a milk fistula after any percutaneous procedure. Although rare, lactating patients should be consented for this. Milk fistulas form because milk will evacuate from the breast through the path of least resistance, which, after a percutaneous procedure, can be through the aspiration or biopsy tract. If persistent, this can promote epithelialization of the procedure tract, forming a fistula. Once established, a milk fistula is difficult to control without cessation of lactation, which is often undesirable for the mother and infant, and in severe

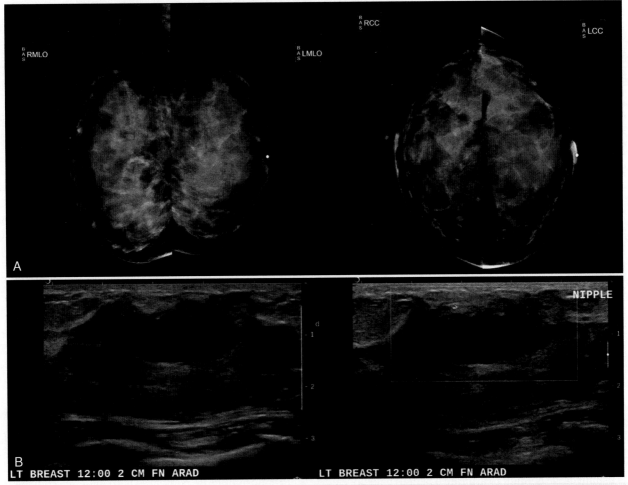

Fig. 19.8 A 38-year-old lactating woman presented with a painful tender palpable lump in the upper central left breast with clinical concern for infection. Mammography was appropriately performed first (A) but was unrevealing. Ultrasound was performed next (B), revealing a complex fluid collection in the area of clinical concern in the left breast at 12 o'clock. Doppler interrogation shows peripheral flow but no internal vascularity. The sonographic and clinical findings together confirm a diagnosis of lactational (or puerperal) abscess. Aspiration was performed, yielding purulent fluid that was sent for culture. The patient was placed on antibiotics and recommended to monitor her symptoms closely with low threshold to return if symptoms worsen.

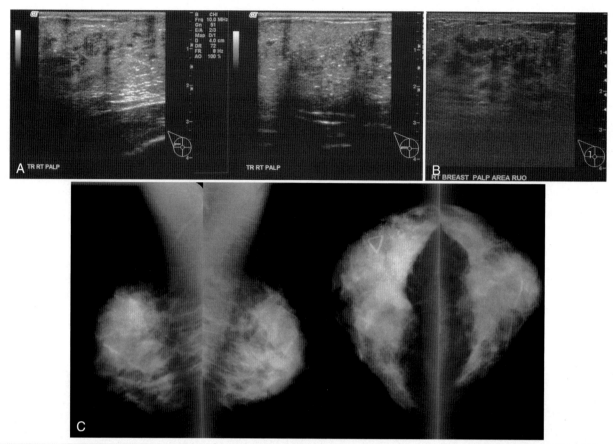

Fig. 19.9 A 27-year-old lactating woman presented with a painless palpable lump in the upper outer quadrant of the right breast. Ultrasound was appropriately performed first (A and B). Images do not reveal a discrete mass; however, there are some vague areas of shadowing and scattered punctate echogenic foci. A diagnostic mammogram (C) was then obtained to assist the evaluation. The breasts are extremely dense. A triangular skin marker in the area of clinical concern demonstrates segmental fine pleomorphic calcifications, corresponding to the echogenic foci seen on ultrasound. Findings were assessed as BI-RADS 4 (suspicious). Pathology demonstrated invasive lobular carcinoma. The addition of a mammogram in this patient under 30, when the ultrasound findings were discordant with the physical examination, improved characterization of the area of clinical concern, increasing the level of suspicion and revealing the necessity for a biopsy recommendation.

Box 19.13   Pregnancy-Associated Breast Cancer (PABC)

- Defined as breast cancer diagnosed during pregnancy, lactation, or within 12 months postpartum.
- Most common malignancy in pregnant women.
- Most common cause of cancer related death in pregnant and lactating women.
- Limited data suggests larger tumors at diagnosis, more often node positive or metastatic disease, and shorter survival than matched non-PABC controls.

cases, surgical intervention may be warranted. Therefore, if diagnostic percutaneous intervention is necessary to differentiate cystic from solid etiologies, aspiration with a narrow-lumen (i.e., larger-gauge) needle, rather than core biopsy, may be more appropriate as the first step. An 18-gauge needle is usually large enough to aspirate a benign galactocele, for example. If the target is solid, consider core biopsy with an 18-gauge or 16-gauge needle. Larger-size (i.e., smaller-gauge) vacuum-assisted biopsy devices, such as those with 8- to 12-gauge needles, may increase the risk of creating

a milk fistula and should be avoided. After biopsy, encourage the patient to pump or breast feed frequently to reduce pressure and decrease breast engorgement until the biopsy site is completely healed. In addition, to avoid unnecessary postprocedure alarm, inform the patient that it is common for blood to appear within the milk for a short time after the biopsy.

PREGNANT OR LACTATING: SUMMARY

- Benign entities cause the majority of breast symptoms in pregnant and lactating patients.
- Current guidelines recommend ultrasound as the initial modality for evaluating focal symptoms in pregnant and lactating patients.
- Mammography is safe for use during pregnancy and lactation and should be performed in addition to ultrasound when appropriate.
- Prognosis of PABC compared with matched controls may be worse, and therefore prompt diagnostic evaluation of symptoms is critical.
- Lactating patients undergoing percutaneous procedures should be consented for the low risk of milk fistula.

Male

Male patients predominately present to the breast imaging clinic for evaluation of a subareolar palpable abnormality with or without associated tenderness, which in the majority of cases represents gynecomastia. Occasionally, male patients harbor other diagnoses, most of which are benign, such as pseudogynecomastia, lipomas, sebaceous cysts, normal lymph nodes, and mastitis or abscess (Figs. 19.10–19.13 and Box 19.14). Although scant, the tissue in the male breast is capable of producing any diagnosis found in the female counterpart. This of course includes breast cancer. Pathology in the male breast is more commonly of ductal origin, as lobule formation and lesions associated with lobules, including cysts and fibroadenomas, are much rarer in the absence of exogenous feminizing hormones.

The normal male breast includes subareolar ducts that are similar in development, concentration, and distribution to prepubertal females. The imaging appearance of the normal male breast is entirely fatty with no parenchymal tissue. Any glandular tissue visible in the subareolar male breast constitutes gynecomastia. Imaging may also demonstrate prominent pectoralis muscles and normal-axillary and low-axillary lymph nodes.

Currently, there are no randomized controlled trial data across large populations to support screening for breast cancer with any imaging modality in male patients at average or high risk for breast cancer (Box 19.15). The National Comprehensive Cancer Network (NCCN) recommends that men with a *BRCA* mutation begin breast self-examinations at age 35 years.

Palpable, unilateral or bilateral, tender, subareolar abnormalities in pubertal males almost uniformly represent gynecomastia, and imaging is not indicated. Reassurance should be provided to the patient and family, and the referring physician should be educated (Box 19.15).

MALE: IMAGING MANAGEMENT

Symptoms of gynecomastia or pseudogynecomastia typically do not require imaging, as these diagnoses are more often established at physical examination. However, imaging may be indicated in indeterminate cases. For male patients with a suspicious physical examination finding, a bilateral full-field two-dimensional, four-view mammogram is generally recommended as the initial imaging study, even for a unilateral concern, as this helps assess symmetry (Fig. 19.14 and Box 19.16). Spot compression views can be difficult to obtain due to the paucity of tissue and are often unnecessary because the breast is predominantly fatty. Magnification views can be performed, however, if the primary finding is microcalcifications.

The ACR Appropriateness Criteria recommends mammography as the initial imaging modality for male patients 25 or older. In younger males (<25) who are unlikely to have breast cancer, they suggest that ultrasound may be useful as the initial imaging modality, though gynecomastia can more easily be confirmed on mammography. Ultrasound should not be performed in patients 25 years or older whose symptoms are explained clinically or mammographically by gynecomastia, as the sonographic features of gynecomastia can be falsely suspicious, including irregular margins and posterior shadowing (Box 19.17). Ultrasound should be performed, however, to evaluate any breast mass deemed indeterminate or suspicious on mammography to assist in clinical management and to guide biopsy.

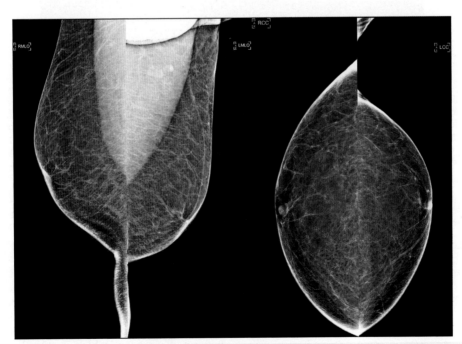

Fig. 19.10 A 46-year-old man reported bilateral breast enlargement. Bilateral mediolateral oblique (MLO) and craniocaudal (CC) diagnostic views demonstrate normal subcutaneous fat without glandular or stromal tissue or other focal abnormalities. Imaging and clinical findings are consistent with pseudogynecomastia.

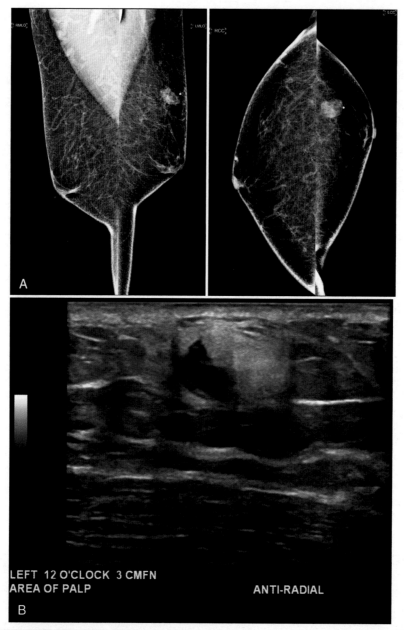

Fig. 19.11 A 62-year-old man presented with a firm, mobile, palpable left breast lump at the site of recent direct trauma. A radiopaque marker (BB) was placed over the clinical area of concern in the upper outer quadrant of the left breast and bilateral mediolateral oblique (MLO) and craniocaudal (CC) mammographic views (A) were obtained. Correlating to the palpable abnormality is an irregular mass with indistinct margins and mixed density. Minimal gynecomastia is also seen incidentally in the subareoar regions bilaterally. Ultrasound (B) at the site of the palpable and mammographic abnormality reveals a predominantly hyperechoic mass with an irregular hypoechoic component. In the setting of reported trauma, this appearance is typical for resolving hematoma or fat necrosis. Follow-up imaging was recommended in 4-6 weeks to assess for resolution of the mass.

Box 19.14   Male: Differential Considerations for a Palpable Lump

- Gynecomastia (most common)
- Breast cancer
- Sebaceous or epidermal inclusion cyst
- Lipoma
- Pseudogynecomastia
- Abscess/mastitis
- Lymph node
- Fat necrosis
- Cyst (rare in the absence of feminizing hormones)
- Fibroadenoma (rare in the absence of feminizing hormones)

MRI is not indicated for male patients, either for screening or for mapping extent of disease. Breast cancer in male patients is treated with mastectomy, which generally obviates the need to map extent of disease with MRI.

MALE: GYNECOMASTIA

Gynecomastia is the benign enlargement of the male breast due to the proliferation of glandular components. It can be caused by an endocrine imbalance between the actions of estrogen, which is stimulatory, and androgen, which is inhibitory, on breast tissue. Gynecomastia is normally observed in neonates secondary to in utero estrogen

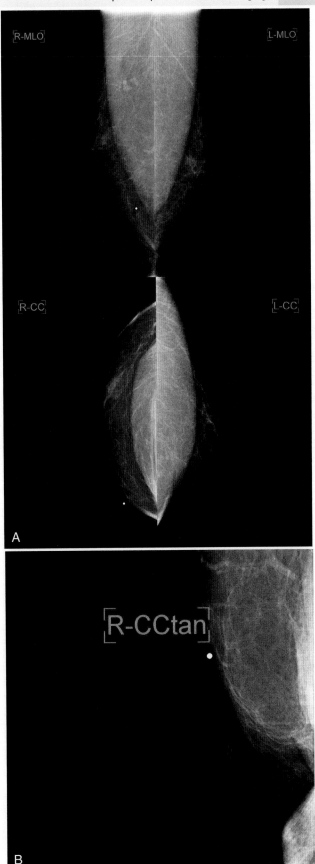

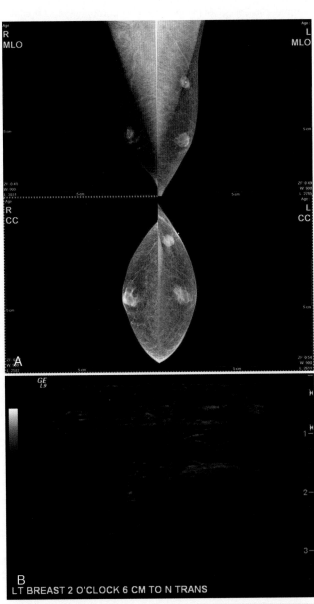

Fig. 19.12 A 56-year-old man presented with a soft, mobile, palpable left breast lump. A radiopaque marker (BB) was placed over the area of clinical concern in the upper outer quadrant of the left breast and bilateral mediolateral oblique (MLO) and craniocaudal (CC) mammographic views (A) were obtained. Correlating to the palpable abnormality is an oval, equal density mass with circumscribed margins. Mild gynecomastia is also seen incidentally in the subareolar regions bilaterally. Ultrasound (B) at the site of the palpable and mammographic abnormality reveals a circumscribed, oval hypoechoic mass with a central hyperechoic hilum, consistent with a lymph node.

Fig. 19.13 A 50-year-old man presented with a soft, mobile, palpable right breast lump. A radiopaque marker (BB) was placed over the area of clinical concern in the lower inner quadrant of the right breast and bilateral mediolateral oblique (MLO) and craniocaudal (CC) mammographic views (A) were obtained. Correlating to the palpable abnormality is a large, circumscribed, oval, fat density mass, consistent with a lipoma. Mild gynecomastia is also seen incidentally in the subareolar regions bilaterally.

Box 19.15   Males: Imaging Management

- Screening: Currently, there is a lack of data across large populations to support screening mammography for average or high-risk males.
- Symptomatic imaging management:
  - Unilateral or bilateral tender subareolar breast masses in pubertal male patients represent gynecomastia and imaging is not indicated. Provide reassurance to the patient and family and educate the referring physician.
  - In adult male patients, gynecomastia is also the most common cause of breast symptoms and is typically a clinical diagnosis not requiring imaging.
  - Imaging is indicated if the physical examination is suspicious or indeterminate.

Box 19.16   Males: Mammography

- In general, begin diagnostic imaging evaluation with a bilateral four-view mammogram, even for unilateral symptoms.
- Gynecomastia is often bilateral even when patients are concerned about only one side.
- Spot compression views can be difficult due to the paucity of tissue and are often unnecessary in the male breast, which is fatty.
- Magnification views should be considered if the primary finding is microcalcifications.

Box 19.17   Male: Ultrasound

- May be used as the initial modality for men under 25 (per American College of Radiology [ACR] Appropriateness Criteria)
- Can be deceiving, because gynecomastia can have falsely suspicious sonographic features, such as irregular margins and posterior shadowing. Mammography more easily confirms the diagnosis of gynecomastia.
- Proceed with ultrasound in the following situations:
  - A suspicious mammographic finding.
  - Suspicious clinical signs or symptoms not explained by the mammogram.
  - Bloody nipple discharge.
  - Erythema and/or fever.
  - Skin changes, such as nonhealing ulcer.
  - Refractory rash of the nipple areolar complex.
  - Nipple inversion or retraction.

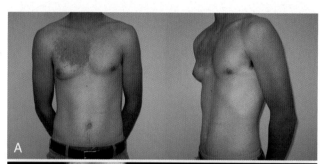

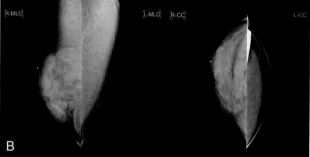

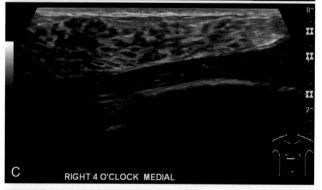

RIGHT 4 O'CLOCK   MEDIAL

Fig. 19.14 A 26-year-old man presented for evaluation of unilateral right breast enlargement. Physical examination confirmed visible asymmetric right breast and areolar enlargement along with asymmetric dermal pigmentation (A). Bilateral mediolateral oblique (MLO) and craniocaudal (CC) mammograms (B) were obtained, showing dense global asymmetry throughout the entire right breast. The left breast was negative. Incidentally noted is mild bilateral axillary skin deodorant artifact. Ultrasound (C) revealed benign glandular tissue in the right breast, indistinguishable from normal, young female dense fibroglandular tissue. The findings confirm unilateral diffuse right gynecomastia. A BI-RADS 2 assessment was given and biopsy was not indicated. Given the severity of the symptoms, the patient was counseled and referred to the plastic surgery service to discuss resection and reconstruction options.

stimulation, in pubertal males secondary to hormonal imbalance, and in older adult males secondary to low testosterone levels. Gynecomastia can also be an iatrogenic side effect of prescribed medicines, alcohol, and marijuana. Other conditions that affect hormonal balance, such as chronic liver disease, hyperthyroidism, and androgen resistance, can also cause gynecomastia (Box 19.18).

There are three common mammographic appearances of gynecomastia: nodular, dendritic, and diffuse (Fig. 19.15). These differences in appearance correlate to differences in the histologic stage. Even when patients report unilateral symptoms, the mammographic findings are often bilateral. Although frequently asymmetric when comparing right to left, the fibroglandular tissue in gynecomastia should be centered in the retroareolar space. Ultrasound should only be performed if the mammographic findings are suspicious or do not explain the patient's symptoms. Gynecomastia on imaging should be assessed as benign (BI-RADS 2).

If the cause is identified and addressed early, gynecomastia can regress partially or completely. However, the fibrosis of long-standing gynecomastia can be permanent. In rare, extreme cases, surgical excision can be performed to relieve severe symptoms or psychological distress related to self-image.

MALE: MALE BREAST CANCER

The incidence of male breast cancer in the United States is 1 in 100,000 with approximately 2000 total cases annually (Box 19.19). Nearly all breast cancers in men are invasive ductal carcinoma. Invasive lobular carcinomas are very rare (less than 2% of male breast cancers) due to the lack of lobular tissue in men. Studies have shown that men with breast cancer have overall poorer survival rates compared with women. Male breast cancer is often linked to family history; approximately 20% of men with breast cancer report a family history of breast or ovarian cancer and approximately 10% have an identifiable genetic mutation, most commonly *BRCA2*. Therefore all men diagnosed with breast cancer should undergo genetic testing. The presentation of male breast cancer, at the median age of 67, includes similar signs, symptoms, and imaging features as female breast cancer.

Because men are not screened for breast cancer, breast cancer is most commonly detected by palpation with masses being the most common imaging feature (Fig. 19.16). Secondary clinical findings of nipple retraction, skin changes, bloody nipple discharge, and palpable axillary nodes are similar to females. In addition to masses, mammographic calcifications, asymmetries, and architectural distortion may be seen. Given that the vast majority of cases present as a palpable and mammographic mass, ultrasound is almost always performed to supplement mammography and can guide tissue sampling (Box 19.20). Ultrasound and mammography can also be used to assess response to neoadjuvant therapy, if needed.

MALE: SUMMARY

- Gynecomastia is the most common cause of a palpable abnormality in the male breast and is most commonly diagnosed on physical examination without the need for imaging.

Box 19.18   Gynecomastia

- Mechanism: imbalance between estrogen (stimulatory) and androgen (inhibitory) action on breast tissue where estrogen is elevated relative to androgen levels.
- Causes:
  - Expected hormonal imbalances seen in neonates, during puberty, and in the elderly.
  - Primary or secondary gonadal failure leading to low testosterone.
- Medical conditions, such as:
  - Androgen resistance syndromes
  - Hyperthyroidism
  - Chronic liver disease
- Medications/substances, such as:
  - Spironolactone
  - Digoxin
  - Cimetidine
  - Bicalutamide
  - Marijuana
  - Many others

Box 19.19   Male Breast Cancer: Demographics

- 1% of all breast cancer
- Approximately 2000 cases per year
- 1 per 100,000 men
- Mean age 67
- Prognosis at comparable stage is similar or worse than females
- Invasive ductal carcinoma is most common
- Lobular cancers are rare, given lack of lobular tissue in males
- Approximately 10% have an identifiable gene mutation, most commonly *BRCA2*

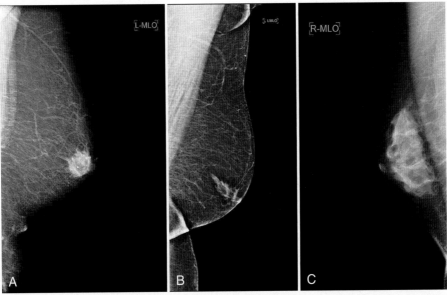

Fig. 19.15 There are three classic appearances of gynecomastia: nodular, dendritic, and diffuse. Nodular gynecomastia (A) can appear as a nodular, rounded, mass-like subareolar density. This is sometimes described as a disc or fan. Nodular gynecomastia is the closest mimic to a true mass. When unilateral, ultrasound, along with clinical examination, is often necessary to exclude malignancy. Dendritic gynecomastia (B) is commonly described as "flame-shaped" and looks similar to subareolar breast tissue commonly seen in women, with scalloped edges and lobules of fat density. Diffuse gynecomastia (C) usually represents long-standing proliferation and may be indistinguishable from a fully developed female breast. If the underlying cause of gynecomastia can be eliminated, nodular and dendritic types may fully regress because they are predominately glandular. However, diffuse gynecomastia includes some fibrosis that is often permanent.

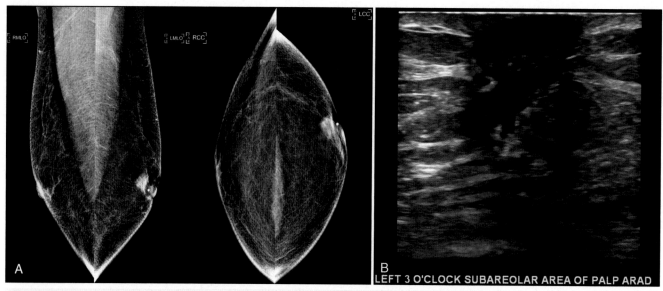

Fig. 19.16 A 57-year-old man presented with a palpable left breast lump. Bilateral mediolateral oblique (MLO) and craniocaudal (CC) diagnostic views (A) demonstrate a left breast subareolar mass with irregular shape and indistinct margins correlating to the palpable abnormality. While the mammographic findings on the left are similar to nodular gynecomastia, the mass is more eccentric in location relative to the nipple, and there is associated nipple retraction. The right breast demonstrates minimal subareolar dendritic gynecomastia. Ultrasound (B) of the left breast palpable abnormality demonstrates a corresponding irregular, hypoechoic, antiparallel mass with angular margins. This mass involves the nipple, which is retracted. Ultrasound guided biopsy was recommended and pathology yielded invasive ductal carcinoma.

Box 19.20   Male Breast Cancer: Imaging Findings

- Imaging features are similar to breast cancer in females
  - Mass (most common)
  - Calcifications
  - Asymmetry or architectural distortion
  - Secondary findings, such as nipple or skin retraction
- Clinical presentation is most often a firm subareolar mass. Other signs/symptoms, include:
  - Nipple retraction
  - Bloody nipple discharge
  - Skin ulceration
  - Axillary adenopathy

- For suspicious clinical symptoms, start with a bilateral diagnostic mammogram.
- Starting with ultrasound may be considered in those younger than 25.
- Perform ultrasound for any suspicious or indeterminate mammographic finding.
- Male breast cancer is rare.
- MRI is not indicated in male patients.

Transgender

The term *transgender* encompasses an expanding group of people whose gender identity or expression differs from that traditionally associated with the sex assigned to them at birth. Transgender includes patients who have altered their outward appearance but not their physical anatomy; for example, a person born female who still has breast tissue but has adopted an outward male appearance. Transgender also includes patients who have altered their anatomy; for example, a person born female who has undergone breast reduction mammoplasty or mastectomy or a person born male who takes feminizing hormones with or without breast augmentation. Regardless of whether a patient has undergone gender-affirming intervention, the term *transgender man* (sometimes referred to as female-to-male transgender person) includes anyone who was assigned female at birth but identifies as a male. The term *transgender woman* (sometimes referred to as male-to-female transgender person) includes anyone who was assigned male at birth but identifies as a female.

As a breast radiologist, it is important to know the patient's history, including natal sex, surgical history, current and past hormonal influences, and genetic risk factors, in order to best direct the appropriate imaging management for both symptomatic and asymptomatic patients seeking breast care.

It is also important to be aware of other factors that can potentially increase breast cancer risk, delay diagnosis or treatment, and even affect navigation through the health care system for transgender patients. These factors may include financial restrictions (including insurance coverage issues), nulliparity, obesity, and mental health issues. Unfortunately, transgender patients who seek health care may sometimes be discriminated against or denied. Therefore transgender patients may avoid the health care system out of fear of discrimination and harassment. Furthermore, transgender patients may feel uncomfortable in the breast center, which often reflects traditional feminine decor. This can be especially daunting for patients who are born female and have breasts or breast tissue, but who identify, dress, and appear as male. Technologists can also feel uncomfortable when they are uncertain how to address a patient or are uncertain where to seat them—whether to seat them in a waiting room with cisgender women or to route them through the standard path for men.

Staff, technologists, and radiologists should be properly trained and work to ensure that all patients, regardless of gender identity or gender expression, feel safe, comfortable, welcome, and respected in the breast imaging facility. When unsure how to address a patient, it is generally best to first address them by their first name, then ask them for their preference.

TRANSGENDER: EXPECTED IMAGING APPEARANCES

There is a range of expected imaging appearances in transgender patients depending on whether they are a transgender man or a transgender woman and what gender-affirming interventions they have undergone.

A transgender woman, for example, may undergo feminizing hormone therapy, with or without orchiectomy, and/or augmentation mammoplasty. It takes approximately 2 to 3 years of hormone therapy to see maximum breast growth. Patients who have undergone augmentation mammoplasty typically have undergone hormone therapy for at least 1 year prior to surgery. Histologically, fibroglandular breast tissue that forms from hormone stimulation in a transgender woman is similar to that seen in the female breast; therefore one can expect to find similar pathologies, both benign and malignant (Fig. 19.17). The imaging appearance of augmentation mammoplasty, including implants and fat grafting, is the same in transgender and cisgender women. Direct silicone injection, while illegal to perform in the United States, may also be encountered.

A transgender man has the option to undergo masculinizing hormone therapy, with or without oophorectomy, and/or reduction mammoplasty or mastectomy (sometimes referred to as top surgery). It takes approximately 2 years of hormone therapy to see masculinizing effects on the breast tissue. Even with hormone therapy, however, one can still expect to find the same pathologies as cisgender females, both benign and malignant, in any remaining breast tissue. The imaging appearance of surgical complications associated with reduction mammoplasty and mastectomies are also the same, regardless of gender.

TRANSGENDER: BREAST CANCER RISK

The breast cancer risk in a transgender woman who has undergone feminizing hormone therapy is higher than in cisgender men but lower than in cisgender women. The risk of breast cancer in a transgender man who has not undergone mastectomy but takes masculinizing hormones is higher than in cisgender men but lower than in cisgender women. Similar to a cisgender woman who has undergone bilateral mastectomy, the risk of breast cancer in a transgender man who has undergone bilateral mastectomy is reduced substantially, by greater than 90%.

TRANSGENDER: SCREENING CONSIDERATIONS

While currently there are no evidence-based screening guidelines, it is suggested that transgender women with risk factors for breast cancer who have undergone feminizing hormone therapy for 5 or more years should undergo

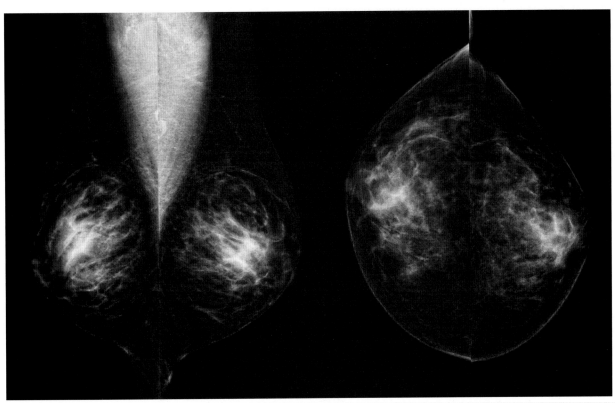

Fig. 19.17 A 68-year-old transgender male-to-female patient with a history of long-term hormone therapy presented for screening mammography. Bilateral mediolateral oblique (MLO) and craniocaudal (CC) screening mammograms demonstrate bilateral heterogeneously dense breast tissue without any suspicious findings.

Table 19.4   Screening Recommendations in Transgender Patients

Transgender woman	With breast cancer risk factors + on hormone therapy ≥5 years	Annual screening mammography
Transgender woman	With breast cancer risk factors + on hormone therapy <5 years or without breast cancer risk factors + on hormone therapy ≥ 5 years	Discuss need for screening with doctor
Transgender woman	Without breast cancer risk factors + on hormone therapy <5 years	Discuss need for screening with doctor; screening is generally not indicated
Transgender man	Status post mastectomy	Screening mammography is not indicated; annual chest wall physical examination is controversial
Transgender man	Not status post mastectomy	Annual screening mammography

Suggested screening recommendations for various transgender patients, based on hormonal and surgical treatments. Data on screening outcomes in transgender patients is limited to nonexistent in each of these scenarios.

routine screening mammography. Those without risk factors for breast cancer or those with risk factors but who have been taking feminizing hormone therapy for less than 5 years should have a discussion with their doctor about whether screening is appropriate for them.

Transgender men who have not undergone a bilateral mastectomy should continue with annual screening mammography, following the same screening guidelines as cisgender women regardless of masculinizing hormone therapy. Those who have undergone bilateral mastectomy should be managed clinically given the technical limitations of mammography after mastectomy (Table 19.4). Some suggest annual chest wall examinations in transgender men after mastectomy, but, in the absence of a personal history of breast cancer, this is controversial, and evidence supporting this is incomplete.

TRANSGENDER: DIAGNOSTIC CONSIDERATIONS

The diagnostic imaging evaluation of a transgender patient who is recalled from screening mammography or who is presenting with a focal symptom should follow the same diagnostic algorithm for a cisgender woman, including starting with ultrasound in any patient presenting with a focal symptom who has undergone mastectomy or who is under the age of 30.

TRANSGENDER: SUMMARY

- Screening mammography recommendations are based on natal sex, surgical history, current and past hormonal influences, and genetic risk factors of the patient.
- Greater than 5 years of feminizing hormone therapy increases the risk of breast cancer in transgender women.
- Evaluation of a suspicious breast symptom or a screen-detected finding should generally follow the same diagnostic imaging protocol as for a cisgender woman.

- All patients should be made to feel welcome, safe, comfortable, and respected in the breast imaging facility.
- When unsure how to address a patient, it is generally best to initially address them by their first name and then ask them for their preference.

KEY POINTS

Special Populations
- Young
  - Breast cancer is rare in patients <30 years old.
  - For patients <30 years old with focal breast symptoms, ultrasound should be the initial imaging modality used.
  - Mammography is not contraindicated and can be considered if sonographic findings are suspicious or do not explain suspicious clinical symptoms.
  - Cancer is extremely rare in the pediatric and adolescent populations; therefore, biopsy is rarely needed, and special caution must be taken to avoid damage to the developing tissue or breast bud.
- Pregnancy and lactation
  - Current guidelines recommend ultrasound as the initial modality for evaluating focal symptoms in pregnant and lactating patients.
  - Mammography is not contraindicated and is safe for pregnant or lactating patients.
  - Radiation dose from a mammogram is well below teratogenic level, with no evidence of harm to the fetus.
  - Lactating patients should pump or breast feed immediately prior to mammography to decrease breast density and improve compression and patient comfort.
  - Pregnancy-associated breast cancer is rare but often aggressive.
  - When a percutaneous procedure is performed in a lactating patient, always allow for the low risk of a milk fistula.
- Male
  - Gynecomastia is the most common cause of breast symptoms and is often a clinical diagnosis not requiring imaging.
  - When symptoms are indeterminate, a bilateral full-field mediolateral oblique (MLO) and craniocaudal (CC) two-dimensional mammogram is usually sufficient to establish the diagnosis.
  - Targeted ultrasound should be performed for any suspicious mammographic findings.
  - Male breast cancer is rare and imaging features are similar to female breast cancer.
- Transgender
  - The breast imaging center should be a comfortable and welcoming environment for all patients, regardless of gender identity.
  - Transgender women on feminizing hormone therapy have a risk of breast cancer higher than cisgender men but lower than cisgender women.
  - Breast cancer screening in transgender women should be directed by presence of risk factors and duration of hormone therapy use.
  - Transgender men on masculinizing hormone therapy who have not undergone mastectomy have a slightly reduced risk of breast cancer than cisgender women.

- Routine screening mammography is recommended in transgender men of screening age in the absence of mastectomy.
- In symptomatic transgender patients, the same diagnostic imaging protocol as for cisgender women should be followed.

Suggested Readings

Abramson L, Massaro L, Alberty-Oller J, Melsaether A. Breast imaging during pregnancy and lactation. *J Breast Imaging*. 2019;1(4):1–10.

Chowdhry DN, O'Connell AM. Breast imaging in transgender patients. *J Breast Imaging*. 2020;2(2):161–167.

Dedelzon K, Katzen JT. Evaluation of palpable breast abnormalities. *J Breast Imaging*. 2019;1(3):253–263.

Expert Panel on Breast Imaging diFlorio-Alexander RM, Slanetz PJ, Moy L, et al. ACR appropriateness criteria: breast imaging of pregnant and lactating women. *J Am Coll Radiol*. 2018;15(11S):S263–S275.

Expert Panel on Breast Imaging Niell BL, Lourenco AP, Moy L, et al. ACR appropriateness criteria evaluation of the symptomatic male breast. *J Am Coll Radiol*. 2018;15(11S):S313–S320.

Gao Y, Heller SL, Moy L. Male breast cancer in the age of genetic testing: an opportunity for early detection, tailored therapy, and surveillance. *Radiographics*. 2018;38(5):1289–1311.

Giess CS, et al. Risk of malignancy in palpable solid breast masses considered probably benign or low suspicion: implications for management. *J Ultrasound Med*. 2012;31(12):1943–1949.

Kaneda HJ, et al. Pediatric and adolescent breast masses: a review of pathophysiology, imaging, diagnosis, and treatment. *AJR*. 2013;200:W204–W212.

Nguyen C, Kettler MD, Swirsky ME, et al. Male breast disease: pictorial review with radiologic-pathologic correlation. *Radiographics*. 2013;33(3):763–779.

Parikh U, Mausner E, Chhor CM, Gao Y, Karrington I, Heller SL. Breast imaging in transgender patients: what the radiologist should know. *Radiographics*. 2020;40(1):13–27.

Sabate JM, et al. Radiologic evaluation of breast disorders related to pregnancy and lactation. *Radiographics*. 2007;27(Suppl 1):S101–S124.

Vashi R, Hooley R, Butler R, Geisel J, Philpotts L. Breast imaging of the pregnant and lactating patient: imaging modalities and pregnancy-associated breast cancer. *AJR*. 2013;200:321–328.

Vashi R, Hooley R, Butler R, Geisel J, Philpotts L. Breast imaging of the pregnant and lactating patient: physiologic changes and common benign entities. *AJR*. 2013;200:329–336.

20 Mammography Quality Standards Act (MQSA) and American College of Radiology (ACR) Accreditation Programs

ELIZABETH S. McDONALD AND SAMANTHA P. ZUCKERMAN

OVERVIEW This chapter reviews the key components of the Mammography Quality Standards Act and American College of Radiology (ACR) accreditation programs, including personnel qualifications, imaging and equipment standards, reporting requirements, and the medical audit.

Mammography Quality Standards Act Origins and Purpose

The Mammography Quality Standards Act (MQSA) was established by the United States Congress as law on October 27, 1992. MQSA's overall goal is to "ensure that all women have access to quality mammography for the detection of breast cancer in its earliest, most treatable stages." MQSA ensures quality mammography through routine inspections by the U.S. Food and Drug Administration (FDA). Upon successful completion of annual inspections, a facility can be certified by the FDA to perform mammograms.

Each facility that performs mammography in the United States (with the exception of Department of Veterans Affairs) is required to:

- Be accredited by an FDA-approved accreditation body (either the American College of Radiology [ACR] or the states of Arkansas and Texas).
- Meet quality standards for personnel and equipment.
- Perform examinations under the maximum allowable radiation dose.
- Perform quality assurance, medical audit and outcome analysis, medical record keeping, and abide by reporting requirements.

Facilities maintain their MSQA certification status by:

- Having an annual survey performed by a licensed medical physicist.
- Undergoing annual inspections conducted by an MQSA inspector.
- Correcting deficiencies found during audits.
- Prominently displaying MQSA certificate in the facility.
- Staying current with inspection fees.

Under federal law, all mammography facilities in the United States are required to comply with the MQSA final regulations. Only facilities with MQSA certification are eligible to receive Medicare/Medicaid payments for screening and diagnostic mammography.

Annual inspections of facilities include the following evaluations:

- Personnel qualification records of physicians, technologists, and physicists
- Minimal equipment requirements and evaluation of equipment performance
- Quality assurance (QA) and quality control (QC) records and tests
- Medical records (mammography reports and images) and lay summaries
- Medical audit and outcome analysis

Personnel Qualifications

The MQSA dictates the minimum requirements for all personnel, including interpreting physicians, technologists, and medical physicists, who are involved in any aspect of the production, processing, and interpretation of mammograms. These requirements are summarized in Boxes 20.1 to 20.3 and are also available as checklists on the ACR accreditation website. The imaging facility must maintain records documenting these personnel qualifications, and these records must be available for review by MQSA inspectors.

Equipment Requirements and Quality Assurance

The MQSA specifies the required standards for mammography equipment. Selected equipment requirements are summarized in Box 20.4. In addition, all mammography facilities must establish and maintain a quality assurance program. The lead interpreting physician, quality control technologist, and medical physicist must ensure that quality assurance records be kept and maintained until the next annual MQSA inspection has been completed. The

Box 20.1 Requirements for Interpreting Physicians.

Initial qualifications (to be met before interpreting mammograms independently):

- Must have a valid state medical license
- Must have 3-month full-time training in mammography interpretation, radiation physics, radiation effects, and radiation protection or be certified by a body approved by the FDA
- Must have 60 hours of documented mammography specific continuing medical education (CME) and 8 hours of training in each modality. Residency training is acceptable for this requirement.
- Must have read 240 examinations in the preceding 6 months under the supervision of a fully qualified interpreting physician

Continued experience and education (maintenance of qualifications):

- Have read 960 mammograms over a period of 24 months
- Have earned at least 15 category 1 CME credits in mammography over a 36-month period, with 6 credits in each modality used
- Have earned 6 CME credits specific to any new imaging modality prior to reading that modality

Reestablishing qualifications:

- Interpreting physicians who failed to maintain continuing experience requirements must either interpret or double read 240 mammograms under direct supervision or bring the total to 960 over a period of 24 months and accomplish these tasks within the 6 months immediately before resuming independent interpretation.

Box 20.2 Requirements for Radiologic Technologists

Have a state license to perform radiographic procedures or be certified by one of the bodies approved by the FDA

Have undergone 40 hours of documented mammography training, with 8 hours of instruction in each modality used, and have completed 25 mammography examinations

Complete 200 examinations in the previous 24 months and complete at least 15 continuing education units (CEUs) in the past 36 months, including 6 in each modality used

Box 20.3 Requirements for Medical Physicists

Have a state license to conduct evaluations of mammography equipment or have certification by one of the accrediting bodies approved by the FDA

Have at least a master's degree or higher in a physical science with at least 20 semester hours of graduate or undergraduate physics

Have at least 20 contact hours of mammography facility survey training

Have the experience of conducting surveys of at least one mammography facility and at least 10 mammography units

Have at least 8 hours of training in the modality before independently performing surveys of mammographic equipment

Have conducted two mammography facility surveys and a total of six mammography unit surveys during the 24 months preceding the annual MQSA inspection

Have taught or completed at least 15 continuing education units in medical physics or mammography during the 36 months immediately preceding the annual MQSA inspection

Box 20.4 Selected Equipment Requirements for Mammography

Mammography units must be specific to mammography.

Compression must be able to be obtained both manually and by machine.

Both 18 × 24 cm and 24 × 30 cm image receptors (screen film) must have moving grids and compression paddles.

The mean glandular dose (mGy) to an FDA-accepted phantom simulating a 4.5-cm thick breast must be less than 3 mGy (0.3 rad).

The mammography unit must be able to angulate 180 degrees from craniocaudal orientation in at least one direction. Once fixed at the desired position, the tube-image receptor assembly shall not undergo unintended motion.

Systems used for noninterventional diagnostic procedures must have magnification capability within the range of 1.4–2.0.

X-ray system must have a post exposure display of x-ray focal spot and target material used during the exposure.

The mammography system must provide an automatic exposure control (AEC) mode that operates in all equipment configurations. There must be flexibility in the positioning or selection of the AEC detector under the target tissue.

Manual selection of mAs shall be available. Following AEC mode use, the system must indicate the actual mAs and kVp used.

Table 20.1 Medical Physicist Quality Control Tests Performed Annually (and After Equipment Changes)

Full-field digital mammography (FFDM) unit assembly evaluation	Breast entrance exposure, mean glandular dose, and radiation output rate
Flat field uniformity test	Assessment of collimation
Artifact evaluation	Evaluation of focal spot condition
Automatic exposure control mode and signal-to-noise ratio check	Assessment of beam quality (half value layer measurement)
Phantom image quality test	Modulation transfer function measurement
Contrast to noise ratio test	kVp accuracy and reproducibility
Image quality of the display monitor	

Table 20.2 Frequency of Quality Assurance Tasks for Full-Field Digital Mammography

Processor quality control	Daily
Dark room cleanliness	Daily
Phantom evaluation[a]	Weekly
Screen and viewbox cleanliness	Weekly
Visual checklist	Monthly
Analysis of fixer retention in film	Quarterly
Repeat analysis	Quarterly
Darkroom fog	Semiannually
Screen-film contact	Semiannually
Compression	Semiannually

[a]Phantom evaluation: Must see four fibers, three speck groups, three masses. Must be free of significant artifacts (Fig. 20.1).

medical physicist quality control tests are summarized in Table 20.1. Selected quality assurance tests performed by the QC technologist and the required frequency of testing are summarized in Table 20.2. These tests include imaging a mammography phantom, which simulates a 4.2 cm compressed breast of average density and has a wax insert containing fibers, specks, and masses (Fig. 20.1).

The above tests are for standard digital mammography. Additional QA tasks are required for film screen mammography and digital breast tomosynthesis for both

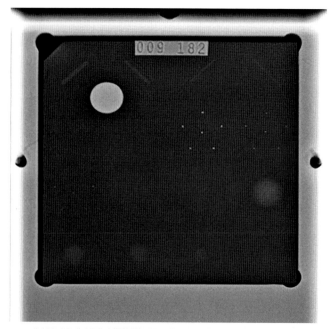

Fig. 20.1 Mammography Phantom Image.

technologists and physicists. Please see the FDA ACR website for further details.

American College of Radiology (ACR) Accreditation

The ACR offers accreditation in multiple modalities including mammography, stereotactic breast biopsy, breast MRI, and breast ultrasound. The ACR is the only nationally approved accrediting body, with the only state-level alternative being Arkansas and Texas. Nearly all mammography facilities in the United States accredit throughout the ACR. ACR accreditation is a self-assessment and peer-reviewed process. It is considered the gold standard in medical imaging accreditation. Accreditation assures patients and providers that the facility in question provides the highest level of imaging quality and safety by meeting requirements for equipment, personnel, and quality assurance. ACR accreditation occurs every 3 years.

Accreditation is a two-part process and includes the following:

Part 1: Initial application includes information regarding practice site characteristics (facility, equipment, and personnel) and payment of the application fee.
Part 2: Online testing package: submission of information regarding policies and procedures, reporting mechanisms, patient outcomes data, personnel, QC results, and example images.

At the end of the accreditation review process, the ACR will issue a confidential report for each facility. The facility will also receive an accreditation certificate and decal for each passing unit at the facility. The name of the accredited facility will be listed on both the ACR and FDA website.

Box 20.5   Mammography Reports: Required Content, Terminology, and Communication

Patient name and additional patient identifier
Examination date
Interpreting physician name
Final assessment category using the following terminology:
- "Negative"
- "Benign"
- "Probably benign"
- "Suspicious"
- "Highly suggestive of malignancy"
- "Known biopsy proven malignancy"
- "Incomplete: Need additional imaging evaluation"

Recommendations to the health care provider about management
Written mammography report must be sent to the referring provider within 30 days of the examination
Written "lay letter" must be sent to the patient within 30 days of the examination

Mammography Reporting and Medical Records Requirements

The MQSA requires that specific information and terminology be provided in the written mammography reports (Box 20.5).

The MQSA also requires that written communication of mammography results summarized in lay terms (i.e., a "lay letter") be sent to the patient within 30 days of the mammographic examination. When the patient has a referring provider, the written mammography report must be sent to that referring health care provider within 30 days of the mammographic examination. For "suspicious" or "highly suggestive of malignancy" assessments, the facility must attempt to communicate the results to the patient and to the referring health care provider as soon as possible.

For medical recordkeeping, the MQSA requires that the mammography facility maintain mammography films and reports in the patient's permanent medical record for a minimum of 5 years, or for a minimum of 10 years if no additional mammograms of the patient are performed at that facility, or longer as mandated by state or local law.

Medical Audit

MQSA requires that each accredited facility have a process to track positive mammograms (screening mammograms that were recalled and diagnostic mammograms that were recommended for biopsy). The ACR endorses this audit but also recommends additional more comprehensive auditing of screening and diagnostic mammograms. Medical audit of both the facility and individual radiologists is compared against national benchmark statistics from the Breast Cancer Surveillance Consortium (BCSC) and acceptable ranges of performance recommended by a panel of breast imaging experts.

Each facility must designate at least one lead interpreting physician to review the medical outcomes audit data at least once every 12 months, and these results must be documented. All interpreting radiologists must be notified of their individual audit results and the facility's aggregate results. If follow-up actions are needed, the nature of the follow-up must also be documented.

Recommended ranges of performance and benchmarks from the 2017 evaluation of BCSC data are summarized in Tables 20.3–20.4.

Definitions of statistics per ACR auditing guidelines are as follows. These definitions assume a 1-year screening interval:

- True positive (TP): positive imaging with a tissue diagnosis of breast cancer within 1 year
- True negative (TN): negative imaging without a breast cancer diagnosis within 1 year

Table 20.3 Screening Mammography Performance Measures*

Screening Measure	Acceptable Range Carney et al.	2017 Breast Cancer Surveillance Consortium (BCSC) Mean Lehman et al.
Screening recall rate	5%–12%	11.6%
Cancer detection rate per 1000 examinations	>2.5	5.1
Sensitivity	>75%	86.9%
Specificity	88%–95%	88.9%
False negative rate per 1000 examinations	N/A	0.8
PPV1	3%–8%	4.4%
PPV2[a]	20%–40%	25.6%
PPV3[a]	N/A	28.6%

PPV, Positive predictive value.
[a]Although included in the benchmarks, if mammographic reporting is done in accordance with American College of Radiology (ACR) Breast Imaging Reporting and Data System (BI-RADS) guidelines, PPV2 and PPV3 would not apply to screening mammography.

Table 20.4 Diagnostic Mammography Performance Measures[a]

Diagnostic Measures	Palpable	All Examinations
Cancer detection rate per 1000 examinations	57.7	30.0
Median size of invasive cancers (mm)	21.8	17.0
Percentage of node negative invasive cancers	56.5%	68.2%
Percentage minimal cancer	15.2%	39.8%
Percentage stage 0 or 1 cancer	37%	60.7%
PPV2	43.7%	31.2%
PPV3	49.1%	35.9%
Sensitivity (if measurable)	87.8%	83.1%
Specificity (if measurable)	92.2%	93.2%

[a]Adapted from D'Orsi CJ, Sickles EA, Mendelson EB, Morris EA, et al. ACR BI-RADS® Atlas, Breast Imaging Reporting and Data System. Reston, VA, American College of Radiology; 2013.

- False positive (FP): positive examination without a breast cancer diagnosis within 1 year
- False negative (FN): negative examination with a tissue diagnosis of breast cancer within 1 year
- Recall rate: proportion of women undergoing screening who are given a positive interpretation (Breast Imaging Reporting and Data System [BI-RADS] 0); (TP + FP)/(all examinations)
- Cancer detection rate (CDR): number of cancers detected by imaging per 1000 patients examined
- Sensitivity: ability of imaging to find cancer when it is present; TP/(TP + FN)
- Specificity: ability of imaging to determine that cancer is absent when a patient is cancer-free; TN/(TN + FP)
- Abnormal interpretation rate: the proportion of examinations interpreted as positive (positive examinations)/(all examinations)
- False negative rate: number of women who have a breast cancer diagnosis within 1 year of a negative examination per 1000 examinations.

For screening mammography, BI-RADS categories 1 or 2 are considered negative examinations and BI-RADS category 0 is considered a positive examination. BI-RADS categories 3, 4, or 5 should not be used at screening mammography.

For diagnostic mammography, BI-RADS categories 1, 2, or 3 are considered negative examinations and BI-RADS categories 4 or 5 are considered positive examinations.

Positive predictive value (PPV) is the proportion of positive examinations with a breast cancer tissue diagnosis within 1 year, or TP/(TP + FP). In breast imaging, there are three separate definitions for PPVs as follows:

- PPV1 (abnormal screening): proportion of all women with positive screening examinations (BI-RADS 0) who are diagnosed with breast cancer; TP/(number of positive screening examinations)
- PPV2 (biopsies recommended): proportion of all examinations with a recommendation for tissue diagnosis (BI-RADS 4 and 5) with a tissue diagnosis of breast cancer; TP/(number of biopsies recommended)
- PPV3 (biopsies performed): proportion of all biopsies performed due to a positive examination (BI-RADS 4 and 5) that result in a tissue diagnosis of breast cancer; TP/(number of biopsies done)

If mammographic reporting is done in accordance of ACR guidelines, PPV1 applies to screening examinations, while PPV2 and PPV3 should apply to only diagnostic examinations (very rarely to screening).

KEY POINTS

- The Mammography Quality Standards Act (MQSA) mandates that all facilities performing mammography be certified by the FDA. Most facilities achieve accreditation through the American College of Radiology (ACR). Arkansas and Texas have their own accreditation process.
- To begin independent interpretation of mammograms, radiologists must fulfill three criteria during their training: 3 months of full-time mammography

interpretation, 60 hours of mammography-specific CME, and supervised interpretation of 240 examinations in a 6-month period within 2 years of completing residency.

- Phantom evaluation should be performed weekly as part of the QA process. Phantom images must include at least four fibers, three speck groups, and three masses.
- The MQSA mandates specific terminology and language to be included in mammography reports. Both a lay letter to the patient and a report to the referring provider must be sent within 30 days of the examination.
- Acceptable screening benchmark measures include recall rate between 5% and 12% and cancer detection rate of at least 2.5 per 1000, noting the mean cancer detection rate in the BCSC is 5.1 per 1000.

Suggested Readings

1. Mammography Quality Standards Act and Program. https://www.fda.gov/radiation-emitting-products/mammography-quality-standards-act-and-program.

2. Destouet JM, Bassett LW, Yaffe MJ, Butler PF, Wilcox PA. The ACR's mammography accreditation program: ten years of experience since MQSA. *J Am Coll Radiol.* 2005;2(7):585–594.

3. ACR accreditation. https://www.acr.org/Clinical-Resources/Accreditation.

4. Personnel requirements on FDA website. https://www.acraccreditation.org/-/media/ACRAccreditation/Documents/Mammography/Forms/PersonnelRequirements.pdf?la=en.

5. Carney PA, Parikh J, Sickles EA, et al. Diagnostic mammography: identifying minimally acceptable interpretive performance criteria. *Radiology.* 2013;267(2):359–367.

6. Sprague BL, Arao RF, Miglioretti DL, et al. National performance benchmarks for modern diagnostic digital mammography: update from the Breast Cancer Surveillance Consortium. *Radiology.* 2017;283(1):59–69. https://doi.org/10.1148/radiol.2017161519.

7. Lehman CD, Arao RF, Sprague BL, et al. National performance benchmarks for modern screening digital mammography: update from the Breast Cancer Surveillance Consortium. *Radiology.* 2017;283(1):49–58. https://doi.org/10.1148/radiol.2016161174.

8. D'Orsi CJ, Sickles EA, Mendelson EB, Morris EA, et al. *ACR BI-RADS® Atlas, Breast Imaging Reporting and Data System.* Reston, VA: American College of Radiology; 2013.

9. Sickles EA, D'Orsi CJ. *ACR BI-RADS® Follow-up and Outcome Monitoring. ACR BI-RADS® Atlas, Breast Imaging Reporting and Data System.* Reston, VA: American College of Radiology; 2013.

21 Mammography Physics 101*

JAMES GORDON MAINPRIZE

OVERVIEW *This chapter covers some of the basic physics of operation of a mammography system including the components of the mammography system, the effects of scatter, radiation dose requirements, magnification, and common artifacts in digital mammography.*

A mammography system is a dedicated radiography system designed and optimized specifically for imaging the breast. Some systems still employ a cassette with a fluorescent screen and x-ray film, although most sites (>99.5%) in the United States use more modern devices that have a digital detector to record the x-ray image. As of March 1, 2020, there are 8696 (8671 with digital) certified mammography facilities with 21,563 accredited mammography systems. A total of 39,840,776 mammography procedures are performed annually (https://www.fda.gov/radiation-emitting-products/mqsa-insights/mqsa-national-statistics).

Image Acquisition

All mammography systems include an x-ray tube, filters, compression paddle, an antiscatter grid, and x-ray image receptor in a rotatable C-arm (Fig. 21.1; Box 21.1). All systems have an automatic exposure control (AEC) system that can detect the lowest signal (densest region) behind the breast and provide feedback to adjust one or more technique factors (kV, filtration, tube current, imaging time; Box 21.2)

to optimize image quality. The AEC may either use a separate x-ray sensitive device or use the image receptor itself to determine the signal level.

A certified breast technologist positions the breast between the compression paddle and the tabletop and applies compression. This reduces the effective thickness of the breast, reducing the radiation dose needed; spreads out the breast tissue so that some overlapping structures can be better seen; and reduces blurring due to patient motion. Note, however, that overcompression may lead to reduced imaging performance, although the mechanism for this loss in performance is not well understood.

The technologist hits the acquire button, and x-rays emitted from the x-ray tube port pass through the breast. Some are absorbed by the breast tissue while others pass through to the image receptor. The amount of x-ray absorption (or conversely transmission) depends on the x-ray energy, the compressed breast thickness, and tissue composition. The image captured by the image receptor is effectively an x-ray "shadow" of the tissue structure in the breast.

The x-ray tube (Fig. 21.2) is powered by the generator, which applies a high potential of 25 to 45 kilovolts (kV) between the anode and cathode inside the x-ray tube. The

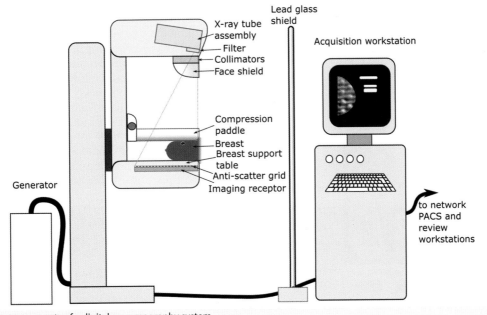

Fig. 21.1 Common components of a digital mammography system.

*The authors gratefully acknowledge the original contributions of *R. Edward Hendrick, Debra M. Ikeda, and Kanae K. Miyake* for figure 21.13b 21.13c, 21.14,21.15 and 21.16 (previously published in Ikeda D, Miyake, KK eds., 2016. *Breast imaging: the requisites.* Elsevier Health Sciences.)

Box 21.1 Components of a Mammography System

Generator	Converts 220 V (from the wall box) to the voltages required for system operation. In particular, the high voltage (25–45 kV) needed to energize the x-ray tube.
X-ray tube	A vacuum glass tube containing a rotating anode and small wire cathode. An accelerated electron beam from the cathode smashing into the anode generates x-rays that exit through the tube port.
Filter	A thin metal plate put into the x-ray field to filter out low energy x-rays.
Collimators	Lead or heavy metal strips near the x-ray tube port that move to limit the size of the x-ray field.
Compression paddle	A plastic semirigid plate that is used to immobilize and compress the breast.
Breast support table	Supports the breast and protects the sensitive detector underneath.
Antiscatter grid	A focused array of lead strips that preferentially block scattered x-rays while allowing unscattered primary radiation through to the detector. Some systems use two-dimensional honeycomb array rather than strips.
Imaging receptor	The x-ray sensitive detector. Usually a two-dimensional flat-panel array of detector elements.
Automatic exposure control (AEC)	The AEC is an electronic module, software control, or combination of both that provides feedback during the first few milliseconds of imaging to adjust the technique factors to achieve a target signal and/or noise level in the final image. The AEC may change the filter, kV, mA, and/or imaging time.
Acquisition workstation	The console from which the breast technologist controls image acquisition and determines image acceptability.
Picture and archiving system (PACS)	The network of computers, storage devices, and related software used to store and catalog images acquired in radiology departments.
Review workstation	A dedicated workstation with specialized high-resolution monitors for reviewing digital mammograms.

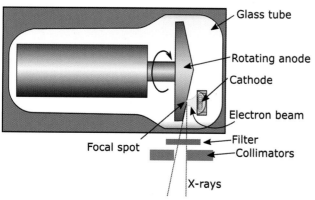

Fig. 21.2 Components of an x-ray tube, cross-section.

Box 21.2 Technique Factors

Tube potential, kV	The high voltage applied between the anode and cathode to accelerate the electron beam.
Tube current, mA	The measure of the current flow of electrons between the cathode and anode.
Tube current-time product, mAs	The total amount of radiation generated is proportional to the tube current (mA) multiplied by the imaging time (s). Radiation dose will be proportional to mAs.

tube potential (often referred to as the "kV") is much lower than other radiography procedures (chest radiography or computed tomography [CT]). This is to take advantage of the differential x-ray absorption between soft tissue, which is increased at lower x-ray energies. This increases the contrast between the adipose (fatty) and fibroglandular (ductal tissue, stroma, and Cooper ligaments) tissues.

Early generators did not produce a constant tube potential and instead had the voltage rippling up and down. In those days, the tube potential was described by the maximum or "peak kV" (kVp). Because modern generators produce stable voltage levels, kV or kVp are used interchangeably.

The generator also controls the electron beam (the flow of electrons from cathode to anode), known as the *tube current*, which is measured in milliamperes (mA). Often, users simply state "mA" when referring to the tube current. Higher tube currents (more electrons) allow for shorter imaging times, but it causes a greater heating of the x-ray tube. The total tube output is the *current-time product* in milliampere-seconds (mAs).

The electron beam originates from the cathode, picks up kinetic energy from the kV applied between the anode and cathode, and the energetic electron beam slams into the anode. A tiny portion of that kinetic energy (~1%) is converted into energy that is released from the anode in the form of x-ray photons. The rest (~99%) is lost as heat to the anode. In a vacuum tube, heat can only dissipate slowly, and if an x-ray tube is used heavily, the tube may be damaged from overheating. Generally, the heating, or "tube loading," of a mammography tube during normal clinical use is not a significant issue. However, when testing, images can be acquired very quickly and the amount of heat may build up. Overheating will damage the x-ray tube.

If the tube potential is 25 kV, then the x-ray photon emitted by the tube can have an energy up to 25 kiloelectronvolts (keV). If the tube potential is increased to 34 kV, then the x-ray photon will energies up to a maximum of 34 keV. An "electron-volt" (eV) is a convenient unit of energy equal to 1.6×10^{-19} Joules (J). The x-rays emitted by an x-ray tube can have any energy from 0 up to the maximum specified by the tube potential. The distribution of energies is referred to as a "spectrum." Example spectra are shown in Fig. 21.3.

TARGET/FILTER COMBINATIONS

X-rays emitted from an x-ray tube are polyenergetic, meaning that each x-ray photon from essentially zero keV to the maximum set by the tube potential. The energy distribution of the x-rays, or spectrum will be dictated by the composition

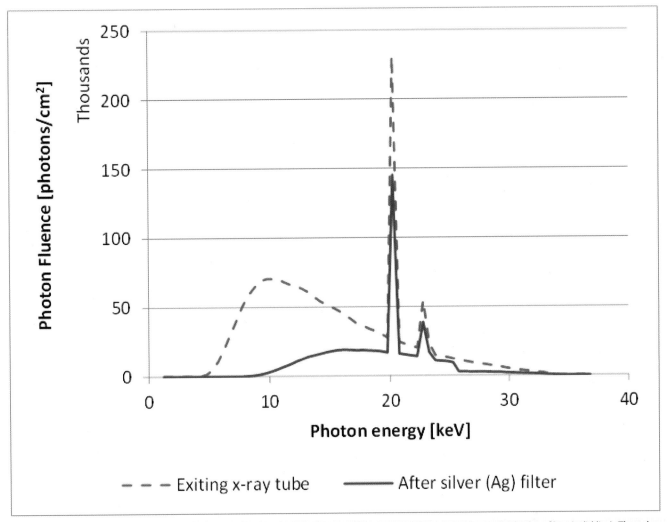

Fig. 21.3 Typical polyenergetic x-ray spectra for a Rh anode x-ray tube (*dotted line*) and after exiting a 25 μm thick silver filter (*solid line*). The tube potential is 34 kV.

Table 21.1 Target/Filter Combinations Used in Digital Mammography

Target (Anode)	Filter	kV Range (Typical)
Mo	Mo	25–27
Mo	Rh	26–28
Rh	Rh	28–30
Rh	Ag	28–34
W	Al	28–32
W	Ag	29–36

of the "target" or anode. Generally, most anodes are composed of tungsten (W), although some anodes have special tracks made of molybdenum (Mo) or rhodium (Rh). A list the most common target/filter combinations for digital mammography is provided in Table 21.1. The unfiltered x-ray spectrum is largely dominated by low-energy x-rays, which are generally highly absorbed by tissue (large organ dose) and provide little signal to the detector. As a result, a filter (a thin sheet of absorbing material, usually a metal of high purity and uniformity) is placed at the tube port to preferentially absorb most of the low-energy x-rays while

letting the higher-energy x-rays through. The selection of the anode and filter are described as the anode/filter or target/filter combinations.

Because of better dynamic range than screen-film mammography, digital mammography systems have moved toward higher-energy beams to provide greater signal at lower organ dose. To optimize these beams, common combinations from the screen-film era (Mo/Mo, Mo/Rh, Rh/Rh) have largely been supplanted by combinations such as Rh/Ag, W/Al, and W/Ag, though some systems still provide the former target/filter combinations for thinner breasts. For systems that offer contrast-enhanced mammography, an emerging technology, a copper filter may also be available for use.

The role of the filter is to remove the low energy x-rays. This is quantified by the "hardness" or penetrating capability of the x-ray beam. This is typically evaluated by a measure known as the half-value layer (HVL) thickness, which is the thickness of material (usually pure aluminum) needed to reduce the x-ray beam exposure by 50%. "Harder" beams will have thicker HVL values. As a rule of thumb, the MQSA regulations require that the HVL should exceed kVp/100 in mm of Al. For example, at 30 kV, the HVL must not be less than 0.30 mm (MQSA regulations

Part B Table 2, therein, available at https://www.fda.gov/radiation-emitting-products/regulations-mqsa/mammography-quality-standards-act-regulations). Harder beams provide more detector signal at reduced dose. However, the intrinsic contrast between adipose and fibroglandular tissue is also reduced. Key points on x-ray tubes and x-ray spectra are listed (Box 21.3).

IMAGING RECEPTORS

There are four main types of mammography systems based on their image receptor (Box 21.4). The image receptor in screen-film mammography (SFM) is the screen-film cassette. The phosphor screen is the x-ray absorber, which emits visible light and exposes the film. The cassette is loaded into a film processor to extract the film and develop it in a chemical bath.

There are a variety of technologies employed for digital mammography. In one approach, computed radiography (CR), the film-screen cassette is replaced with a photostimulable phosphor plate inside a cassette. The phosphor plate absorbs the x-rays just like the screens used in SFM, but that energy is "trapped" by energizing the electrons in the phosphor crystals. The CR cassette is then taken to a reader or processor, inside of which a red laser light is scanned across the phosphor plate. The energy is released from the traps in the form of blue light, which is measured by a blue light sensitive photodetector.

The CR cassettes can be used in older SFM systems with little modification; however, studies have shown that the image quality is lower than other digital systems, higher doses are needed, and cancer detection rates can be impacted.

Most digital mammography (DM) systems (Box 21.5) use a dedicated flat-panel detector that consists of a large two-dimensional array of detector elements that capture the signal from an x-ray (converter) layer. There are two types of x-ray detectors: indirect-conversion and direct-conversion systems (Fig. 21.4). For indirect-conversion systems, the x-ray sensitive portion is a fluorescent material, or phosphor, that converts a portion of the x-ray energy to visible light photons. These photons are captured by the flat-panel detector array underneath it, which converts the light signal to an electronic charge that is subsequently read out and digitized into a numeric value. In the phosphor, the light photons are emitted in all directions, and careful selection and optimization of the phosphor material is required to limit the spread of the light before it reaches the detector.

Box 21.3 X-Ray Tubes and X-Ray Spectra

- The target or anode is the large rotating disk inside the x-ray tube on which the electron beam is focused.
- Emission of x-rays from the target consists of bremsstrahlung (broad spectrum) and characteristic x-rays (narrow energy peaks, unique energy specific to anode material).
- The filters are selected to remove low-energy x-rays and improve penetration of the x-ray beam at the breast.
- The "hardness" of the x-ray spectrum is measured by the half-value layer (HVL).
- Harder spectra can reduce dose and improve image signal-to-noise but reduce tissue contrast.
- Harder spectra and higher kV are used for thicker and/or denser breasts.

Box 21.4 Mammography Systems

Screen-film mammography (SFM)	Older technology. Uses a phosphor screen as x-ray conversion layer, emitted light exposes film inside a removable cassette. Film must be developed in a chemical bath. Film mammograms are reviewed on a light box.
Computed radiography (CR)	Uses a cassette containing a storage phosphor. Phosphor is "read-out" using a laser scanner and digital image is recorded. Image quality is inferior to most digital mammography systems.
Digital mammography (DM)	Fully electronic image receptor. Usually integrated into the gantry. Usually, the image receptor is a flat-panel array that is 24 cm × 30 cm (9" × 12") in size.

Box 21.5 Full-Field Digital Mammography Systems

In the literature, digital mammography is often referred to as full-field digital mammography (FFDM). This is to distinguish them from smaller format x-ray detectors that were first used in breast biopsy systems. FFDM or DM are both common abbreviations for digital mammography.

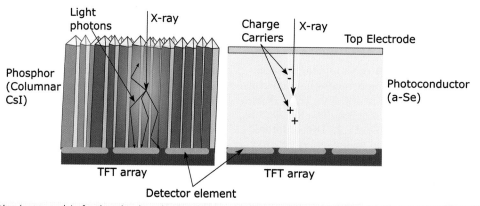

Fig. 21.4 Cross-section (not to scale) of a phosphor-based indirect conversion flat-panel detector (*left*) and a photoconductor-based direct conversion detector (*right*). *TFT*, Thin-film transistor.

This light spread leads to blurring or unsharpness that can limit the detail visible in the final image. Direct-conversion detectors have a photoconductor plate directly deposited on the flat-panel array. Here, the x-ray energy is converted directly to electronic charges that are collected at the detector array. Unlike phosphors, however, the electronic charge is confined by an applied electric field and does not spread before it reaches the detector. As such, direct conversion detectors generally have resolution limits imposed only by the physical size of each detector element.

Every column in a flat-panel can be switched or "addressed" so that the signal can be read-out by a digitizer for the entire column at one time. The digitizer converts a voltage signal to a computer binary number. Most DM systems convert the signal to a value representing a binary number in 12 to 14 bits. This corresponds to a dynamic range of 0 to 4095 or 0 to 16,383 digital units.

SCATTER AND GRID

X-rays at mammographic energies interact with matter either by the "photoelectric effect" in which the photon energy is completely absorbed by the material or by "scattering," in which the photon is deflected or scattered randomly in a direction that is different from the original primary beam. Scattered x-rays that reach the detector create a diffuse background signal that can degrade image quality. A similar effect is seen when driving in foggy conditions with high-beam headlights on, and the resulting glare makes it difficult to see objects ahead of the car.

Antiscatter grids (Fig. 21.5) can be used to block the scattered x-rays preferentially. Usually, the grid is composed of strips of an attenuating material (usually lead) with spaces in between. The strips are angled toward the x-ray source such that the primary beam (unscattered) x-rays can pass through the spaces whereas any scattered x-ray photons traveling along different directions will be blocked by the strips. To avoid the grid appearing in the image, the grid is usually moved during imaging to blur out the strips uniformly. Special care must be taken to ensure that the grid motion is appropriate for the imaging time or a "grid artifact" will appear in the image. Grid artifacts generally require corrective action.

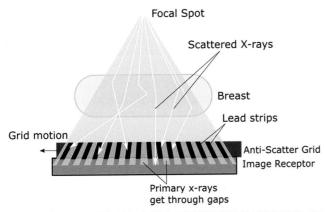

Fig. 21.5 Illustration (not to scale) of the operation of the antiscatter grid to preferentially allow unscattered primary x-rays through and block scattered radiation from reaching the detector. The breast support plate between the breast and the rest of the assembly is not shown.

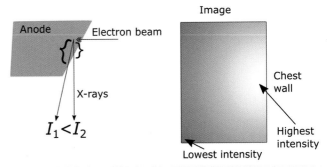

Fig. 21.6 Heel effect. Illustration (*left*) of the x-rays exiting the anode, where the pathlength (indicated by braces) is dependent on the exit angle. The pathlength toward the anode is greater, resulting is greater attenuation of the x-ray and lower intensity compared with the x-rays on closer to the cathode. X-ray intensity map due to the heel effect at seen by the image receptor (*right*).

As described later, the antiscatter grid is not used when obtaining magnification views, in which scatter is reduced with the air-gap technique.

HEEL EFFECT

The surface of the anode is aligned obliquely to the tube port (Figs. 21.2 and 21.6), with x-rays emitted in straight lines from the anode and exit through the tube port and collimators. Some x-rays are emitted from the surface of the anode, but some are emitted deeper in the anode or must travel through different thicknesses of anode material. As a result, the x-ray spectrum and the number of x-rays are dependent on the exit angle of the x-ray. This leads to a nonuniform variation across the x-ray field (Fig. 21.6), with higher field intensity toward the cathode than toward the anode. The effect of this nonuniform x-ray field on the image is mitigated through patient positioning. In mammography, the chest wall should be positioned toward the cathode side while the nipple should be positioned toward the anode.

FOCAL SPOT AND MAGNIFICATION VIEWS

In the x-ray tube, the electron beam is focused to a tiny area on the anode. This area, called the focal spot, is the location from which x-rays are generated. The focal spot has a finite size, for mammography tubes, these are nominally 0.3 mm for the large focal spot or 0.1 mm for the small focal spot that is used in magnification imaging. Because the focal spot is not a single point, a penumbra is created around objects in the image (Fig. 21.7A). Focal spot blurring (the penumbra in Fig. 21.7A) can be minimized by using the small focal spot or by ensuring the object being imaged is close to the image receptor.

Unlike visible light, x-rays cannot be focused using lenses, so one cannot zoom in on an area of interest as would be done with a telephoto lens or a microscope. Instead, geometric magnification is used (Fig. 21.7B). Because x-rays travel in a straight line from the x-ray tube focal spot to the detector, the x-rays field is described as a diverging beam. To achieve geometric magnification, the object is moved closer to the x-ray tube and further from the image detector. The degree of magnification is equal to the

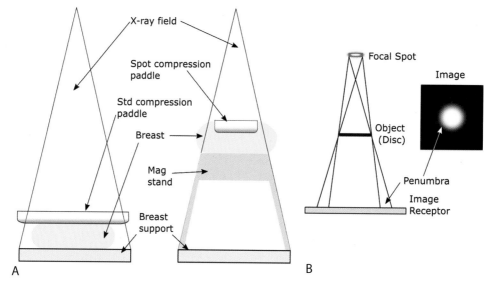

Fig. 21.7 Comparison of contact mammography and magnification mammography (A). The diverging beam geometry makes the breast tissue appear larger at the image receptor, but only a portion of the breast will be visible. Illustration (not to scale) of the penumbra caused by an extended focal spot and the corresponding blurred image of a disc (B).

source-image-distance (SID) divided by the source-object-distance (SOD). For example, if the object is moved halfway between the focal spot and image receptor, then the image would appear two times larger. If the object was placed one-third the distance from the focal spot to the receptor, then the image would appear three times larger. However, the penumbra effect from the finite-size focal spot becomes more apparent the further the object is from the detector. Because of this, the small focal spot is always used for magnification imaging.

In a magnification view, only a portion of the breast will be visible in the image. Smaller, spot compression paddles are used to immobilize and compress a portion of the breast. Spot compression views are used to characterize abnormalities, get better views of microcalcifications, or rule out tissue superposition. Note that less x-ray scatter reaches the image receptor in magnification mode due to the air gap, and the antiscatter grid is not used. MSQA regulations require that a mammography system must provide at least one fixed geometric magnification mode between 1.4× and 2×.

Radiation Dose

When x-rays interact with matter, they interact with the electrons in the atoms of the object. Either some (by scatter) or all (by photoelectric effect) of its kinetic energy is transferred to the electron. If that kinetic energy exceeds the binding energy of the electron, it can knock that electron from the atom resulting in an ion (a particle with a net charge) or break chemical bonds. The freed electron may have gained sufficient kinetic energy to interact with other electrons potentially liberating more electrons and breaking chemical bonds. At mammographic energies (~15–40 keV), this cascade of ionizations may cause several hundred or thousands of breaks.

If this ionization occurs near the DNA of the cell, the DNA molecule may be damaged either by these ionization events or by the reactive free ions (also called radicals) liberated by the x-ray energy. These free radicals can cause oxidative reactions that result in further DNA damage. This is in addition to the naturally present oxidative reactions and free radical generation during the normal metabolism of the cell. Fortunately, there are complex chemical repair mechanisms that continually repair and renew the cellular DNA. Only when these repairs fail is the DNA permanently altered (mutated). Even then, only certain mutations have the potential to transform the cell into cancer.

The amount of radiation delivered to an object or person is measured in grays (Gy), which is equal to 1 Joule deposited per kilogram of the (1 Gy = J/kg). Older references may indicate radiation dose in units of "rads" (100 rad = 1 Gy). Although radiation-induced cancer risk is well determined for high doses (from such studies as the Lifetime Survival Study after the atomic bomb attacks in Japan), the risk at low doses is difficult to determine. Conservatively, the risk at high dose is extrapolated to low doses using a linear no threshold (LNT) approach meaning that radiation risk is assumed to be linear with radiation dose and that there is no dose level below which the risk falls to zero. While the LNT model is commonly used to calculate the risk of radiation-induced cancer at high doses, its accuracy at low doses is unknown and some argue that it may overestimate risk.

For drugs, the dose is colloquially associated with the total amount of medicine administered (e.g., 400 mg of drug A). However, radiation dose is not an amount and is more like a concentration (of energy per unit body mass or J/kg). As such, if a woman receives 2 mGy from one mammogram on each breast, then she receives 2 mGy to each breast, *not* 4 mGy in total. However, if two repeated views were performed on one breast, then the total dose delivered to that breast would be 4 mGy. If the views are different (e.g., craniocaudal [CC] and mediolateral oblique [MLO] views) where the radiation is delivered to slightly different parts of the one breast, then the total dose to that breast would be *roughly* 4 mGy.

For mammography, we specifically refer to the dose delivered to the glandular tissue, which is the most susceptible to radiation (higher risk tissue) in the breast. Adipose tissue, stroma, and other tissues in the breast are generally considered to be more resistant (lower risk) to radiation exposure. As such, the dose to the breast is more properly referred to as the glandular dose. A common measure is the mean glandular dose (MGD) or average glandular dose (AGD), which are synonymous.

Radiation risk is inversely related to age; younger people are at higher risk of radiation-induced cancer, with the risk falling rapidly and tailing when approaching middle age. The radiation may induce cancer several years after exposure (5–30 years). For a typical MGD of 3.7 mGy for a two-view mammography examination, young women (age 20) may have a 4 in 100,000 risk of developing fatal radiation-induced cancer. At age 50, it drops to approximately 0.7 in 100,000 and down to 0.2 in 100,000 at age 70 (Hendrick, 2010). In a similar analysis (Yaffe and Mainprize, 2011), for 25 screens over a lifetime, the total combined risk of a fatal radiation-induced cancer was estimated to be 10 per 100,000 women.

In any risk analysis for an intervention, this should be compared against the benefit of the intervention. Lifetime risk of breast cancer is approximately 1 in 9 (or ~11,000 in 100,000) and the risk of a breast cancer fatality is approximately 1 in 30 (or ~3300 in 100,000). Estimates of the benefit of screening are between 15% and 45% based on various randomized controlled trials and observational screening studies. Assuming a moderate mortality reduction of 20% (660 deaths averted), then the benefit-to-risk ratio for 25 screens is approximately 66:1. Key points for radiation dose and risk (Box 21.6).

MQSA Dose Requirements

As part of the requirements, the MQSA stipulates that the radiation dose to a test phantom (Box 21.7) representing a "standard breast" shall not exceed 3 mGy in a single view. Typically, the test phantom is the American College of Radiology (ACR) *Mammography Accreditation Phantom* or a plastic phantom equivalent to a 4.2 cm compressed breast composed of 50% adipose and 50% glandular tissue.

Box 21.6   Radiation Dose and Risk

- The mean glandular dose (MGD) is a common measure of radiation delivered to the breast.
- Typical MGD are 1–6 mGy per mammogram, dependent on breast thickness and breast density.
- The glandular tissue is the most sensitive tissue in the breast to radiation (x-rays).
- Radiation risk is greatest in young women, such as those in their teens and 20s.
- Radiation risk is inversely proportional to age at exposure, and very low in screening aged women.

Box 21.7   Quality Control Phantoms

- The American College of Radiology (ACR) has two Quality Control (QC) phantoms for mammography.
  - A smaller mammography accreditation phantom (MAP) that is in widespread use. Originally for screen-film mammography (SFM), but still used in many manufacturer's digital mammography (DM) and digital breast tomosynthesis (DBT) QC routines.
  - A larger digital mammography phantom (DMP) for DM and for DBT that is gradually being adopted.
- Either phantom may be used as a standard breast for dose measurements.
- Less than 3 mGy per view is stipulated by MQSA to a standard (4.2 cm) breast phantom.
- Image quality is assessed by experienced readers and must pass QC requirements.
  - Mammography accreditation platform (MAP): must be able to see at least four fibers, three speck groups, and three masses
  - Digital mammography platform (DMP): must be able to see at least two fibers, three speck groups, and two masses

---

Note that this requirement is only for the standard breast and that the dose delivered to a patient may be significantly lower or higher depending on breast thickness and composition (breast density).

Image Processing

The image data collected from the detector goes through several processing steps. First, a "gain-and-offset correction" or "flat-fielding" step is performed to adjust for variations in sensitivity and signal levels for each detector element. The flat-fielding correction is determined by imaging a uniform phantom several times during a special calibration procedure. Second, a map of the detector element defects (see section Detector-Based Artifacts) is also used to correct for dead detector elements by replacing the bad values with a weighted average of the signal from adjacent elements. The resulting image should have nearly uniform sensitivity across the whole area. This image is stored as a raw or "for processing" DICOM image (Fig. 21.8A). This image may be used for computer aided detection (CAD) or automated breast density analysis. However, the raw image is typically not reviewed by the radiologist.

Special image processing algorithms are used to enhance the mammogram appearance. These processing steps may include: peripheral equalization (to reduce the appearance of the changing breast thickness at the edge of the breast), contrast enhancement (to increase the contrast between fibroglandular and adipose tissues), and image sharpening or denoising to improve the appearance of fine structures. The resulting output is a "for presentation" or processed mammogram. The for presentation mammograms are displayed to the radiologist for review (Fig. 21.8B).

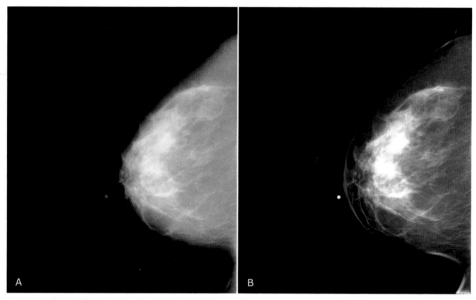

Fig. 21.8 Comparison of raw or "for processing" (A) and processed or "for presentation" (B) mammograms. Note improved soft tissue contrast and better skin edge visualization.

Image Quality

Image quality refers to the characteristics of an image that can potentially help (or impede) the imaging tasks desired. Image quality includes attributes such as image sharpness, signal, contrast, and noise in the image. Image quality also includes artifacts (undesired structures or patterns in the image that distract or limit image perception). Optimizing image quality for mammography is dependent on the choice of x-ray detector, use of antiscatter grids, selection of x-ray technique factors (kV, mAs, and target/filter combinations), and radiation dose limits. Often, improving image quality comes with a corresponding increase in radiation dose.

IMAGE UNSHARPNESS

Mammography requires very high spatial resolution to visualize microcalcifications, subtle architectural distortion, and margins of masses. Resolution is limited by image unsharpness or blurring, caused by three main factors: blurring in the detector, x-ray focal spot unsharpness, and patient motion.

Blurring in the detector is a fundamental and intrinsic characteristic of the x-ray converter and the detector element size.

Focal spot unsharpness is generally not a problem with the breast in the standard nonmagnification view because the penumbra created by the 0.3 mm focal spot is very small. If, however, imaging was performed with the 0.3 mm focal spot, instead of the standard 0.1 mm focal spot, for the magnification view, the focal spot blurring would be significant.

Patient motion is reduced by shorter imaging acquisition times (less time to move) and proper breast compression (immobilizing the breast). Examples of patient motion blurring are shown in the artifact section.

Resolution may be measured by special bar patterns with equal size bars and spaces called line pairs (lp). Higher resolution means that smaller line pairs can be visualized in the image. The limiting resolution for nonmagnification or "contact mammography" is generally 5 to 10 lp/mm and is almost entirely due to the detector blurring and detector element size. For a detector with a pitch (center-to-center) distance of 0.1 mm (or 100 μm), the smallest line pair (line and space) that can be seen is 0.2 mm, or 5 lp/mm. At 85 μm, the limiting resolution would be 5.88 lp/mm. Note, however, that because of other sources of unsharpness (e.g., blurring in the image receptor, focal spot blurring), the limiting resolution may be lower than expected for a given detector element spacing.

CONTRAST

Contrast is a description of the differential signal between an object and its background in the image. The intrinsic contrast is the difference in x-ray absorption between the object and the background. In general, intrinsic contrast decreases with increasing x-ray energy. In mammography, contrast between adipose and fibroglandular tissue is important but nevertheless is quite low. Microcalcifications, primarily composed of calcium and denser than tissue have much higher contrast despite their small size. Larger calcifications, metallic clips, and other foreign objects (e.g., pacemakers) have even higher intrinsic contrast. Contrast resolution refers to the ability to distinguish between differences in intensities within an image. Because the soft tissue components of the breast have intrinsically low contrast, lower energy (kV) x-rays are generally used increase contrast resolution in mammography compared with imaging of other body parts like the chest or extremities.

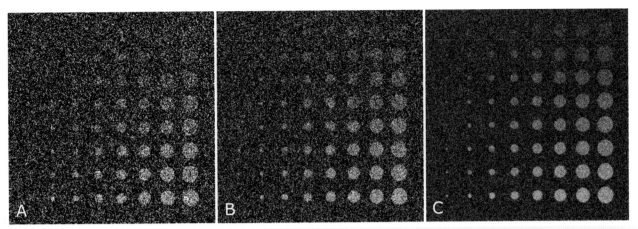

Fig. 21.9 Simulated contrast-detail phantom of small disks of varying diameter, 2.5–20 pixels (columns) and contrast levels, 2.5%–20% (rows). Images are made with $n = 64$ x-rays / pixel (A), $n = 128$ x-rays/pixel (B) and $n = 256$ x-rays/pixel (C). The pixel signal-to-noise ratio (SNR) is $\sqrt{n} = 8$, 11.3, and 16, respectively. Smaller detail and lower contrasts are easier to see as the pixel SNR improves. Relative radiation dose in (B) and (C) are two and four times higher. Display window and level have been set to match for all three examples

SIGNAL-TO-NOISE

X-ray interactions are random, and x-ray imaging is affected by this randomness. Even under uniform irradiation of the detector, each detector element will actually record variable signal proportional to different numbers of x-rays. This randomness is dictated by a probability distribution referred to as a Poisson distribution. Under Poisson statistics, the standard deviation, σ, in the distribution is always equal to the square root of the mean value. For example, if the mean number of x-rays measured in a detector element was 100, the standard deviation, would be $\sigma = \sqrt{100} = 10$ x-rays. A common measure of image quality is the pixel signal-to-noise ratio or pixel signal-to-noise ratio (SNR) $= n/\sigma$. In this example, the pixel SNR would be $n/\sigma = 100/\sqrt{100} = 10$. The Rose Criterion (named after Albert Rose) suggests that to detect a high contrast object equal to the detector element size, the SNR should be greater than 5 for reliable (>99%) detection. For low contrast objects, the pixel SNR needs to be even higher. Larger objects (bigger than one pixel) are easier to see and the pixel SNR can be lower. This can be demonstrated with a contrast-detail phantom, which consists of an array of objects of different size and contrast (Fig. 21.9). Higher pixel SNR allows for the detection of smaller and/or lower contrast objects. Note that mammograms also have blurring and other noise sources (e.g., electronic noise). As a result, the SNR and object detection relationship is more complicated. Nevertheless, in general, better pixel SNR leads to better detection performance.

The SNR is dictated by the number of x-rays reaching the detector. This, in turn, is dictated by the choice of x-ray spectra (anode/filter and kV), the detector characteristics, breast thickness, and breast density. The AEC will attempt to optimize kV, mAs, and/or the anode/filter selection to obtain a consistent minimum SNR in the mammogram. As breast thickness increases or as breast density increases, the radiation dose required to achieve a certain SNR at the detector increases. Using harder x-ray spectra can help reduce the dose/SNR trade off, although soft-tissue

Box 21.8   Signal and Noise in X-Ray Images

- The variation in the number of x-rays captured in each pixel is described by Poisson statistics.
- The mean pixel signal is proportional to the mean number, $\bar{n}$, of x-rays at the detector.
- The standard deviation in the number of x-rays is equal to $\sigma = \sqrt{\bar{n}}$.
- The pixel signal-to-noise ratio (SNR) is $\bar{n}/\sigma = \sqrt{\bar{n}}$.
- If the number of x-rays is doubled, the pixel SNR improves by $\sqrt{2} \sim 1.41$. The radiation dose will double.
- At very low exposures, electronic noise in the detector and readout electronics will reduce the SNR.

contrast may be reduced. Key points on signal and noise (Box 21.8)

ARTIFACTS

Detector-Based Artifacts

Perhaps surprisingly, flat-panel detectors in digital mammography systems can have a significant variation in sensitivity and may have a few defects; dead or stuck detector elements are common, and even partial or whole lines may be nonfunctional or unstable. As the detector ages, even more defects can occur, where single pixels in the image, lines, or even blocks of the image become unstable or dead (Fig. 21.10). In many cases, if the defects are isolated, these can be corrected by performing the flat-fielding procedure again. However, large clusters of new defects may indicate an imminent failure of the detector.

Ghosting is another phenomenon that can occur in which the image receptor response changes slightly depending on what parts of the detector received more (or less) radiation. In subsequent images, the sensitivity of the parts of a detector is may be slightly different than other parts and

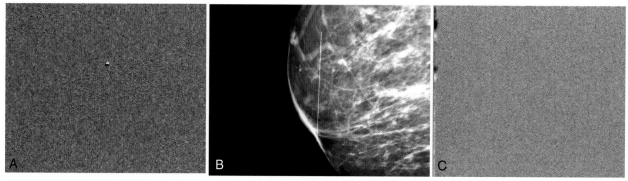

Fig. 21.10 Detector artifacts. Dead pixels (bright or dark) are seen in zoomed image (A). These may be mistaken for microcalcifications in a clinical image. A line defect appeared in a right craniocaudal mammogram (B). New line defects are sometimes correctable by flat-fielding but often require detector replacement. Failing detector section near the chest wall is seen in a uniform phantom image (C).

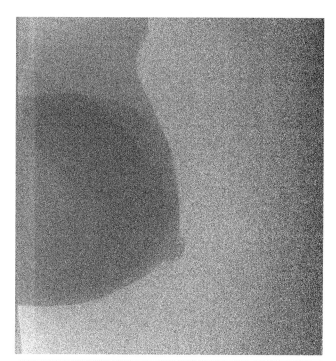

Fig. 21.11 Ghosting. Several outlines of previous breasts are visible in an image of a uniform phantom. The ghosts are most noticeable at high-contrast edges (air/skin boundary, edges of thick phantoms, or metal plates) and after high-dose exposures. Generally, these ghosts are very low signal and are only detectable on images of uniform phantoms and when the display window/level is set to a very narrow range.

an apparent ghost of the previous image might be visible. If imaging happens fairly quickly, then several ghost outlines may be apparent (Fig. 21.11). Many detectors have some level of ghosting, but only rarely are the levels high enough to be of clinical significance. However, special care is required when flat-fielding is performed to avoid capturing the ghosts in the correction. Usually this is achieved by ensuring that flat-fielding is performed either early in the day or hours after clinical imaging is completed.

Machine-Based Artifacts

Like detector artifacts, machine-based artifacts are generally reproducible from image to image. These include problems like dust or scratches on the breast support table, compression paddle, or even in the tube port (Fig. 21.12). Sometimes, dust particles are present during the flat-fielding process and then are subsequently cleaned or moved, leaving a negative "shadow" of the object. In such cases, cleaning and repeating the flat-fielding procedure is usually recommended.

Grid line artifacts commonly occur due to incorrect motion of the grid during exposure (Fig. 21.13). If grid lines become apparent in clinical images, corrective action is required.

Patient-Based Artifacts

Patient-related artifacts are specific to the patient. These include foreign objects, patient motion, and positioning artifacts. Any object in the x-ray field can obscure the breast tissue (Fig. 21.14), such as accidentally included body parts (e.g., fingers, chin, hair, nose, ears) and foreign objects (pacemakers, surgical clips, jewelry, tattoos). An improperly positioned breast may cause skin folds (Fig. 21.15) to appear as linear or slightly curved structures in the image that may obscure or distort the breast tissue. Despite immobilization during compression, patient motion (Fig. 21.16) can occur and degrade image quality. This is most likely to occur when imaging acquisition times are long.

KEY POINTS

- Mammography systems are specialized radiography units designed for the detection of breast cancer.
- Most mammography systems in the United States are digital, often referred to as full-field digital mammography (FFDM).
- Most detectors use a two-dimensional flat panel array. The array is bonded to the x-ray sensitive component which is a phosphor (indirect conversion) or a photoconductor (direct conversion).
- Mammography operates at lower kV than general radiography and CT to improve soft tissue contrast.
- X-ray spectra are optimized by anode and filter choice to maximize signal to noise at the detector, while minimizing patient dose.
- The small focal spot is used for magnification imaging to reduce the effect of focal spot blurring.

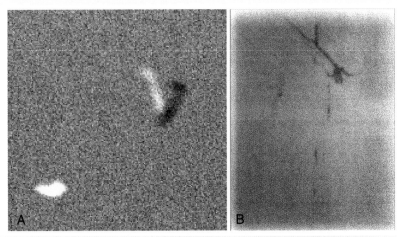

Fig. 21.12 Machine-based artifacts. Dust or speck artifacts in a uniform phantom image, zoomed (A). The sharper appearing speck on the lower left is likely on the breast support or paddle. The unsharp speck in the upper right was present during flat-fielding and subsequently moved slightly. The "burned-in" negative shadow would remain until the flat-field is redone. This speck was thought to be somewhere in the tube port, perhaps on the filter. Damaged filter in uniform phantom image (B). The filters in the tube port are quite thin and can be easily damaged

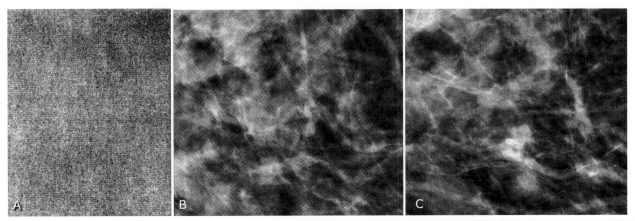

Fig. 21.13 Grid-line artifacts. Grid lines (*horizontal*) appearing on a uniform plastic phantom images (A). Grid lines occur when the grid motion is altered and appear superimposed on the image. Cellular grid lines on digital mammography on a right craniocaudal view (B) are removed after correction (C).

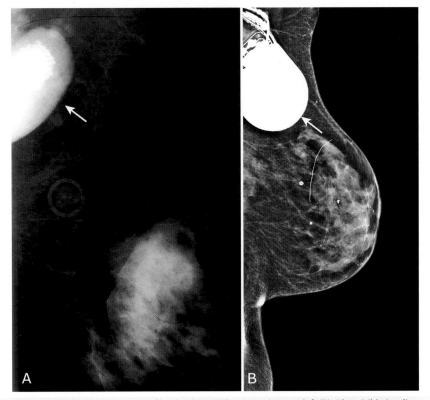

Fig. 21.14 Foreign objects. Patient's finger (*arrow*) seen on film (A). Pacemaker (*arrow*) upper left (B). Also visible is a linear scar marker showing the location of a previous biopsy

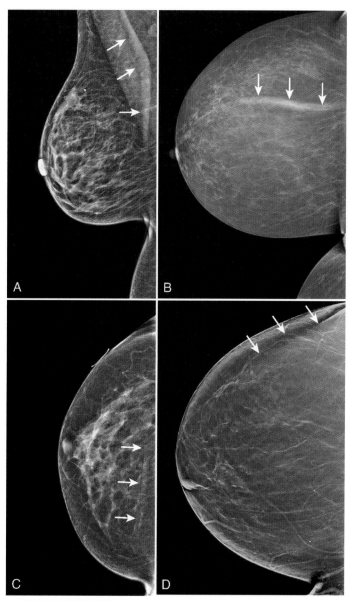

Fig. 21.15 Skin folds (A–D; *arrows*). Substantial skin folding usually appear as linear white lines (A, B). Minimal skins folds can also appear as dark lines (C, D)

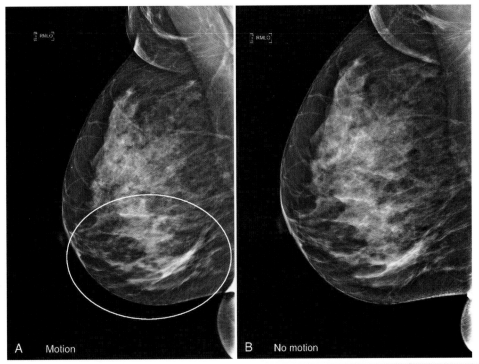

Fig. 21.16 Motion artifact on digital mammography. (A) Right mediolateral oblique (MLO) view shows blurred breast tissue (*circle*). (B) On a corrected right MLO, the breast tissue and Cooper ligaments appears sharper against the background. Long exposure times can lead to patient motion.

- The mean glandular dose is a measure of the radiation energy absorbed in the glandular tissue of the breast.
- Risk of a radiation-induced fatal cancer in screening-aged women is very low (<1/100,000) and decreases with age.
- Artifacts may be detector, machine, or patient-based. Artifacts that are noticeable in clinical images and negatively impact interpretation require corrective action.

Suggested Reading

General Mammography Physics

1. Markey MK, ed. *Physics of Mammographic Imaging*. Boca Raton, FL; CRC Press; 2012.
2. Séradour B, Heid P, Estève J. Comparison of direct digital mammography, computed radiography, and film-screen in the french national breast cancer screening program. *AJR*. 2014;202(1):229–236.
3. Burgess AE. The Rose model, revisited. *J Opt Soc Am A*. 1999;16:633–646.
4. Radiographic and Mammographic Systems for Radiology Residents (2018), RSNA/AAPM Online Physics Modules, www.rsna.org/education/trainee-resources/physics-modules Accessed Jun 6, 2020.

X-Ray Tubes and X-Ray Spectra

5. Radiology Masterclass Basics of X-ray Physics. X-ray production. https://www.radiologymasterclass.co.uk/tutorials/physics/x-ray_physics_production. Accessed Jun 6, 2020.

Radiation Dose and Risk

6. Hendrick RE. Radiation doses and cancer risks from breast imaging studies. *Radiology*. 2010;257(1). https://pubs.rsna.org/doi/pdf/10.1148/radiol.10100570.
7. Yaffe MJ, Mainprize JG. Risk of radiation-induced breast cancer from mammographic screening. *Radiology*. 2011;258:98–105.
8. Peck D, Samei E. How to Understand and Communicate Radiation Risk. https://www.imagewisely.org/Imaging-Modalities/Computed-Tomography/How-to-Understand-and-Communicate-Radiation-Risk. Accessed Jun 6, 2020.

Breast Positioning and Compression

9. Popli MB, Teotia R, Narang M, Krishna H. Breast positioning during mammography: mistakes to be avoided. *Breast Cancer (Auckl)*. 2014;8:119–124. https://doi.org/10.4137/BCBCR.S17617.
10. Holland K, Sechopoulos I, Mann RM, den Heeten GJ, van Gils CH, Karssemeijer N. Influence of breast compression pressure on the performance of population-based mammography screening. *Breast Cancer Res*. 2017;19(1):126. https://doi.org/10.1186/s13058-017-0917-3.

Image Quality, Quality Control and Accreditation

11. Mammography Image Quality and Dose (2018). Radiological Society of North America (RSNA). https://www.rsna.org/education/trainee-resources/physics-modules. Accessed Jun 6, 2020.
12. MQSA Program, FDA. https://www.fda.gov/radiation-emitting-products/mammography-quality-standards-act-and-program. Accessed Jun 6, 2020.
13. Mammography Accreditation, American College of Radiology, https://accrediationsupport.acr.org/suppport/solutions/11000003436. Accessed Jun 6, 2020.

Artifacts in Mammography

14. Ayyala RS, Chorlton MA, Behrman RH, Kornguth PJ, Slanetz PJ. Digital mammographic artifacts on full-field systems: what are they and how do i fix them? *RadioGraphics*. 2008;28(7):1999–2008.
15. Choi JJ, Kim SH, Kang BJ, Choi BG, Song B, Jung H. Mammographic artifacts on full-field digital mammography. *J Digit Imaging*. 2014;27(2):231–236. https://doi.org/10.1007/s10278-013-9641-4.
16. Geiser WR, Haygood TM, Santiago L, et al. Challenges in mammography: Part 1, artifacts in digital mammography. *Am J Roentgenol*. 2011;197:1023–1030.

Index

Pages followed by *b*, *t*, or *f* refer to boxes, tables, or figures, respectively.